Understanding Antibacterial Action and Resistance

Understanding Antibacterial Action and Resistance

SECOND EDITION

A. D. RUSSELL
I. CHOPRA

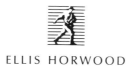

ELLIS HORWOOD

London New York Toronto Sydney Tokyo Singapore
Madrid Mexico City Munich

First published 1990
This second edition published 1996 by
Ellis Horwood Limited
Campus 400, Maylands Avenue
Hemel Hempstead
Hertfordshire, HP2 7EZ
A division of
Simon & Schuster International Group

Typeset by Keyset Composition, Colchester, Essex
Printed and bound in Great Britain by
Redwood Books, Trowbridge, Wiltshire

Library of Congress Cataloging-in-Publication Data

Available from the publisher

British Library Cataloguing in Publication Data

A catalogue record for this book is available from
the British Library

ISBN 0-13-124827-8

1 2 3 4 5   00 99 98 97 96

Contents

7   *Mechanisms of spore resistance to biocides*   243

8   *Impact on society of bacterial resistance to antibiotics and biocides and ways of counteracting it*   257

Preface to the second edition

In the six years that have elapsed since the first edition was written there have been many advances in our knowledge of the ways in which antibiotics and biocides work and the molecular basis of resistance to these agents. In addition, the public health problems associated with increased emergence of antibiotic-resistant bacteria have assumed even greater significance since the publication of the first edition, adding greater urgency to the need to introduce strategies to circumvent, or control, resistance. The second edition describes these recent developments, utilizing the concepts set out in the first edition as a foundation. Consequently, in the second edition we have retained the same format as that adopted in the first edition. However, inclusion of the new developments has meant that many parts of the book have been rewritten, or substantially revised. The references recommended in Further Reading have also been updated to reflect the publication of new material.

We would like to express our thanks to Mrs Helen Baden Powell for her invaluable assistance in the preparation of the manuscript and to colleagues at SmithKline Beecham for helpful advice.

CHAPTER ONE

Introduction

1
General nature and development of antibacterial agents

Bacteria comprise a large group of unicellular, prokaryotic, microorganisms some of which are also able to form spores, i.e. dormant forms produced under adverse conditions, but with the potential to germinate or revert to the cellular, replicating, bacterial form in a favourable environment. Some bacterial activities are beneficial to humans while others, notably the capacity to cause disease, are detrimental. Undoubtedly one of the most important scientific achievements of this century has been humanity's ability to control the detrimental activities of bacteria by the judicious use of antibacterial agents. This relates not only to the prevention of bacterial growth *per se* but also to the destruction of bacterial spores. The impact on society has been felt in many ways. For example, the era of antibacterial chemotherapy, heralded by the introduction of the sulphonamides and penicillin in the 1930s, has led to a dramatic decline in the incidence of numerous life-threatening bacterial infections such as endocarditis, meningitis and pneumonia, and the use of disinfectants and antiseptics has removed the hazards of infection during surgery. Although the types of antibacterial agents and their mechanisms of action will be considered in more detail in Chapters 2 and 3, it will be useful at this stage to make various general statements about the inhibitors.

Antibacterial agents comprise a large group of substances that inhibit bacterial growth (bacteriostatic agents), cause bacterial death (bactericidal agents), or destroy spores (sporicidal agents). Some bactericidal agents are also sporicidal and vice versa, but bacteriostatic agents are ineffective against resting spores. Antibacterial agents include disinfectants, antiseptics, preservatives and antibiotics. The various terms are now described more fully.

By tradition, bactericidal agents which are used on inanimate objects are termed 'disinfectants'. Disinfectants include antibacterial agents that are usually too toxic, irritant or corrosive to be applied to body surfaces or tissues, but are suitable for disinfection of equipment or the inanimate environment. Antiseptics include bacterial inhibitors that are sufficiently free from toxic effects to be applied to body surfaces or exposed tissues and are agents which should assist and not impair natural defence systems of the body. Although antiseptics have greater selective activity against bacteria than disinfectants, they are not suitable for the treatment of infections by systemic administration. Preservatives are frequently added to pharmaceutical, cosmetic and food products to inhibit bacterial contamination and proliferation and hence prevent infectivity or spoilage. Some, but not all, of the chemicals used as disinfectants and antiseptics may also act as preservatives. However, there are additional antibacterial agents which are used only as preservatives. The term 'biocide' is a general term that encompasses antiseptic, disinfectant and preservative activity and denotes a non-chemotherapeutic agent that kills microorganisms.

The term 'antibiotic' includes a variety of naturally occurring and synthetic organic molecules many of which have sufficient selective activity against bacteria to permit systemic administration as chemotherapeutic agents for the treatment of bacterial infections. The establishment of an infection in humans and animals by a pathogenic bacterium usually involves the following steps: (a) attachment to the epithelial surfaces of the respiratory, alimentary or urogenital tracts; (b) penetration of the epithelial surfaces by the pathogen; (c) interference with, or evasion of, host defence mechanisms; (d) multiplication in host tissues; (e) damage of the host's tissues. Steps (a) and (b) do not occur if the bacterium is introduced into the host directly through the skin by trauma or vector bite. Antibiotics usually prevent step (d) either by killing the pathogens or by slowing their growth to the point where host defence mechanisms can clear the infection.

It could be assumed that antibiotics which kill bacteria are superior in combating infections to those which merely prevent bacterial growth and rely largely on the host's immune defence mechanisms to eradicate the infection. However, numerous bacteriostatic drugs have been successfully used for many years as chemotherapeutic agents and only in a relatively small number of infectious conditions is it essential that bactericidal antibiotics are used.

Although the basis of selectivity varies from one antibiotic to another it usually results from one, or both, of the following: (a) the target inhibited is only found in bacteria so that host (animal) cells remain insusceptible to the drug, (b) the antibiotic is concentrated within the bacterial cell, but not in the host cell. Therefore, although the antibiotic may potentially inhibit both bacterial and host cell targets, the higher concentration in bacteria ensures selectivity. However, it should be remembered that not all antibiotics are suitable for the chemotherapy of infections because some of them fail to meet the criteria for selectivity outlined above. Although such antibiotics (e.g. puromycin) may be useful biochemical tools, we will not specifically consider them here since we wish to address only antibiotics of value in the chemotherapy of infectious diseases. Readers wishing to learn more about the antibiotics that lack selectivity should consult the texts by Gale *et al.* (1981) and Franklin and Snow (1989) listed at the end of this chapter.

The development process from discovery to product launch for a new antibacterial agent is lengthy, particularly for an antibiotic which has the potential of chemotherapeutic application in humans. The procedure for an antibiotic, which

Table 1.1 The development process for a new antibiotic (based on Gootz, 1990)

Stage or phase	Studies	Approximate period to complete (years)
Preclinical	Mode of antibacterial action. Pharmacokinetic and pharmacodynamic studies in animals. Acute and chronic toxicology tests in animals.	1
Phase I	Evaluation of safety and pharmacokinetic profile in healthy human volunteers.	1
Phase II	Initial controlled trials for efficacy and safety. Dose and duration for specific infections. Additional pharmacological data.	2
Phase III	Demonstration of safety and efficacy for multiple therapeutic indications in expanded controlled clinical trials.	3
Regulatory authority review	Assessment–review of data prior to market approval.	1

can take eight years to complete, is designed to characterize the mechanism of action of the drug and to assess extensively its safety and efficacy in both humans and animals. The development process (Table 1.1) comprises preclinical studies and three clinical testing phases (phases I–III) prior to market approval. Progression of a new antibiotic from one phase to the next depends upon satisfying the various criteria set at each stage.

Effective antibacterial agents inactivate bacteria or their spores by interacting with susceptible targets within these structures. It is therefore appropriate at this stage to provide a brief outline of the structure and composition of bacteria and spores to prepare the reader for the more detailed approach to antibacterial targets in Chapters 2 and 3.

2
Structure of bacteria

2.1 Introduction

Bacteria can be divided into two main classes, Gram positive and Gram negative, on the basis of their differential abilities to retain an iodine–crystal violet stain

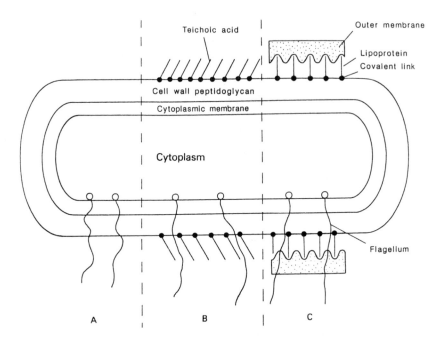

Fig. 1.1 Diagram of the bacterial cell: A, the generalized structure of the bacterial cell; B, Gram-positive structure; C, Gram-negative structure. (Reproduced, with permission, from Hugo & Russell (1992).)

when treated with organic solvents (e.g. alcohol or acetone). Bacteria that retain the stain are termed Gram positive and those that do not Gram negative. The staining response depends primarily on the morphology and composition of the bacterial cell wall, in particular the possession by Gram-negative bacteria of an outer membrane within the wall. Apart from the outer membrane the compositions of Gram-positive and Gram-negative bacteria are fundamentally similar and Fig. 1.1 shows the generalized structures of Gram-positive and Gram-negative bacteria. However, there are differences in detailed structural and compositional features between different bacterial species and even between strains of the same species. A description of cellular components now follows.

2.2　Cell wall

2.2.1　General structure

The cell wall surrounds the inner, cytoplasmic membrane. It maintains the shape of the cell and protects the mechanically fragile cytoplasmic membrane from rupture due to the high internal osmotic pressure generated by the cytoplasm. As noted, wall composition differs fundamentally between Gram-negative and Gram-positive

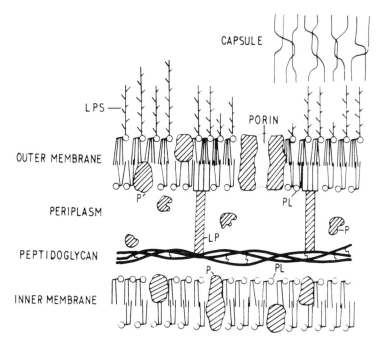

CAPSULE

LPS

PORIN

OUTER MEMBRANE

P'

PL

PERIPLASM

LP

P

PEPTIDOGLYCAN

P

PL

INNER MEMBRANE

Figure 1.2 The cell envelope of a Gram-negative bacterium: LP, lipoprotein; LPS, lipopolysaccharide; P, protein; PL, phospholipid. Flagella are not illustrated. (Reproduced, with permission, from Hancock & Poxton (1988).)

organisms. In Gram-negative bacteria (Fig. 1.2) the inner region of the wall is a thin layer of peptidoglycan. The outer region of the wall in some respects resembles the cytoplasmic membrane and is therefore commonly called the outer membrane. The region between the inner and outer wall layers is termed the periplasm and found only in Gram-negative bacteria. In Gram-positive bacteria (Fig. 1.3) the wall also contains peptidoglycan, but in addition it contains 'accessory' or secondary wall polymers, e.g. teichoic acids, polysaccharides and proteins that are covalently linked to the peptidoglycan throughout its thickness. The walls of Gram-positive bacteria can also contain loosely associated lipocarbohydrates (Fig. 1.3). In Gram-positive cells the wall is not bounded by the outer membranous layer that is found in Gram-negative bacteria, and hence there is no periplasm. Various surface appendages such as pili, capsules and flagellae may also be attached to the wall. These frequently play a role in the pathogenesis of bacterial infections, for example pili mediate adhesion of pathogens to epithelial surfaces, capsules can prevent phagocytosis and flagellae, by virtue of chemotactic responses, can propel bacteria through mucus layers that overlie epithelial surfaces.

Capsules, which are discrete, tightly bound, polysaccharide layers, are quite distinct from the extracellular mucoid substance (glycocalyx or mucoexopolysac-charide), loosely associated with the surface of some types of bacteria, e.g.

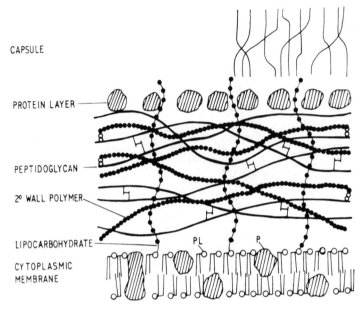

CAPSULE

PROTEIN LAYER

PEPTIDOGLYCAN

2° WALL POLYMER

LIPOCARBOHYDRATE

CYTOPLASMIC MEMBRANE

PL   P

Figure 1.3 The cell envelope of a Gram-positive bacterium. Note that not all the components shown occur in every strain of Gram-positive bacterium. P, protein; PL, phospholipid. Flagella are not illustrated. The secondary wall polymer is frequently teichoic acid. (Reproduced, with permission, from Hancock & Poxton (1988).)

Pseudomonas aeruginosa. The glycocalyx, composed of fibrous polysaccharides or globular glycoproteins, plays an important role in bacterial adhesion, both to sister cells and to other strata to produce microcolonies in the form of biofilms. The formation of biofilms may protect organisms from inhibition by antibacterial agents.

2.2.2 Peptidoglycan

Peptidoglycan, which contributes to the mechanical stability of cell walls, is a polymer consisting of a disaccharide repeating unit of two different *N*-acetylated amino sugars, to one of which is attached a short peptide chain. Individual glycan strands are cross-linked through peptide bonds between the peptide chains to create a covalent network with great mechanical strength. The same types of cross-link also serve to join together sheets of peptidoglycan in bacteria that have multiple sheets. Fig. 1.4 shows the structure of *Escherichia coli* peptidoglycan illustrating a repeating *N*-acetylglucosamine-*N*-acetylmuramic acid disaccharide unit, a tetrapeptide side chain and one of the frequent types of cross-link found, i.e. the carboxyl group of D-alanine residue 4 in one primary chain is linked directly to another amino acid, mesodiaminopimelic acid, at the third position of a neighbouring chain. There is considerable diversity among bacteria in the nature and frequency of the

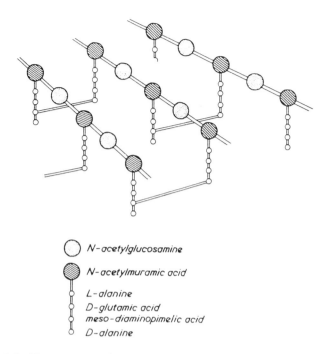

N-acetylglucosamine
N-acetylmuramic acid
L-alanine
D-glutamic acid
meso-diaminopimelic acid
D-alanine

Figure 1.4   The structure of *E. coli* peptidoglycan showing one of the frequent types of cross-link. (Reproduced, with permission, from Hammond *et al.* (1984).)

cross-linking bridges as well as the composition of the tetrapeptides, particularly at positions 2 and 3. Until recently the traditional view of bacterial peptidoglycan structure has emphasized that in any particular bacterial species only one type of cross-link is found, e.g. the well-known tetrapeptide–tetrapeptide pattern in *E. coli* (Fig. 1.4). However, the recent introduction of sophisticated methods for bacterial peptidoglycan analysis reveals that other types of cross-linkages can also occur alongside the well-recognized ones, e.g. in *E. coli* cross-links involving two diaminopimelic acid residues have now been identified.

The peptidoglycan layer is not covalently attached to the underlying cytoplasmic membrane but, in the case of Gram-negative bacteria, it is firmly bound to the outer membrane of the wall by covalent linkage of occasional side chains to an abundant outer membrane protein called murein lipoprotein (Figs 1.2 and 1.5). Nearly all bacteria have an absolute requirement for peptidoglycan in their walls in contrast to mammalian cells which are surrounded only by a cytoplasmic membrane which does not contain peptidoglycan. Peptidoglycan synthesis therefore constitutes a good selective target for antibiotic action and we shall see later (Chapter 2) that there are indeed many clinically useful compounds that inhibit peptidoglycan synthesis at various stages in its production. Without doubt the most important of these antibiotics are the β-lactams.

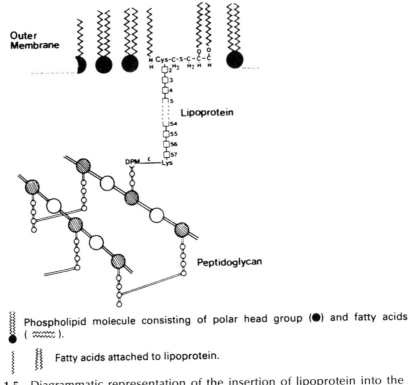

Figure 1.5   Diagrammatic representation of the insertion of lipoprotein into the
/outer membrane. The diagram shows a lipoprotein molecule linked to the
diaminopimelic acid residue (DPM) of peptidoglycan by its terminal lysine. The
symbols used for peptidoglycan structure are as in Fig. 1.4. (Reproduced, with
permission, from Hammond *et al.* (1984).)

2.2.3   *Outer membrane of the Gram-negative cell wall*

The outer membrane of the Gram-negative cell wall has a bilayer structure (Fig.
1.2) but, in contrast to the cytoplasmic membrane (see below), only the inner
leaflet contains phospholipid molecules. The lipid content of the outer leaflet
derives exclusively from lipopolysaccharide, a molecule unique to the outer
membrane. The lipopolysaccharide molecule consists of three regions (Figs 1.6
and 1.7). The lipid moiety of the lipopolysaccharide, called lipid A, is integrated
into the outer membrane bilayer with its fatty acid residues projecting towards the
centre. The core polysaccharide with its attached *O*-polysaccharide side chain (O
antigen) projects outwards.

If the outer leaflet of the outer membrane was composed only of lipopolysaccharide very few molecules (e.g. essential solutes) would be able to cross it to
reach the cytoplasmic membrane. However, interspersed throughout the outer

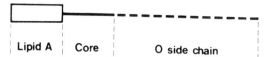

Figure 1.6 Representation of the three regions of bacterial lipopolysaccharides (LPSs). The lipid A region is embedded in the phospholipid bilayer, the core and O side chain polysaccharide extending outwards from the cell. (Reproduced, with permission, from Hammond *et al.* (1984).)

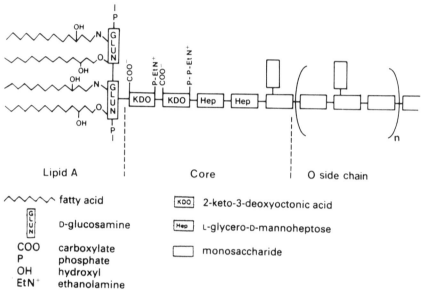

Figure 1.7 Generalized structure of bacterial lipopolysaccharide. The structure of the lipid A region is highly conserved amongst a wide range of Gram-negative bacteria. Similarly, little variation is found in the inner core (KDO–heptose) region. Considerable variation is present in the monosaccharides that constitute the outer core and O side chain regions and consequently they have been left as empty blocks. (Reproduced, with permission, from Hammond *et al.* (1984).)

membrane are a number of proteins, in particular the porins, that considerably modify its permeability characteristics. The *E. coli* proteins OmpC, OmpF and PhoE (and their counterparts in other species) form abundant non-specific transmembrane pores that allow the diffusion of small hydrophilic molecules (including antibiotics) within a limited size range (generally up to 600 Da), across the membrane. PhoE channels are particularly involved with the passage of negatively charged molecules (e.g. compounds containing carboxylate, sulphate or phosphate residues). The OmpC and F channels contain three Omp protein molecules each of which opens at the surface of the outer membrane (Fig. 1.8).

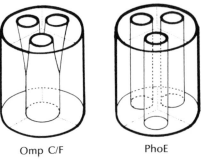

Omp C/F   PhoE

Figure 1.8 Schematic three-dimensional representations of the structures of different porin proteins. The porins are oriented such that the top of the figure is the portion exposed in the external environment, whereas the bottom is the portion extending into the periplasm. The plane of the outer membrane would run horizontal to these channels. (Reproduced, with permission, from Hancock (1987).)

However, the three separate openings merge into a single channel near the mid-point of the membrane (Fig. 1.8). In contrast, individual PhoE protein molecules can form transmembrane channels in their own right, but tend to aggregate in groups of three within the outer membrane (Fig. 1.8). Some molecules that pass through the outer membrane do so by routes that do not involve diffusion through the non-specific pores mentioned above. Many of the less abundant proteins of the outer membrane are specific transport proteins or receptors that mediate the entry of molecules unable to pass through the regular porins. These proteins are responsible for the entry of ferric iron chelates, maltose and maltodextrins, nucleosides and vitamin B12. In some cases these transport proteins form specialized pores, but in other cases the molecular mechanism by which transmembrane transport is achieved is unknown.

Certain chelating agents, e.g. ethylenediamine tetraacetic acid (EDTA) at alkaline pH, are particularly active against *Ps. aeruginosa* and *Neisseria* spp. This is attributable to effects on the structural integrity of the outer membrane. For example, EDTA, by virtue of its chelating properties, causes release of Mg^{2+} and Ca^{2+} from the outer membrane resulting in secondary loss of up to 50% of the lipopolysaccharide (see also permeabilizing agents, Chapter 3).

2.2.4 Cell walls of mycobacteria

Although mycobacteria are difficult to stain, they do, nevertheless, give a Gram-positive staining response. However, the cell walls of the mycobacteria differ considerably from those of the more typical Gram-positive bacteria described above. Since the unusual nature of the cell wall in these organisms is responsible for intrinsic resistance to certain antibiotics and biocides, a brief description of wall structure is presented here.

The mycobacterial cell wall is a complex structure (Fig. 1.9: see also Chapter

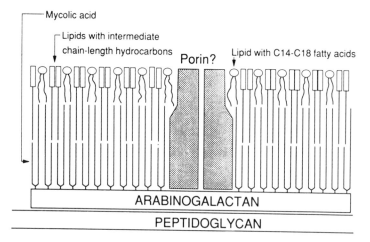

Figure 1.9 A model for the structure of the mycobacterial cell wall. Each residue of mycolic acid contributes two hydrocarbon chains of unequal lengths. Consequently, the outer leaflet must also contain intermediate-length hydrocarbons, in order to fit with the staggered surface of the inner leaflet. Such lipids have been found in mycobacteria. The model also shows the hypothetical shape of the porin protein, whose presence has recently been established. (Reproduced, with permission, from Nikaido *et al.* (1993).)

6). Its basal layer is peptidoglycan covalently linked to arabinogalactan (a polysaccharide copolymer of arabinose and galactose) which is esterified to the mycolic acids. The mycolic acids are high-molecular-weight (60–90 carbon atoms) 3-hydroxy fatty acids with an alkyl side chain at the 2-position. Many types of mycolic acids, with a variety of different oxygen functions and skeletal features, have been identified in mycobacteria and their distribution within the mycobacteria displays some degree of species specificity. *Mycobacterium tuberculosis* contains α, keto and methoxy mycolic acids (Fig. 1.10). Within the α series there are acids with *cis* double bonds, *cis* cyclopropane rings or *trans* double bonds with adjacent methyl branches (Fig. 1.10). Mycobacterial cell walls also contain complex lipids, lipopolysaccharides and proteins.

Until recently the lipids found in the mycobacterial cell envelope were considered to form an amorphous, unorganized wax. However, recent evidence points to a more organized structure with the hydrocarbon chains of the various lipids lying perpendicular to the plane of the cell wall (Fig. 1.9). This arrangement undoubtedly acts as a barrier to the penetration of hydrophilic molecules, including antibiotics. However, mycobacteria must take up nutrients, which are mostly hydrophilic molecules, from the outside medium. Recent evidence points to the presence of porin (protein) channels in the mycobacterial cell envelope (Fig. 1.9) through which nutrients could diffuse. Thus there are obvious similarities in the organization of cell walls in mycobacteria and Gram-negative bacteria.

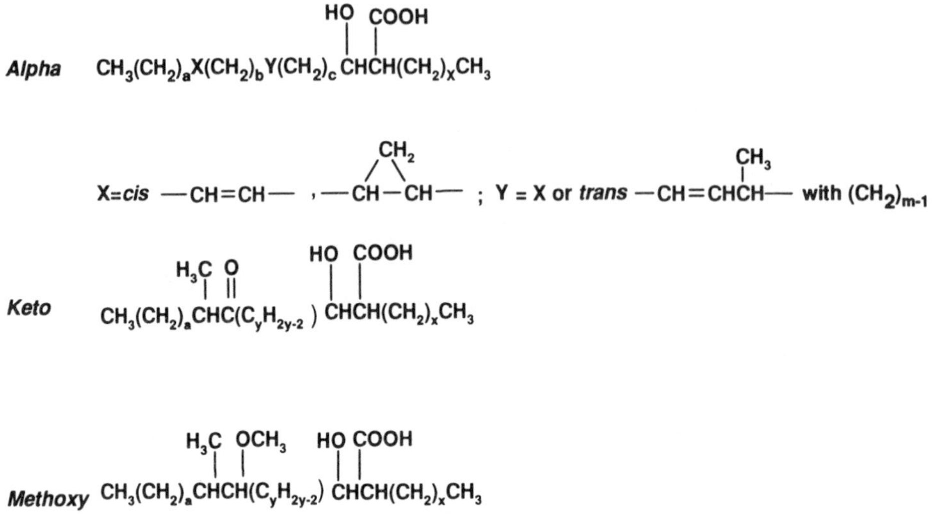

$$HO \quad COOH$$
$$| \quad |$$
Alpha $CH_3(CH_2)_aX(CH_2)_bY(CH_2)_c CHCH(CH_2)_xCH_3$

$$CH_2$$
$$/ \ \backslash$$
X=*cis* —CH=CH— , —CH—CH— ; Y = X or *trans* —CH=CHCH— with $(CH_2)_{m-1}$

$$\qquad\qquad CH_3$$
$$\qquad\qquad |$$

$$H_3C \quad O \qquad HO \quad COOH$$
$$| \quad \parallel \qquad | \quad |$$
Keto $CH_3(CH_2)_aCHC(C_yH_{2y-2}) CHCH(CH_2)_xCH_3$

$$H_3C \quad OCH_3 \quad HO \quad COOH$$
$$| \quad | \qquad | \quad |$$
Methoxy $CH_3(CH_2)_aCHCH(C_yH_{2y-2}) CHCH(CH_2)_xCH_3$

a = 15, 17, 19; b = 14, 16; c = 11, 13, 15, 17; x = 19, 21, 23; y = 31 - 39

Figure 1.10   Structure of mycolic acids found in *Mycobacterium tuberculosis*.

Uptake of antimicrobial agents across the mycobacterial cell wall will be considered in more detail in Chapter 2 and the role of the wall in resistance to biocides in Chapter 6.

2.3 Cytoplasmic membrane

The cytoplasmic membrane lies directly outside the cytoplasm (Fig. 1.1). It acts as a selective permeability barrier between the cytoplasm and the cell environment and is also the site at which many important and indispensable cellular activities occur. Cytoplasmic membranes primarily consist of phospholipids and proteins, although the exact membrane composition depends on the cell of origin. The phospholipid molecules are arranged in a bilayer with polar groups directed outwards on both sides (Figs 1.2, 1.3). The membrane proteins are enzymes and carrier proteins, the latter mediating specific transport of nutrients and ions. Membrane enzymes perform the following reactions: (a) energy generation through electron transport and oxidative phosphorylation, (b) synthesis of complex lipids, (c) the final stages of peptidoglycan synthesis, (d) synthesis of external envelope components such as lipopolysaccharides and capsular polysaccharides, (e) transduction of sensory signals for motility and chemotaxis and (f) secretion of exo proteins.

The bacterial cytoplasmic membrane is a vital cellular component since it provides the matrix by which metabolism is linked to solute transport, flagellar movement and the generation of ATP (Fig. 1.11). The electron transport system, the cytochromes, quinones, iron sulphur proteins and flavine adenine dinucleotides are embedded in the cytoplasmic membrane, which acts as an insulator. During metabolism, protons are extruded to the exterior of the bacterial cell, the net result being acidification of the cell exterior which also becomes positively charged relative to the interior. This combined potential, the concentration or osmotic effect of the proton and its electropositivity, is the electrochemical potential of the proton (μ_{H^+}), which can be quantified and expressed in terms of electrical units (mV). It is this potential, termed the proton-motive force (PMF), which drives those ancillary activities described above.

The net result of electron transfer or ATP hydrolysis is the generation of gradients of electrical or membrane potential ($\Delta\psi$) and chemical potential (ΔpH). The PMF, denoted by Δp, is described by the equation $\Delta p = \Delta\psi - Z\Delta$pH, where Z represents $2.303\,RT/F$ and has a value of 61 millivolts at 37°C; Δp is also expressed in millivolts. The pH difference (ΔpH) measures the contribution to Δp of the osmotic gradient due to the proton concentration potential.

Several antibacterial compounds affect the cytoplasmic membrane. They include the polymyxin group of antibiotics, the ionophorous antibiotics and various types of antiseptics, disinfectants and preservatives. The polymyxins, which disrupt cytoplasmic membrane integrity, have some limited uses in antibacterial chemotherapy (Chapter 2), but the ionophores, e.g. valinomycin which is a specific conductor of K^+, interact with both bacterial cytoplasmic membranes and mammalian membranes and therefore cannot be used clinically. The various antiseptics, disinfectants and preservatives that act at the level of the bacterial cytoplasmic membrane (Chapter 3) may inhibit specific membrane-bound enzymes or perturb homeostatic mechanisms by (a) inducing leakage of intracellular constituents, (b) inducing lysis, or (c) dissipating the PMF. The cytoplasmic membrane might be a primary site of action of the cross-linking agent glutaraldehyde (used as a chemical sterilizing agent for specific purposes). Although this compound rapidly inhibits DNA, RNA and protein synthesis (and indeed combines with these macromolecules) its antibacterial activity is likely to occur via aldehyde–protein reactions in the cell wall or membrane which 'seal' the surface thereby preventing uptake of macromolecular precursors into the cell.

2.4 Cytoplasm

The cytoplasm (or cytosol) is the region lying within the bacterial cytoplasmic membrane. It contains DNA, RNA and protein synthesizing complexes, a variety of enzymes, macromolecular precursors and other low-molecular-weight metabolites. Together these components participate in a variety of catabolic and anabolic processes (e.g. see Fig. 1.12) that are essential for bacterial growth. We shall concentrate in particular on the structure and synthesis of nucleic acids and

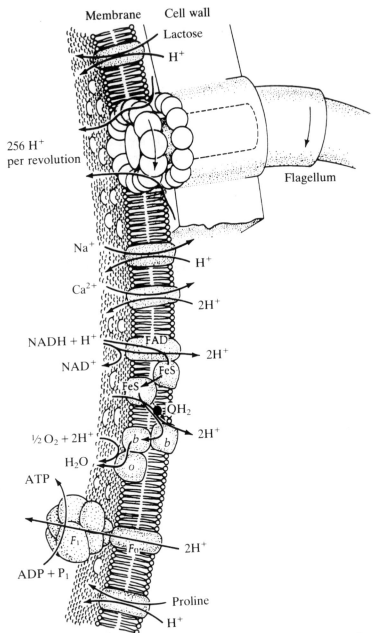

Figure 1.11 Chemiosmosis and the bacterial membrane. A proton gradient is generated by the operation of the respiratory chain. The passage of protons down this gradient can be coupled to ATP synthesis, active transport and flagellar motion. FeS, iron sulphur protein; QH_2, hydroquinone; b, o, cytochromes b and o; F_1, F_0, components of ATPase. (Reproduced, with permission, from Hinkle & McCarthy (1978).).

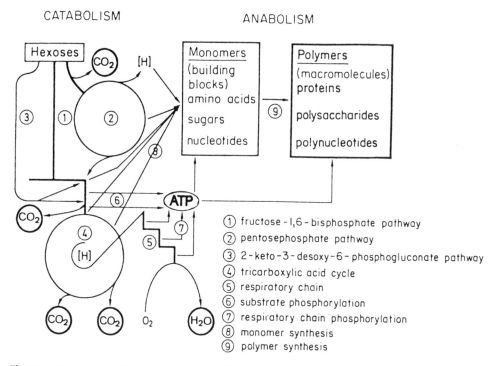

Figure 1.12 Metabolic map of aerobically respiring cells catabolizing hexoses. (Reproduced, with permission, from Schlegel (1986).)

proteins since many clinically useful antibiotics interfere with these processes in bacteria, and some biocides combine strongly with these macromolecules. The biocides are not suitable for consideration as internal chemotherapeutic agents because of their lack of selective toxicity. Some are, however, important disinfectants or sterilizing agents (aldehydes, ethylene oxide), hydrogen peroxide is used as a disinfectant for cleansing wounds, and many find use as antiseptics or preservatives.

2.4.1 *Chromosome structure and DNA replication*

The bacterial chromosome is a single circular DNA molecule consisting of two very long helical polynucleotide chains coiled around a common axis. It is not surrounded by a membrane and has no defined shape. Because DNA contains the genetic information of the cell, its replication and division must precede cell division so that the chromosome is distributed to the two new cells. Although the concept of DNA replication developed by Watson and Crick in the 1950s is of course still generally valid, the process is now known to be highly complex in that at least 18 different gene products participate directly in the replication of the *E.*

coli chromosome. One of these gene products, the enzyme DNA gyrase, is a target for the quinolone antibiotics (see Chapter 2). Although mammalian cells have a similar enzyme, quinolones developed to date for medical use inhibit this enzyme only at concentrations that are two to three orders of magnitude above that required for antibacterial activity. The action of quinolones will be considered in more detail in Chapter 2. The acridines, which are biocides rather than chemotherapeutic agents, also inhibit DNA synthesis. In this case, however, inhibition results from intercalation of acridines into DNA molecules.

Although DNA synthesis can be blocked at the level of replication by quinolones and acridines, other antibacterial agents interfere with the synthesis of the nucleotides required for the formation of the polynucleotide chain in DNA. Antibiotics that interfere with the synthesis of tetrahydrofolate act in this manner because this compound acts as a donor of one-carbon units in several steps of nucleotide biosynthesis. Interruption of the supply of tetrahydrofolate soon brings nucleotide and nucleic acid synthesis to a halt. The reaction most severely affected is thymine synthesis, and hence DNA synthesis is particularly susceptible to inhibition of tetrahydrofolate production. Although tetrahydrofolate is an essential coenzyme for all cells, the ability to synthesize it from simple constituents is restricted to bacteria (Fig. 1.13). Since mammalian cells are unable to synthesize folic acid (Fig. 1.13), it therefore becomes an essential vitamin for humans and is obtained from the diet. Most pathogenic bacteria are unable to take up preformed folic acid derivatives from the environment and require the enzyme dihydropteroate synthetase (DHPS) to meet their need for tetrahydrofolic acid (Fig. 1.13). This enzyme (DHPS) is inhibited by a group of antibiotics known as the sulphonamides. Since DHPS is absent from mammalian cells, human tissues are unaffected by sulphonamide drugs. The action of sulphonamide and other antifolate agents will be considered in more detail in Chapter 2.

2.4.2 *Synthesis of RNA and protein and the nature of ribosomes*

DNA coding regions in the chromosomes are termed 'genes'. Genes govern the synthesis of proteins, ribosomal and transfer RNAs. Proteins are made under the direction of structural genes by the coupled processes of transcription and translation. Transcription (messenger RNA synthesis) involves the copying of one strand of DNA into mRNA which is then decoded or translated into protein at the ribosome in participation with aminoacyl-tRNA molecules (see below). A single enzyme, RNA polymerase, is responsible for all mRNA synthesis. Ribosomal and transfer RNAs are also made by the same polymerase that makes mRNA.

Ribosomes are the complex organelles that catalyse the translation of information encoded in mRNA into protein. Polypeptide elongation is a cyclic process whereby aminoacyl-tRNA molecules bind to the ribosome as dictated by the mRNA. In growing bacteria approximately 80–90% of ribosomes are attached to mRNA and are actively engaged in protein synthesis. The structure for synthesizing protein, i.e. mRNA with attached ribosomes, is termed a polysome. Proteins that

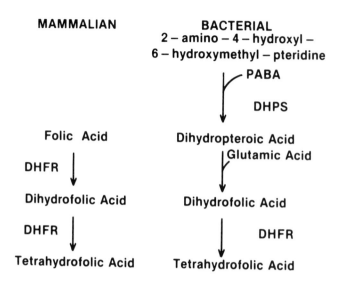

Figure 1.13 The tetrahydrofolic acid biosynthetic pathway in mammals and bacteria: PABA, p-aminobenzoic acid; DHPS, dihydropteroate synthetase; DHFR, dihydrofolate reductase.

are to pass into or through the bacterial cytoplasmic membrane are invariably synthesized on polysomes that become attached by their nascent polypeptides to the inner surface of the cytoplasmic membrane, whereas cytoplasmic proteins are synthesized on polysomes that are not membrane associated.

An individual bacterial ribosome is a complex ribonucleoprotein particle which is designated as a 70S ribosome since it sediments in centrifugation studies with a velocity of 70 Svedberg (S) units. The molecular structure of bacterial ribosomes, particularly those from *E. coli*, is well understood and a system of nomenclature to describe them was adopted a number of years ago (Fig. 1.14). The 70S ribosome comprises two subunits, the so-called 50S and 30S subunits. Each subunit contains RNA and protein (Fig. 1.14). The small subunit contains one RNA molecule (16S) and 21 different proteins numbered S (small subunit) 1–21. The large subunit contains two RNA molecules (5S and 23S) and 32 different proteins numbered L (large subunit) 1–34. Subsequently it was discovered that L8 is an aggregate of proteins L7–L12–L10 and that L26 is identical to S20. Furthermore, L7 and L12 differ only by the presence in L7 of an acetyl group at the amino terminus of the protein.

Bacterial RNA synthesis can be selectively inhibited by the group of antibiotics known as rifamycins (Chapter 2). These antibiotics bind to and inhibit bacterial RNA polymerases but are without effect on the corresponding mammalian enzyme. Many antibacterial substances directly inhibit protein synthesis (Chapter 2). In most cases this is due to prevention of processes which take place on ribosomes. As we shall see, the specificity of clinically useful inhibitors of protein

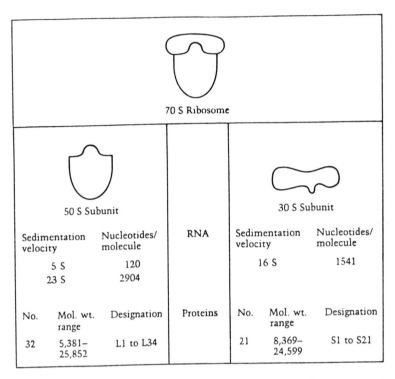

Figure 1.14 The molecular structure of ribosomes from *E. coli*: based on the molecular weights of 19 proteins from the small subunit and 29 proteins from the large subunit, the primary structures of which are known. The discrepancy between numbers of proteins (32) in the large subunit and their designation (up to L34) derives from the fact that one protein, L8, which was thought to be unique when numbered as a spot on a chromatogram, is now known to be an association of L7, L12, and L10 and that another, L26, is identical to S20. Only small amounts of L26 remain associated with the large subunit on dissociation of the 70S ribosome. (Reproduced, with permission, from Ingraham *et al.* (1983).)

synthesis arises principally from their binding to bacterial 70S ribosomes, while mammalian ribosomes (80S particles) are left unaffected because the drugs usually fail to bind to this class of ribosome. The disinfectant hydrogen peroxide reversibly dissociates 70S ribosomes into 50S and 30S subunits. Peroxide does, however, have effects elsewhere in the cell which also contribute to its bactericidal activity.

3
Structure of spores

Currently 13 bacterial genera are recognized as endospore formers, although several of these are heterogenous in the context of their DNA base composition.

The most important spore formers are members of the genera *Bacillus* and *Clostridium*, but certain other bacteria, e.g. *Sporosarcina*, *Desulfomaculum* and *Sporolactobacillus* can also form spores. True endospores are also produced by thermophilic actinomyces, e.g. *Thermoactinomyces vulgaris*. Only spores produced by *Bacillus* spp. and *Clostridium* spp. will be considered here and subsequently.

The structure (Figs 1.15 and 1.16) and composition (Table 1.2) of spores differ fundamentally from those of vegetative cells. The germ cell (protoplast or core) and germ cell wall are surrounded by the cortex. The cortex itself is surrounded by spore coats, the outer coat being the most dense. In some spores, e.g. *B. polymyxa*, a layer known as the exosporium exists outside the spore coats, whereas in other spores, e.g. *B. cereus*, an exosporium surrounds only one dense spore coat. Under certain conditions, spores will germinate and outgrow to produce vegetative cells, which have the typical form and composition of non-sporing bacteria.

Bacterial spores are among the most resistant of all microbial forms to inactivation by chemical or physical (e.g. heat, radiation) agents. This aspect will be dealt with in considerably more detail in Chapter 7, and suffice to state here that the outer coats and to some extent the cortex also appear to present a barrier to the intracellular penetration of many biocides, whereas the comparatively dry interior of the spore is associated with resistance to heat and radiation. Since spores develop from vegetative cells that are themselves sensitive to most chemical and physical processes, it follows that resistance will be expressed during sporulation. However, during the germination and/or outgrowth stages, the organisms may, like vegetative cells, be susceptible to inhibitors. These aspects are also considered in depth in Chapter 7. The remainder of the present section is devoted to a description of spore structure and the sequence of changes during endospore formation and germination.

3.1 Spore core (protoplast)

In terms of its macromolecular constituents, the core is a relatively normal cell and most, if not all, spore enzymes are structurally similar to the corresponding enzymes in germinated cells. However, when located inside the spore, enzymes are protected from denaturation by heat. The core is the location of DNA, RNA and protein.

Some 10–20% of the protein in the dormant spore is in the form of a group of small acid-soluble proteins (SASPs). These exist as two types:

(a) α,β types, associated with spore DNA, the products of a multigenic family and synthesized around the third hour (t_3) of sporulation;
(b) γ types, not associated with any macromolecule, the products of a single gene and also synthesized at around t_3 of sporulation.

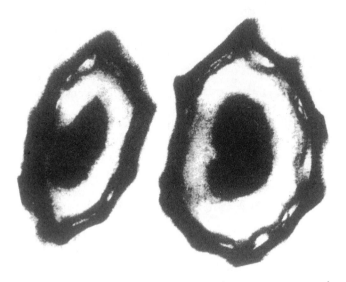

Figure 1.15 *Bacillus subtilis* spores showing the core, cortex and spore coats. Magnification, ×80 000.

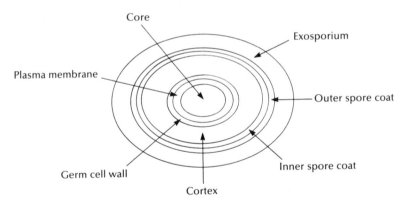

Figure 1.16 A diagrammatic representation of a typical bacterial spore.

During germination, these proteins are rapidly degraded. SASPs are essential for spore resistance to ultraviolet radiation and spores deficient in $\alpha\beta$-type SASP ($\alpha^-\beta^-$ spores) are much more sensitive to hydrogen peroxide than are mature spores: see Chapters 4 and 7.

The spore core is a comparatively dry compartment with a low water activity (A_w value). Therefore the environments surrounding DNA in spores and vegetative cells differ. The biologically important form of DNA in vegetative cells is the B form, in which there are ten base pairs for each turn of the double helix.

Table 1.2 Chemical composition of spore structures

Spore structure	Chemical composition	Comment
Outer spore coat (OSC)	Predominantly protein: a preponderance of disulphide (−S−S) bonds in cystine-rich protein	Alkali-resistant, the OSC may be removed by disulphide bond-disrupting agents
Inner spore coat (ISC)	Predominantly protein: mainly acidic polypeptides	Alkali-sensitive, the acidic polypeptides can be dissociated to unit components by treatment with SDS[a]
Cortex	Mainly peptidoglycan	Presence of internal amide (muramic lactam: see Fig. 1.18)
Core	Protein, DNA, RNA, DPA, divalent metals	DNA in B form. Presence of SASP[b], α/β types of which associated with DNA

[a]SDS, sodium dodecyl sulphate.
[b]SASP, small, acid-soluble proteins (see also text and Chapters 3 and 7).

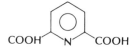

Figure 1.17 Chemical structure of dipicolinic acid.

However, within the comparatively dry spore, the bases tilt to produce a more compact structure, the A form, where there are eleven base pairs per turn. Interestingly, compared with DNA in vegetative cells, the DNA in spores responds differently to ultraviolet and ionizing radiations, but DNA extracted from spores shows the same *in vitro* response as vegetative cell DNA. The core contains much less free water than do vegetative cells: in fact, the amount actually free in the core could well be zero because much of the water is likely to be intimately associated with macromolecules or with small molecules.

Dipicolinic acid (DPA, Fig. 1.17) is a unique spore constituent the majority of which is associated in a chelated form with calcium, thereby preserving electrical neutrality. For many years DPA was considered to be a component of the spore cortex, but more recent evidence demonstrates that DPA is located in the core and not in the cortex. DPA is lost during germination and its specific role in the spore remains a subject of conjecture. DPA is no longer considered to be a major contributory factor to the high heat resistance of spores.

Major differences between the dormant spore core and the interior of a vegetable cell reside in their complement of small molecules. Thus, a cell has high ATP, ADP, glutamic acid, NAD, NADH, NADP and NADPH but low DPA, calcium, magnesium, manganese and 3-phosphoglycerate (3-PGA). In contrast, a spore core has high DPA, metals and 3-PGA but a low content of ATP, ADP, etc.

3.2 Spore membranes

During sporulation, two membranes surround the forespore. These are

(a) the inner forespore membrane (IFSM), which eventually becomes the cytoplasmic membrane of the germinating spore, and
(b) the outer forespore membrane (OFSM) which persists in the spore integuments i.e. outer spore layers.

Initially, the ISFM and OSFM are extensions of the mother cell membrane, but later they are differentiated both in composition and function and the specialized spore integument is formed between the two.

3.3 Spore cortex

The cortex lies between the core and the coat(s). It consists largely of peptidoglycan which is similar to, but not identical with, that found in vegetative cell forms. A dense inner layer of the cortex known as the germ cell wall (also termed the spore cell wall, primordial cell wall, or cortical membrane) develops into the cell wall of the emergent cell when the cortex is degraded during germination and outgrowth. The germ cell wall has the chemical structure of vegetative rather than spore peptidoglycan. In disrupted spores, the cortex and usually the germ cell wall are degraded by lysozyme and the repeating unit of peptidoglycan depicted in Fig. 1.18 has been obtained following analysis of the digestion products of several *Bacillus* spp.

The osmotically dehydrated nature of the mature spore is maintained by means of the electronegatively charged peptidoglycan and positively charged counterions in the cortex. Heating in the presence of acids results in protonation of the peptidoglycan with a consequent fall in its osmotic effectiveness.

3.4 Spore coats

Spore coat synthesis commences fairly early in sporulation, but completion is a much later event, occurring at the same time as the development of refractility. The spore coats play an important role in the resistance of bacterial spores to

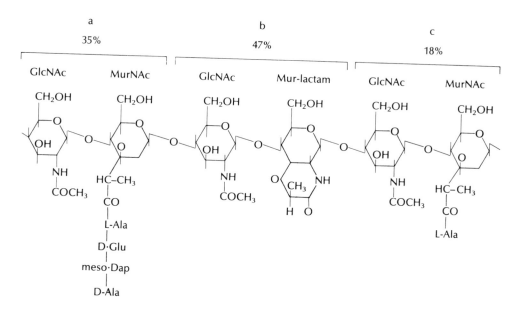

Figure 1.18 Chemical structure of spore peptidoglycan: part a corresponds to vegetative cell peptidoglycan; part b consists partly of muramic lactam (Mur-lactam); part c contains an incomplete peptide. GlcNAc, *N*-acetylglucosamine; MurNAc, *N*-acetylmuramic acid.

disinfectants and preservatives. They constitute a major portion of the spore, occupying about 50% of the spore volume, and consist mainly of protein and inorganic phosphorus with smaller amounts of complex carbohydrates and lipid. Proteins in the inner and outer coats differ quite substantially. An alkali-soluble fraction resides in the inner coat and consists predominantly of acid polypeptides, whereas the outer coat contains an alkali-resistant fraction associated with the presence of cystine-rich protein. The removal of spore coats by various procedures (described in Chapter 7, section 2.4) has been used to define their role as barriers to the intracellular penetration of chemical agents.

3.5 Sporulation, germination and outgrowth

Sporulation is a complex process which commonly takes about 8 h from the end of vegetative growth to the release of a mature spore (Table 1.2). In contrast, germination is more rapid (Table 1.3) and is followed by an outgrowth phase in which macromolecular synthesis takes place leading to the development of a vegetative cell culture. The stages involved in sporulation and germination and their influence on the activity of biocides will be considered in detail in Chapter 7.

Table 1.3 Sequence of major changes accompanying endospore formation and germination[a]

Spore formation[b]	Spore germination[c,d]
End of vegetative growth	Addition of germinants
Chromatin filament formed	Heat resistance lost
Spore protease excreted	
Forespore septum formed	Calcium and DPA excreted
Forespore protoplast engulfed	Temporary rise in resistance to ultraviolet
Heat-resistant catalase formed	irradiation
Peptidoglycan cortex synthesized	Refractility loss observable by contrast
Dipicolinic acid (DPA) synthesized	microscopy (see Chapter 4)
Spore becomes refractile	
Uptake of calcium	Resistance to stains lost
Spore coats assembled	Release of fragments of hydrolysed pep-
Resistance to organic solvents acquired	tidoglycan
Resistance to heat acquired	Fall in optical density of spore suspen-
Resistance to some biocides	sions
Mother cell lyses to release mature	Onset of metabolism
spore	Fall in ultraviolet resistance

[a]Based on G. W. Gould (1984). In *The Revival of Injured Microbes* (eds M. H. E. Andrew and A. D. Russell). Academic Press, London.
[b]Spore formation, time scale about 8 h. Resistance to biocides is discussed in Chapter 7.
[c]Spore germination, time scale about 5 min. Effect of biocides is discussed in Chapter 4.
[d]See also comments about 3-phosphoglycerate (3-PGA) and small, acid-soluble proteins (SASPs) in Chapter 4.

Sporulation (*spo*) and germination (*ger*) mutants have been of considerable value in mapping the changes that occur in these processes. The former have also been employed in relating structural changes during sporulation with resistance to biocidal agents (Chapter 7).

4
Summary

This chapter has outlined the structure and metabolism of bacteria and their spores and indicated those targets that are susceptible to inhibition or destruction by antibacterial agents. It has been noted that some antibacterial agents are also inhibitory to mammalian systems, and are therefore used primarily to disinfect inanimate objects. Other agents with a low level of toxicity can be used as antiseptics or preservatives, while agents (i.e. antibiotics) with a high degree of selectivity towards bacteria are used systemically as chemotherapeutic agents. In general, antibacterial agents that interfere with peptidoglycan synthesis, cytoplasmic membrane integrity or enzymic processes in nucleic acid synthesis are bactericidal, while those which interfere with metabolic pathways or protein synthesis may either be bacteriostatic or bactericidal. The material that has been presented in this chapter is intended primarily to provide a general background for the more detailed discussion of bacterial targets to be found in Chapters 2 and 3.

Further reading

Bacterial structure and metabolism

Books

Hammond, S. M., Lambert, P. A. & Rycroft, A. N. (1984). *The Bacterial Cell Surface*. Croom Helm, London and Sydney.

Hancock, I. & Poxton, I. (1988). *Bacterial Cell Surface Techniques*. John Wiley & Sons, London.

Ingraham, J. L., Maaloe, O. & Neidhardt, F. C. (1983). *Growth of the Bacterial Cell*. Sinauer Associates Inc., Sunderland, USA.

Mandelstam, J., McQuillen, K. & Dawes, I. (1982). *Biochemistry of Bacterial Growth*. Third edition. Blackwell Scientific Publications, Oxford.

Rogers, H. J. (1983). *Bacterial Cell Structure*. Aspects of Microbiology, Volume 6. Van Nostrand Reinhold, Wokingham.

Schlegel, H. G. (1986). *General Microbiology*. Sixth edition. Cambridge University Press.

Review articles

Hancock, R. E. W. (1987). Role of porins in outer membrane permeability. *Journal of Bacteriology* **169**: 929–933.

Hinkle, P. C. & McCarthy, R. E. (1978). How cells make ATP. *Scientific American* **238**: 104–123.

Inderlied, C. B., Kemper, C. A. & Burmudez, L. E. M. (1993). The *Mycobacterium avium* complex. *Clinical Microbiology Reviews* **6**: 266–310.

Lambert, P. A. (1988). Enterobacteriaceae: composition, structure and function of the cell envelope. *Journal of Applied Bacteriology (Symposium Supplement)* **65**: 21S–34S.

McMacken, R., Silver, L. & Georgopoulos, C. (1987). DNA replication. In *Escherichia coli and Salmonella typhimurium, Cellular and Molecular Biology*, Volume 1 (ed. F. C. Neidhardt) pp. 564–612. American Society for Microbiology, Washington.

Minnikin, D. E. (1991). Chemical principles in the organization of lipid components in the mycobacterial cell envelope. *Research in Microbiology* **142**: 423–427.

Research papers

Nikaido, H., Kim, S.-H. & Rosenberg, E. Y. (1993). Physical organization of lipids in the cell wall of *Mycobacterium chelonae*. *Molecular Microbiology* **8**: 1025–1030.

Trias, J., Jarlier, V. & Benz, R. (1992). Porins in the cell wall of mycobacteria. *Science* **258**: 1479–1481.

The nature of spores

Books

Dring, G. J., Ellar, D. J. & Gould, G. W. (1985). *Fundamental and Applied Aspects of Bacterial Spores*. Academic Press, London.
Hurst, A. & Gould, G. W. (1984). *The Bacterial Spore*. Second edition. Academic Press, London.

Review articles

Errington, J. (1993). *Bacillus subtilis* sporulation: regulation of gene expression and control of morphogenesis. *Microbiological Reviews* **57**: 1–33.
Mandelstam, J. (1976). Bacterial sporulation: a problem in the biochemistry and genetics of a primitive developmental system. *Proceedings of the Royal Society of London, Series B* **193**: 89–106.
Setlow, P. (1988). Small, acid-soluble spore proteins of *Bacillus subtilis*: structure, synthesis, genetics, function and degradation. *Annual Review of Microbiology* **42**: 319–338.
Setlow, P. (1994). Mechanisms which contribute to the long-term survival of spores of *Bacillus* species. *Journal of Applied Bacteriology (Symposium Supplement)* **76**: 49S–60S.
Warth, A. D. (1978). Molecular structure of the bacterial endospore. *Advances in Microbial Physiology* **17**: 1–38.

Research paper

Fairhead, H., Setlow, B. & Setlow, P. (1993). Prevention of DNA damage in spores and *in vitro* by small, acid-soluble proteins from *Bacillus* species. *Journal of Bacteriology* **175**: 1367–1373.

Antibacterial compounds, their action and development

Books

Ayliffe, G. A. J., Coates, D. & Hoffman, P. N. (1994). *Chemical Disinfection in Hospitals*. Second edition. Public Health Laboratory Service, London.
Block, S. S. (1991). *Disinfection, Sterilization and Preservation*. Fourth edition. Lea & Febiger, Philadelphia.
Franklin, T. J. & Snow, G. A. (1989). *Biochemistry of Antimicrobial Action*. Fourth edition. Chapman & Hall, London.
Gale, E. F., Cundliffe, E., Reynolds, P. E., Richmond, M. H. & Waring, M. J. (1981). *The Molecular Basis of Antibiotic Action*. John Wiley & Sons, London.

Greenwood, D. (1989). *Antimicrobial Chemotherapy.* Second edition. Baillière Tindall, London.

Greenwood, D. & O'Grady, F. (1985). *The Scientific Basis of Antimicrobial Chemotherapy.* Symposium 38 of the Society for General Microbiology. Cambridge University Press.

Hugo, W. B. & Russell, A. D. (1992). *Pharmaceutical Microbiology.* Fifth edition. Blackwell Scientific Publications, Oxford.

Lorian, V. (1986). *Antibiotics in Laboratory Medicine.* Second edition. Williams & Wilkins, Baltimore.

Russell, A. D. (1982). *The Destruction of Bacterial Spores.* Academic Press, London.

Russell, A. D., Hugo, W. B. & Ayliffe, G. A. J. (1992). *Principles and Practice of Disinfection, Preservation and Sterilization.* Second edition. Blackwell Scientific Publications, Oxford.

Review article

Gootz, T. D. (1990). Discovery and development of new antimicrobial agents. *Clinical Microbiology Reviews* **3**: 13–31.

CHAPTER TWO

Mode of action of antibiotics and their uptake into bacteria

1
Introduction

In the previous chapter the modes of action of antibacterial antibiotics were outlined. In this chapter the molecular basis of their action and the mechanisms by which the drug molecules reach their intracellular target sites are dealt with more extensively.

It is convenient to consider the majority of antibiotics in groups as inhibitors of (a) nucleic acid synthesis, (b) protein synthesis, (c) peptidoglycan synthesis, and (d) membrane integrity. However, those antibiotics that are specific antimycobacterial agents will be considered separately.

2
Inhibitors of nucleic acid synthesis

2.1 Introduction

The growth and division of bacterial cells depend, amongst other factors, on DNA and RNA syntheses. Antibiotics that interfere with these syntheses fall into three main categories:

(a) compounds that interrupt nucleotide metabolism, usually by interference with nucleotide synthesis or nucleotide interconversion;
(b) compounds that interfere with the role of DNA as a template in replication and transcription, either by reacting with it directly to form a complex, or by causing structural alterations such as strand breakage or removal of bases;
(c) agents which directly inhibit enzymic processes in nucleic acid synthesis.

Although many antibiotics are capable of inhibiting bacterial nucleic acid synthesis by these mechanisms, relatively few of the inhibitors are used clinically as antibacterial agents because most of them do not distinguish between nucleic acid synthesis conducted by the host and that by the pathogen. However, even though some of these antibiotics may not be appropriate for the treatment of infectious

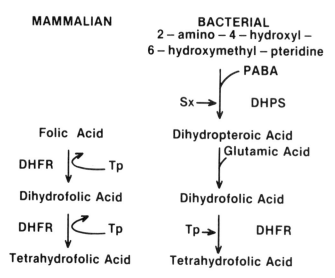

Figure 2.1   The tetrahydrofolic acid biosynthetic pathway in mammals and bacteria: PABA, *p*-aminobenzoic acid; DHPS, dihydropteroate synthase; DHFR, dihydrofolate reductase; Sx→, sulphamethoxazole inhibits; Tp→, trimethoprim inhibits; Tp ⤴, trimethoprim does not inhibit. (Reproduced, with permission, from Smith & Amyes (1984) *British Medical Bulletin* **40**: 42–46.)

diseases they can be used as anticancer drugs. Since anticancer drugs fall outside the scope of this book, attention will be focused only on the relatively few inhibitors that have sufficient selectivity of action ('selective toxicity') to be used for antibacterial chemotherapy.

2.2 Compounds that interrupt nucleotide metabolism

2.2.1 Introduction

Antibiotics that interfere with the biosynthesis of tetrahydrofolic acid (THFA) are powerful indirect inhibitors of nucleotide biosynthesis because THFA is required as a donor of one-carbon units at several stages in purine and pyrimidine synthesis. Synthesis of THFA in bacteria proceeds as shown in Fig. 2.1 and its production is subject to inhibition by two groups of compounds, the sulphonamides (e.g. sulphamethoxazole, Sx) and the 2,4-diaminopyrimidines (e.g. trimethoprim, Tp).

2.2.2 Sulphonamides

Sulphamethoxazole and other sulphonamides (Fig. 2.2) are structural analogues of *p*-aminobenzoic acid (PABA) (Fig. 2.2) acting as alternative substrates that bind

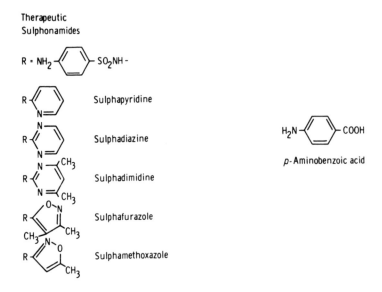

Figure 2.2   Structure of sulphonamide antibiotics, trimethoprim (a 2,4-diaminopyrimidine antibiotic) and the naturally occurring molecules *p*-aminobenzoic acid and dihydrofolate.

more tightly to dihydropteroate synthase (DHPS) than PABA itself. This results in the formation of inactive folate-like analogues. As noted in Chapter 1, DHPS is absent from mammalian cells (see also Fig. 2.1) thereby explaining the selective activity of sulphonamides towards bacteria.

2.2.3   *2,4-Diaminopyrimidines*

The second group of compounds that inhibit synthesis of bacterial THFA are the 2,4-diaminopyrimidines, e.g. trimethoprim (Fig. 2.2) and tetroxoprim which competitively inhibit bacterial dihydrofolate reductase (DHFR) (Fig. 2.1). Although mammalian cells possess DHFR enzymes, these drugs are highly selective towards the bacterial enzymes, e.g. Tp and tetroxoprim are respectively 80 000 and 50 000 times more active against *E. coli* DHFR than against mammalian DHFR.

2.2.4 Sulphonamide–2,4-diaminopyrimidine combinations

Since sulphonamides and 2,4-diaminopyrimidines inhibit sequential stages in THFA synthesis it was initially believed that administration of a combination of appropriate inhibitors (e.g. Sx plus Tp, the combination known as cotrimoxazole) would offer therapeutic advantages over the single agents, through double blockade of the folate pathway (Fig. 2.1). However, this concept has not been entirely borne out in practice. Thus, although some laboratory studies demonstrate synergy between the two components when each is present at sublethal concentrations, other *in vitro* experiments have failed to detect synergy, especially when the concentration of Tp alone is inhibitory. Synergy therefore depends on exposure of bacteria to an optimal ratio of Sx:Tp, a situation apparently rarely achieved in the body owing to differences in the pharmacokinetic properties of the two compounds. Other studies also support the view that laboratory synergy is irrelevant *in vivo* and the continued use of sulphonamide–2,4-diaminopyrimidine combinations for therapy is probably no longer appropriate.

2.3 Compounds that interfere with DNA template functions

A variety of antibiotics interfere with DNA template functions, but they do not have sufficient selective toxicity to be considered as therapeutic antibacterial agents.

2.4 Agents that inhibit enzymic processes in nucleic acid synthesis

2.4.1 Inhibitors of RNA polymerase

The rifamycins constitute a group of closely related antibiotics of which rifampicin (known as rifampin in the USA) (Fig. 2.3), a semisynthetic compound, is the most widely known member of the group. Rifampicin binds to and specifically inhibits bacterial DNA-dependent RNA polymerase, by inhibiting the initiation process. If added after initiation of polymerization it is without effect. Rifampicin has no effect on nuclear or mitochondrial DNA-dependent RNA polymerases from mammalian cells and thus has a selective action against bacteria.

RNA polymerases catalyse the initiation and elongation of RNA molecules using DNA as a template. The reaction performed by the enzyme is

$$(RNA)_n \text{ residues} + \text{ribonucleoside triphosphate}$$

$$\Updownarrow$$

$$(RNA)_{n+1} \text{ residue} + PPi$$

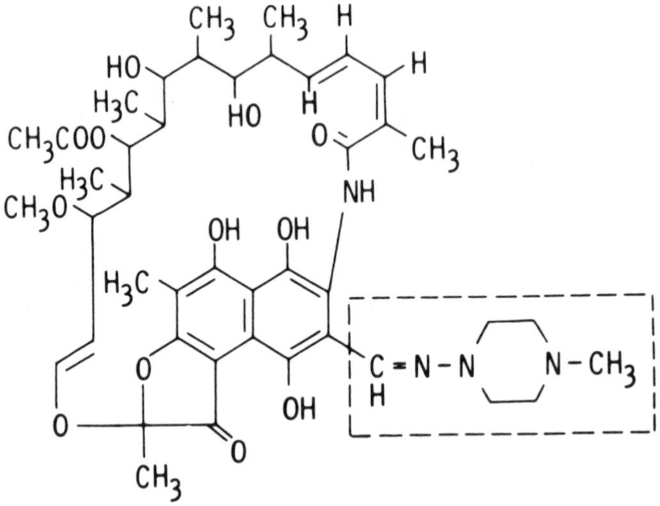

Figure 2.3 Structure of rifampicin. This antibiotic is a semisynthetic member of the rifamycin group; the synthetic side chain is enclosed by the broken line.

The RNA polymerase from *E. coli* consists of two major components, the core (containing four polypeptide chains: 2α, β, and β') which associates with another subunit, the σ factor. The complete (holo) enzyme participates in selection of promoter sites on the DNA template and in initiation of RNA synthesis, whereas the core participates in elongation. Rifampicin binds to the β subunit and in so doing interferes with the ability of the holoenzyme to initiate RNA synthesis. Binding of RNA polymerase to the DNA template is not blocked and inhibition probably results from interference with the formation of the first phosphodiester bond in the RNA chain.

2.4.2 Inhibitors of DNA gyrase

2.4.2.1 Introduction

The principles of DNA replication were established in the 1950s, i.e. at the replication point the double-stranded DNA molecule separates and nucleotides pair with their complementary bases on the two exposed single strands and are then linked by polymerization. Although subsequent studies have confirmed that DNA replication does indeed proceed in this manner, they have revealed that the process is biochemically complex. For instance, in *E. coli* at least 18 different gene products have been identified that participate directly in the replication of the bacterial chromosome.

One of the enzymes involved in bacterial DNA replication, DNA gyrase (a type II DNA topoisomerase) is of particular interest in the context of the action of quinolone antibiotics (Section 2.4.2.2). Replication of the bacterial chromosome, a circular duplex DNA molecule, requires separation of the two highly intertwined parental strands from one another. However, separation of strands wound in a helix generates loops, termed positive supercoiled twists, in the single strands. Unless prevented, positive superhelicity would increase until the rising torsional strain prevented further unwinding of parental DNA at the replication fork. DNA gyrase relaxes positively supercoiled DNA by periodically breaking a phospho-diester bond in one of the strands of the double helix, then introducing negative supercoils and finally resealing the nick.

E. coli DNA gyrase is composed of four subunits: two gyrase A subunits (each containing 857 amino acids with a total molecular weight of 97 000) and two gyrase B subunits (each containing 804 amino acids with a total molecular weight of 90 000). The active enzyme is therefore an A_2B_2 holoenzyme with a molecular weight of 374 000, i.e. $2 \times 97\,000$ plus $2 \times 90\,000$. The A and B subunits are the products of the gyrA and gyrB genes located at 48 min and 83 min respectively on the E. coli chromosome. All activities of the enzyme appear to require both subunits, but certain domains mediate different functions. The A subunits of gyrase are involved in the DNA breakage and resealing events associated with supercoil-ing, while the B subunits are responsible for ATP hydrolysis, which reflects the fact that negative supercoils are energetically unfavourable and require an energy-consuming process for their generation.

Various studies have recently addressed the molecular basis of gyrase interaction with DNA. The enzyme is a heart-shaped structure (Fig. 2.4). Interactions with DNA occur in the upper portion of the heart with tyrosine residues at position 122 in the gyrase A subunits forming transient phosphotyrosine linkages with broken DNA strands (Fig. 2.4). Binding of ATP to the gyrase B subunit causes a conformational change in the protein accompanied by a single round of negative supercoiling. Hydrolysis of ATP returns DNA gyrase to its original conformation. Strand passage followed by further rounds of negative supercoiling and eventual DNA resealing then occurs. Various genetic studies, involving the generation of conditional lethal mutations in gyrA and gyrB, indicate that DNA gyrase is essential for DNA replication.

2.4.2.2   Quinolones

Various quinolone derivatives (Fig. 2.5) inhibit bacterial DNA gyrase. The current 4-quinolones (predominantly 6-fluoro-4-quinolones) were developed from nalidixic acid and its earlier analogues (e.g. cinoxacin, oxolonic, pipemidic and piromidic acids) that had been discovered in the 1960s. The oldest, or so-called first-generation, quinolone analogues, such as nalidixic acid, possess a limited antibacterial spectrum and consequently have not been used extensively in clinical practice. Newer quinolones with improved potency and antibacterial spectrum have been synthesized by modifying the original two-ring quinolone nucleus with different side chain substituents and introducing a fluorine at the 6-position (Fig. 2.5). The second generation of quinolones, developed during the 1980s,

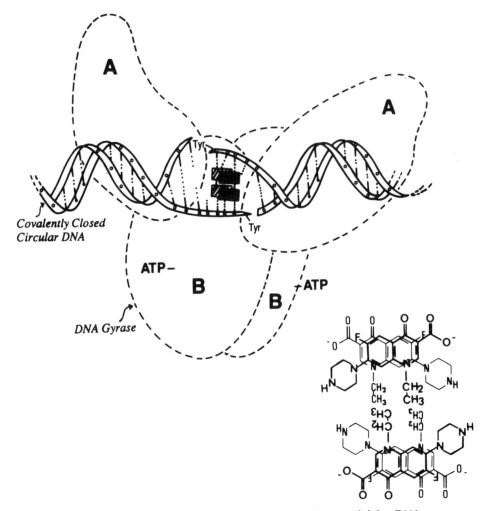

Figure 2.4 Proposed quinolone–DNA cooperative binding model for DNA gyrase inhibition. Filled and hatched boxes denote the quinolone molecules that self-assemble to form a supermolecule inside the gyrase-induced DNA pocket; the drug binds to the unpaired bases via hydrogen bonds (dotted lines). Details of the proposed mode of self-association are illustrated at lower right. The binding pocket is believed to be induced during the intermediate gate-opening step of the DNA supercoiling process. Gyrase A subunits form covalent bonds between tyrosine 122 and the 5′ end of the DNA chain, and the subsequent opening of the DNA chains along the 4-bp-staggered cuts results in a locally denatured DNA bubble that is an ideal site for the drug to bind to. When relaxed DNA substrate (represented by the double-helical ribbon in the diagram) is used, ATP is required for the induction of this specific drug-binding site. Broken curves mimic the shape of the DNA gyrase, a tetramer composed of two A subunits and two B subunits, as revealed by the electron microscopic image of the *Micrococcus luteus* enzyme. (Reproduced, with permission, from Hooper & Wolfson (1993).)

includes ciprofloxacin, enoxacin, norfloxacin, ofloxacin and pefloxacin. More recently, a third generation of quinolones has been developed which includes compounds such as fleroxacin, lomefloxacin, sparfloxacin and tosufloxacin.

Second-generation quinolones are substantially more potent and have broader antibacterial spectra than nalidixic acid and other first-generation compounds. Although nalidixic acid is orally absorbed, second-generation agents possess additional advantageous pharmacokinetic properties permitting twice-daily oral dosing. Differences in spectra of activity exist amongst these antibiotics, but second-generation agents in general exhibit striking potency against enteric Gram-negative bacilli and moderate activity against non-enteric Gram-negative bacilli and staphylococci, but only marginal activity against streptococci and anaerobes. Third-generation quinolones have maintained many of the favourable properties of the second generation. However, some compounds (e.g. fleroxacin and lomefloxacin) have sufficiently favourable pharmacokinetic properties to permit once-daily dosing; others (e.g. sparfloxacin and tosufloxacin) have improved activity against staphylococci, streptococci and anaerobic bacteria compared with second-generation agents. It is beyond the scope of this book to discuss in greater detail the clinical application of the second- and third-generation quinolones. However, further information may be obtained by consulting the text edited by Hooper and Wolfson (1993) listed at the end of this chapter.

The molecular basis of quinolone action is not fully understood but involves interaction of the drugs with gyrase and DNA, followed by a cytotoxic event that leads to bacterial cell death. Quinolones do not bind directly to either the gyrase A or B subunits, or to the intact enzyme (A_2B_2), but do bind significantly to DNA. Furthermore, gyrase stimulates the binding of quinolones to double-stranded DNA. These and other data have led to a model for the interaction of quinolones with gyrase and DNA (Fig. 2.4). In this model gyrase cleaves double-stranded DNA to produce exposed single-stranded regions that constitute binding sites for the antibiotics. The unpaired DNA bases participate in hydrogen bonding to the 3-carboxy and 4-oxo groups that are common to quinolone antibacterials (Fig. 2.5). Drug binding is probably cooperative with at least four molecules binding per site, associating with each other by ring stacking and hydrophobic interactions (Fig. 2.4). Interaction with DNA-associated gyrase is proposed to occur via the group at the C-7 position of the quinolone, but whether contacts are just with the A subunit or with the B subunit as well is not currently clear. In conclusion, the primary binding site for quinolones is therefore the gyrase–DNA complex, with contacts between the drug and both the DNA and the enzyme.

Following the formation of the quinolone–DNA–gyrase complex, an event (or events) must occur that initiates bacterial cell death. Obviously this could be the inhibition of supercoiling by gyrase leading directly to cessation of DNA synthesis. However, quinolone concentrations that inhibit the DNA supercoiling activity of purified DNA gyrase are often 10- to 100-fold higher than concentrations that inhibit bacterial growth. Such findings are unexpected as the isolated target (DNA–gyrase complex) is predicted to be more, not less, sensitive than the intact

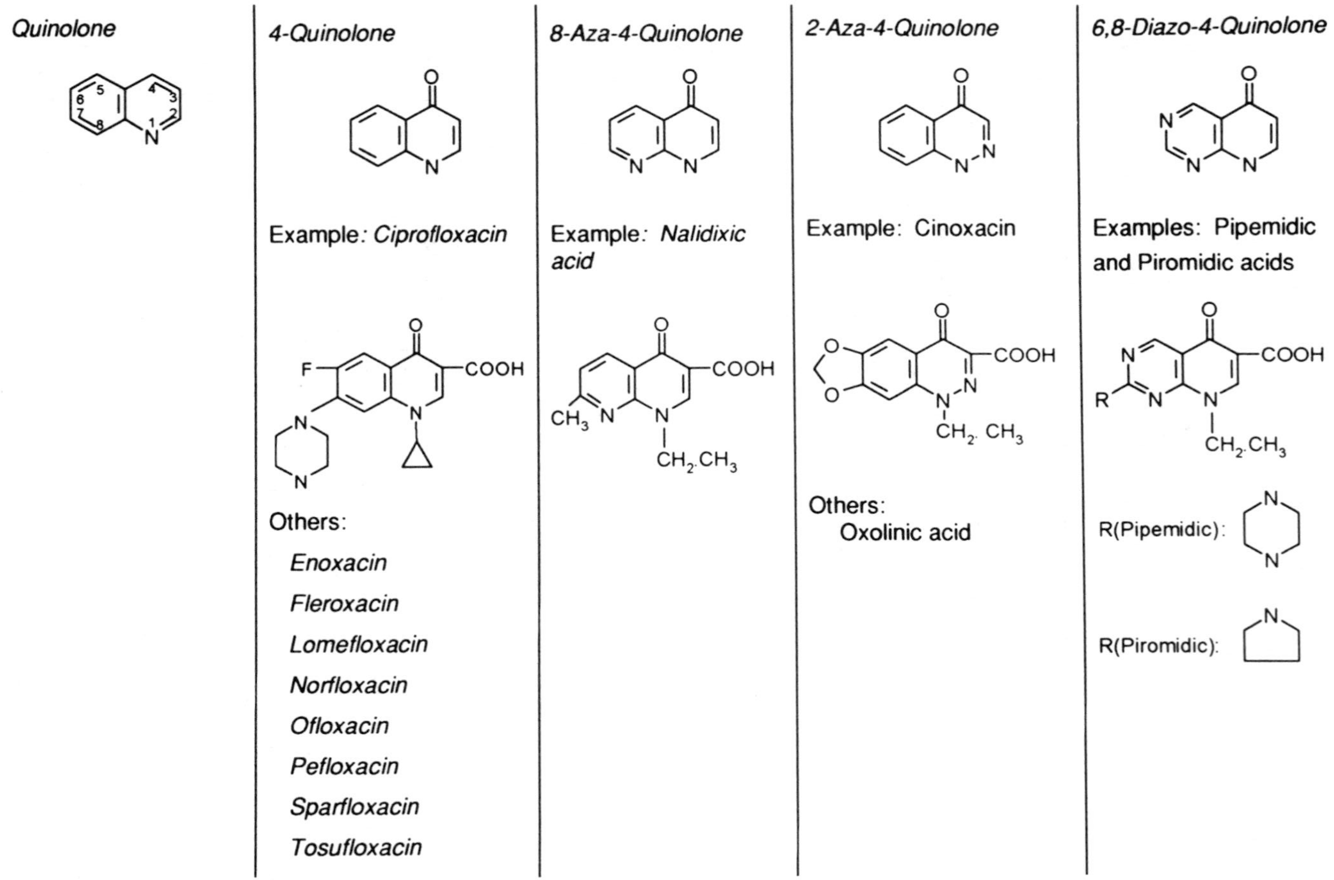

Figure 2.5 Antibacterial quinolones. Note that 4-oxo, $>=$ $_4$, and 3-carboxy, $3>-$ COO⁻ , groups are involved in H bonding to DNA (see Fig. 2.4 and text).

bacterium. A number of suggestions have been made to explain these discrepancies. For example the growth-inhibitory event within the cell may be a subtle perturbation of gyrase activity leading only to a slight reduction of negative supercoiling of DNA that may nevertheless be lethal. Alternatively, the quinolone–gyrase–DNA complex may form a barrier to the passage of DNA and RNA polymerase molecules along the DNA template. According to this hypothesis cell death would not result directly from inhibition of gyrase activity, but would be a secondary consequence of inhibition of transcription or DNA replication. Clearly, more experimental work is required to elucidate the killing mechanism of quinolone antibiotics.

Eukaryotic topoisomerase II displays enzymic activities that are analogous to those mediated by bacterial gyrase. In addition to their similar biochemical mechanisms, bacterial DNA gyrase and eukaryotic topoisomerase II also share significant homology at the amino acid level. However, the eukaryotic enzyme differs in overall structure from bacterial gyrase, being a dimer of two identical subunits. The structural differences between bacterial and mammalian topoisomerase II enzymes presumably account for the observed selective action of the antibacterial quinolones against bacterial DNA gyrase.

3
Inhibitors of protein synthesis

3.1 Introduction

Protein synthesis is inhibited by several antibiotics, some of which are selectively toxic towards bacteria. Although these antibiotics have obvious chemotherapeutic application, it should be noted that other inhibitors of protein synthesis are selectively toxic for eukaryotes rather than bacteria. The latter are not considered here. As mentioned in Chapter 1, the selectivity of clinically useful inhibitors of bacterial protein synthesis arises principally from their ability to bind selectively to bacterial rather than mammalian ribosomes. In contrast to earlier views, a consensus is now emerging that ribosomal RNA is the primary target for a number of antibacterial drugs, rather than ribosomal protein.

Table 2.1 provides a summary of the mode of action of antibiotics that inhibit bacterial protein synthesis. However, in order to understand how antibiotics are inhibitory, it is necessary to consider ribosomal structure and the nature of protein synthesis in more detail than presented in Chapter 1.

3.2 Structure of bacterial ribosomes

As noted in Chapter 1, *E. coli* 30S ribosomal subunits contain one molecule of 16S RNA and 21 proteins (designated S1, S2, etc.) whereas 50S subunits contain

Table 2.1 Antibiotic inhibitors of protein synthesis

Antibiotic	Mechanism of action
Mupirocin	Inhibits isoleucyl-tRNA synthetase
Streptomycin	Inhibits initiation and causes misreading of mRNA by binding to 30S ribosomal subunit
Neomycins Kanamycins Gentamicins Amikacin Tobramycin Spectinomycin	Inhibit translocation by binding to 30S ribosomal subunit
Chloramphenicol	Inhibits peptidyl transferase activity of 50S ribosomal subunit
Fusidic acid	Inhibits translocation by forming stable complex with EF-G, GDP and the ribosome
Lincosamides	Inhibit peptidyl transferase activity of 50S ribosomal subunit
Macrolides	Stimulate dissociation of peptidyl-tRNA from ribosomes by binding to 50S ribosomal subunit
Streptogramin A	Blocks peptide bond formation by distorting ribosomal A site
Streptogramin B	Blocks translocation of growing polypeptide from the A site to the P site
Tetracyclines	Bind to 30S ribosomal subunit and inhibit binding of aminoacyl-tRNAs to ribosomal acceptor site

one molecule each of 5S RNA and 23S RNA together with 32 proteins (designated L1, L2, etc.). Fig. 2.6 shows models of the *E. coli* ribosomal subunits and the 70S ribosome which have been constructed from electron microscopic studies. The groove formed between the two subunits in the 70S ribosome (Fig. 2.6(c)) probably accommodates the mRNA. Other important functional sites on the 70S ribosome are the aminoacyl tRNA and peptidyl tRNA binding sites, also referred to respectively as the A and P sites.

At present primary structures are known for all three ribosomal RNA molecules and reliable secondary structure models have been deduced (e.g. Fig. 2.7 shows a model of 16S ribosomal RNA secondary structure). The nature of tertiary folding in these molecules is also beginning to emerge together with identification (at least at the secondary structure level) of some regions that interact with ribosomal proteins. For instance it is now known that proteins S8 and S15 bind to the central domain of 16S RNA at positions 583–610 + 623–653 and 654–672 + 733–756 (Figs 2.7, 2.8). The general regions in 16S RNA to which other S proteins bind are also

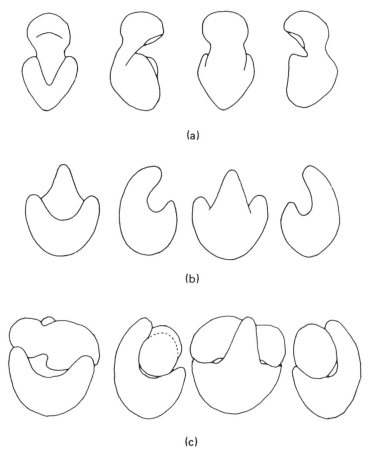

(a)

(b)

(c)

Figure 2.6 Models of the *E. coli* (a) 30S ribosomal subunit, (b) 50S ribosomal subunit and (c) 70S ribosome with the 30S subunit lying on the 50S subunit. The four views are derived by successive rotation through an angle of 90°. (Reproduced, with permission, from Chopra (1985).)

known (Fig. 2.8) but, to date, the precise binding sites have been elucidated only for S8 and S15.

3.3 Stages in protein synthesis

3.3.1 Synthesis of aminoacyl-tRNAs

Prior to incorporation into polypeptides, amino acids are attached to specific tRNA molecules. Each amino acid is converted by a specific aminoacyl-tRNA synthetase

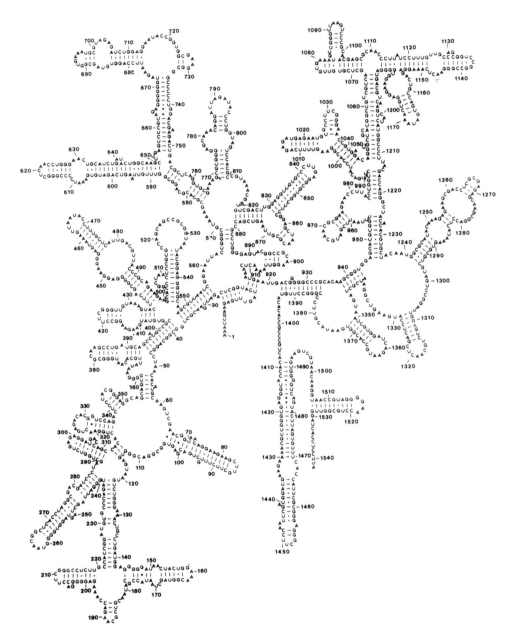

Figure 2.7 Secondary structure of *E. coli* 16S rRNA. (Reproduced, with permission, from Noller *et al.* (1987).)

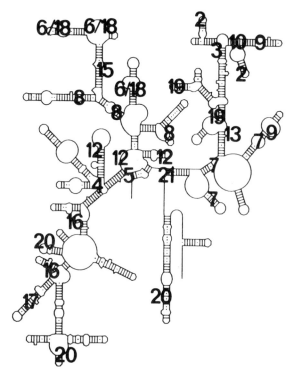

Figure 2.8 Location of 16S rRNA regions with which ribosomal proteins are associated. The number of each protein is centred on regions where significant protein interactions are observed. (Reproduced, with permission, from Noller *et al.* (1987).)

to an aminoacyladenylate–enzyme complex which then interacts with an amino-acid-specific tRNA to form an aminoacyl-tRNA molecule. These steps can be represented as follows:

$$\text{enzyme}_x + \text{amino acid } (aa)_x + ATP \rightleftharpoons \text{enzyme}_x - (aa)_x - AMP + PPi$$
$$\text{enzyme}_x - (aa)_x - AMP + tRNA_x \rightleftharpoons (aa)_x - tRNA_x + AMP + \text{enzyme}_x$$
$$\text{overall: } (aa)_x + ATP + tRNA_x \rightleftharpoons (aa)_x - tRNA_x + AMP + PPi$$

Aminoacyl-tRNA molecules are then linearly ordered by interacting with mRNA bound in the ribosome.

3.3.2 *Initiation of protein synthesis (Fig. 2.9, Section (A), Steps I–IV)*

Initiation of protein synthesis involves a series of reactions during which the following take place.

(1) The 30S ribosomal subunit binds to the region of the mRNA containing the initiation codon AUG.

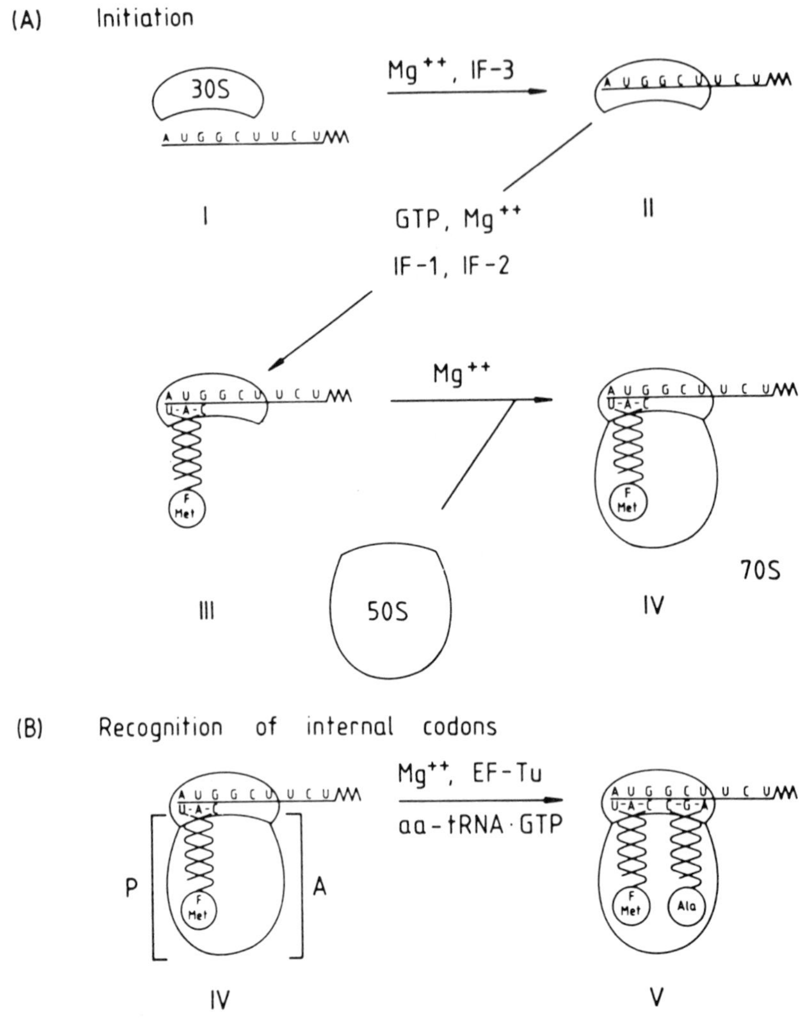

(A)   Initiation

(B)   Recognition of internal codons

Figure 2.9   Schematic summary of protein synthesis in *E. coli*. Details of the individual steps are described in the text and the nature of the soluble protein factors (IF-1, IF-2 etc.) in Table 2.2. P, peptidyl site; A, acceptor site. A third site E for exit of deacetylated tRNA is not illustrated. (Reproduced, with permission, from Chopra (1985).)

(2) Formylmethionyl tRNA (f-Met-tRNAfMet) is attached to the 30S–mRNA complex in response to the codon AUG. The resultant complex is called the '30S initiation complex'.
(3) The 50S ribosomal subunit is added to form the '70S initiation complex'.

Several initiation factors (Table 2.2), i.e. proteins playing an important role in

(C)   Peptide   bond   formation,   translocation

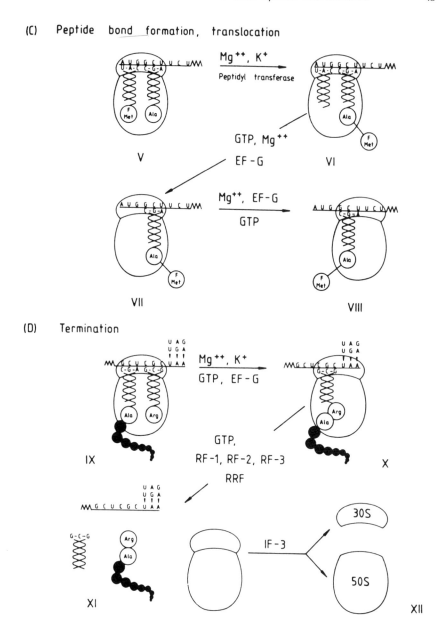

(D)   Termination

initiation but only transiently bound to the ribosome, are involved in the above steps.

Although the codon AUG acts as the initiation signal for translation of mRNA, the AUG codon is not itself the initiation codon recognized by ribosomes. Obviously the sequence AUG often occurs in and out of phase in a message, and

Table 2.2 Soluble protein factors involved in the synthesis of *E. coli* polypeptides

Name of factor[a]	Molecular weight (Da × 10³)	Function
IF-1	8	Promotes IF-2 and IF-3 activity
IF2 alpha	97	Hydrolyse GTP and promote fMet-tRNA
IF2 beta	78˙	binding to 30S subunits
IF3	21	Responsible for formation of mRNA.30S complex. Acts as anti-dissociation factor to prevent formation of 70S ribosomes
EF-Tu	43	Hydrolyses GTP and promotes aminoacyl-tRNA binding to 70S ribosomes
EF-Ts	30	Regeneration of EF-Tu·GTP complex
EF-G	77.4	Hydrolyses GTP and promotes translocation
RF-1	36	Promote release of completed peptidyl residues from the ribosome by recognizing
RF-2	38	UAA, UAG and UGA
RF-3	46	Hydrolyses GTP and stimulates RF-1 and RF-2
RRF	23.5	Ejection of mRNA and tRNA from ribosomes

[a]IF, initiation factor; EF, elongation factor; RF, release factor; RRF, ribosome release factor.

the proper AUG corresponding to the beginning of the gene transcript has to be selected. Recognition involves a pyrimidine-rich sequence at the 3′ end of 16S ribosomal RNA that pairs directly with a polypurine stretch found 10–14 nucleotides upstream of the starter AUG codon. The so-called 'Shine–Dalgarno' sequences in prokaryotic mRNA comprise stretches of three to seven nucleotides which are complementary to the region HO A–U–U–C–C–U–C–C–A (5′) of the 16S RNA. In addition to the Shine–Dalgarno region, nucleotides upstream from this area are probably important for the binding of mRNA to ribosomes. These nucleotides probably stabilize the 30S–mRNA complex by interaction with ribosomal protein. In *E. coli* the proteins S1, S4, S12, S18 and S21 are particularly important in this context.

3.3.3 Recognition of internal codons (Fig. 2.9, Section (B), Steps IV, V)

On addition of the 50S ribosomal subunit the 70S initiation complex is prepared for recognition of internal codons. The P site is occupied by fMet-tRNAfMet and the A site is vacant. The codon present in the A site determines the binding of cognate aminoacyl-tRNA to the ribosome. The affinity of aminoacyl-tRNA itself for the A site is low and the aminoacyl-tRNA binding reaction involves the protein elongation factor EF-Tu (Table 2.2). Aminoacyl-tRNA becomes bound to the A site in the form of the ternary complex EF-Tu·aminoacyl-tRNA·GTP. fMet-tRNAfMet does not react with EF-Tu·GTP so that individual formylmethionine residues never enter the ribosomal A site.

Codon–anticodon interaction in the A site is accompanied by hydrolysis of one molecule of GTP for every molecule of aminoacyl-tRNA bound. This reaction results in release of EF-Tu·GDP from the ribosome. The binary complex itself cannot bind aminoacyl-tRNA, but regeneration of EF-Tu·GDP to EF-Tu·GTP is mediated by the elongation factor EF-Ts (Table 2.2). Thus GTP and GDP are allosteric effectors of EF-Tu. The EF-Tu·GDP complex cannot bind aminoacyl-tRNA and cannot be retained in the ribosome, whereas the EF-Tu·GTP complex binds aminoacyl-tRNA to form a ternary complex which interacts with the ribosomal A site.

3.3.4 Peptide bond formation and translocation (Fig. 2.9, Section (C), Steps V–VIII)

Following release of the EF-Tu·GDP complex from the ribosome, the formyl-methionine residue (or peptidyl residue in subsequent chain elongation cycles) is cleaved from its tRNA in the P site and transferred to the aminoacyl-tRNA in the A site. The reaction is catalysed by peptidyltransferase which is located in the 50S subunit. The P site is now occupied by a deacylated tRNA and the A site contains peptidyl-tRNA that has been elongated by one aminoacyl residue. Several coordinated processes now occur known collectively as 'translocation'.

(1) Deacylated tRNA is transferred from the P to the E site (not illustrated).
(2) The peptidyl-tRNA moves from the A to the P site, where it remains linked to the mRNA via codon–anticodon interaction.
(3) Movement of mRNA and ribosome with respect to each other causes a new codon to enter the A site.

The starting-point for recognition of a further internal codon is therefore reached and the sequence of events (V–VIII, Fig. 2.9) repeated.

Maximum rates of translocation depend on elongation factor EF-G (Table 2.2) and GTP, which is converted to GDP during translocation. Translocation may occur as a result of binding of EF-G to the ribosome and hydrolysis of GTP may be needed to release EF-G for its recycling. Thus GTP may also be an allosteric effector of elongation factor EF-G.

3.3.5 Termination of protein synthesis (Fig. 2.9, Section (D), Steps IX–XII)

Termination involves the arrival of termination codons (UAG, UGA or UAA) in the A site and the release factors RF-1, RF-2 and RF-3 (Table 2.2). RF-1 (in the presence of UAG or UAA) and RF-2 (in the presence of UGA or UAA) promote cleavage of the completed peptidyl residue from tRNA by activating peptidyl transferase. The polypeptide leaves the ribosome, eventually to become an active protein, or to become a subunit in an active protein. At this stage deacylated tRNA and mRNA are released from the 70S ribosome. This involves hydrolysis of GTP by RF-3 and the additional factor RRF (ribosome release factor) (Table 2.2). Initiation factor IF3 (Table 2.2) prevents association of subunits to form 70S ribosomes, thus permitting the start of another initiation cycle.

3.4 Antibiotic inhibitors of protein synthesis and their mechanisms of action

3.4.1 Mupirocin

Mupirocin (Fig. 2.10) is an antibiotic structurally unrelated to any other recognized antibiotic group. It consists of a short fatty acid side chain linked to a larger molecule, monic acid, the tail end of which mimics the amino acid isoleucine (Fig. 2.10). Mupirocin, which is bacteriostatic, competitively inhibits isoleucyl tRNA synthetase (Fig. 2.10), preventing formation of the aminoacyladenylate enzyme complex. By preventing incorporation of isoleucine into growing polypeptide chains the antibiotic stops protein synthesis. Although mupirocin exhibits selective action against bacterial isoleucyl tRNA synthetase, its use is restricted to topical applications, e.g. for treatment of skin infections. This situation arises because the antibiotic is metabolized to the inactive monic acid and its fatty acyl side chain in the body.

3.4.2 Aminoglycoside-aminocyclitol group

3.4.2.1 Introduction

The aminoglycoside–aminocylitol (AGAC) group of antibiotics includes a large number of clinically useful drugs. These antibiotics can be divided into three groups on the basis of their structures:

(1) 4,5-disubstituted deoxystreptamines (e.g. neomycin B; Fig. 2.11),
(2) 4,6-disubstituted deoxystreptamines (e.g. kanamycin A, amikacin, tobramycin, gentamicins; Fig. 2.11),
(3) others (e.g. streptomycin, spectinomycin; Fig. 2.11).

3.4.2.2 Streptomycin

Streptomycin, a bactericidal antibiotic, prevents initiation of protein synthesis and causes misreading of proteins being translated. It binds irreversibly to a single site in the bacterial 30S ribosomal subunit, causing localized structural distortion. This site (Fig. 2.12) is located close to the interface with the 50S particle in the intact 70S ribosome.

Binding of streptomycin to free 30S ribosomal subunits about to initiate protein

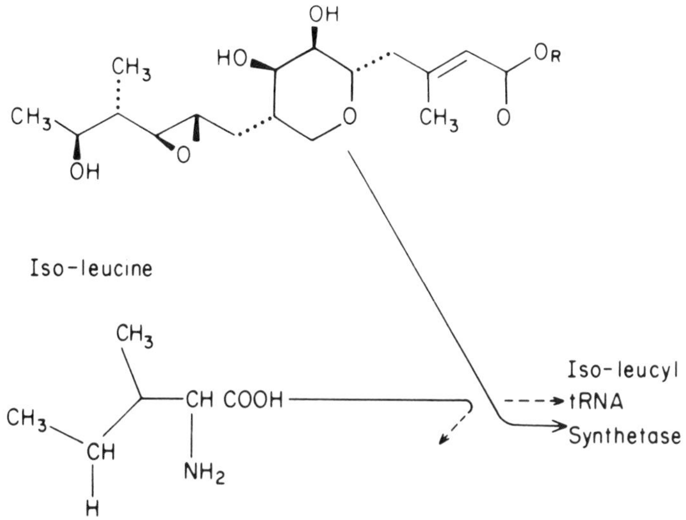

Figure 2.10 Structure and mode of action of mupirocin. R=(CH$_2$)$_8$ COOH, mupirocin (pseudomonic acid); R=H, monic acid. (Reproduced, with permission, from Casewell & Hill (1987).)

synthesis blocks their further progress. The initiation complexes which form with these ribosomes are non-productive. Seemingly aminoacyl tRNA cannot bind to the distorted acceptor site and f-Met-tRNAfMet is released. This irreversible block on protein synthesis, mediated at the level of protein initiation, ultimately leads to cell death.

The anti-initiation and misreading activities of streptomycin relate to perturbation of ribosomal RNA structure following binding of the antibiotic to its single site in the 30S ribosomal subunit. The streptomycin binding site (Fig. 2.12) includes adenosine residues 913–915 of the 16S RNA, a region to which protein S12 also binds (Fig. 2.8). Although streptomycin binds to ribosomal RNA, its affinity for the site in 16S RNA is influenced by protein S12.

3.4.2.3 *Neomycins, gentamicins, kanamycins, amikacin and tobramycin*

In contrast to streptomycin, these bactericidal aminoglycosides bind to bacterial ribosomes at multiple sites, probably reflecting the fact that they are structurally distinct from streptomycin. Binding to the 30S subunit is slightly tighter than binding to the 50S subunit, but none of these antibiotics utilizes the streptomycin-binding site on the 30S subunit. Again, in contrast to streptomycin, these aminoglycosides inhibit translocation by preventing the binding of EF-G to the ribosome. The inhibitory activity of the antibiotics probably depends on direct binding to ribosomal RNA, and bases at positions 1408 and 1494 in 16S RNA (Fig. 2.7) have been implicated as binding sites for neomycins, gentamicins and kanamycin.

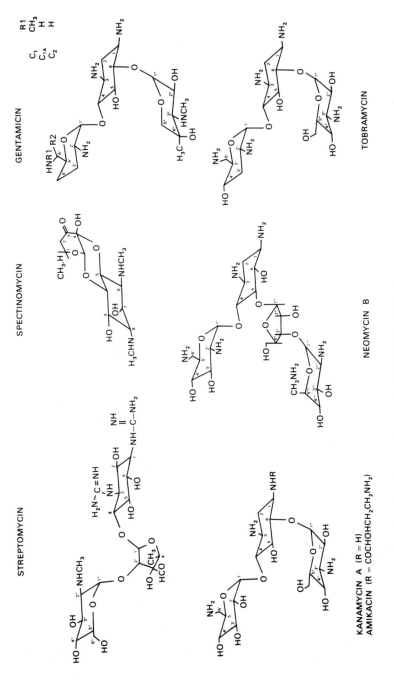

Figure 2.11 Structure of aminoglycoside–aminocyclitol (AGAC) antibiotics.

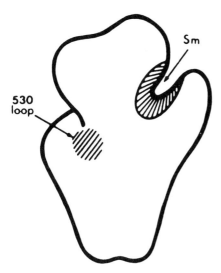

Figure 2.12   Site of streptomycin binding in the *E. coli* 30S ribosomal subunit. Binding of the antibiotic causes distortion of ribosomal RNA in the so-called '530' loop region (see text for further details). (Reproduced, with permission, from Melancon *et al.* (1988), *Nucleic Acids Research* **16**: 9637.)

3.4.2.4   Spectinomycin

This aminocyclitol antibiotic is bacteriostatic and interacts reversibly with the 30S ribosomal subunit. Spectinomycin inhibits translocation possibly by preventing the relative movement between ribosomes and mRNA that occurs at this stage in polypeptide elongation. As with other AGAC antibiotics the inhibitory activity of spectinomycin seems to be related to binding to 16S ribosomal RNA, in particular to bases at positions 1063 and 1064 (Fig. 2.7).

3.4.3   Chloramphenicol

Chloramphenicol (Fig. 2.13) is a broad-spectrum bacteriostatic agent that binds to 70S (bacterial) ribosomes but not the 80S type. The antibiotic prevents peptide bond formation by inhibiting the peptidyl transferase reaction. Recent work suggests that peptidyl transferase activity is mediated by 23S ribosomal RNA, and there is evidence that chloramphenicol binds directly to ribosomal RNA, in particular to bases at positions 2451 and 2505 in 23S rRNA. Chloramphenicol therefore may act either by perturbing an RNA tertiary structure essential for peptidyl transferase activity or by hampering correct alignment of the peptidyl and aminoacyl substrates at the peptidyl transferase catalytic site. Hence the inhibitory activity of chloramphenicol probably relates to direct binding to ribosomal RNA.

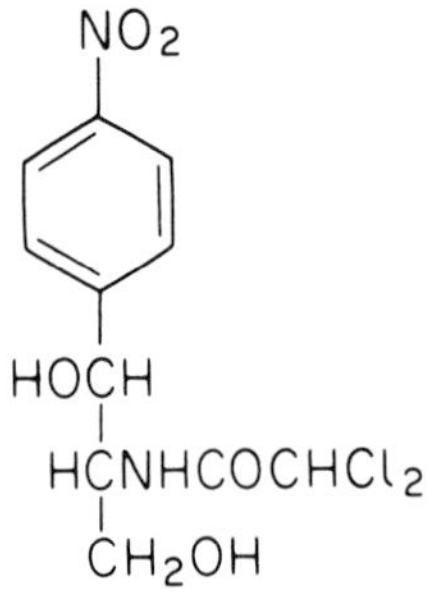

NO₂

HOCH

HCNHCOCHCl₂

CH₂OH

Figure 2.13   Structure of chloramphenicol.

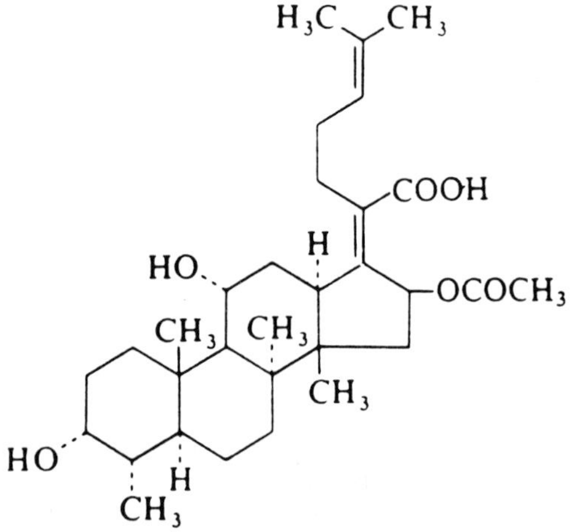

H₃C   CH₃

.COOH

H

HO.

-OCOCH₃

CH₃ CH₃

CH₃

HO

H

CH₃

Figure 2.14   Structure of fusidic acid.

3.4.4 *Fusidic acid*

Fusidic acid is a narrow-spectrum steroidal antibiotic (Fig. 2.14) that inhibits protein synthesis in prokaryotic and eukaryotic subcellular systems. The antibiotic forms a stable complex with EF-G (or EF-2 in eukaryotes), GDP and the ribosome which is unable to release EFG for a further round of translocation. The lack of toxicity of fusidic acid against mammalian cells is probably explained by its poor accumulation in cells of this type.

3.4.5 *Lincosamides*

Lincomycin and its chlorinated derivative clindamycin (Fig. 2.15) are members of the lincosamide group of antibiotics. They inhibit the peptidyl transferase function

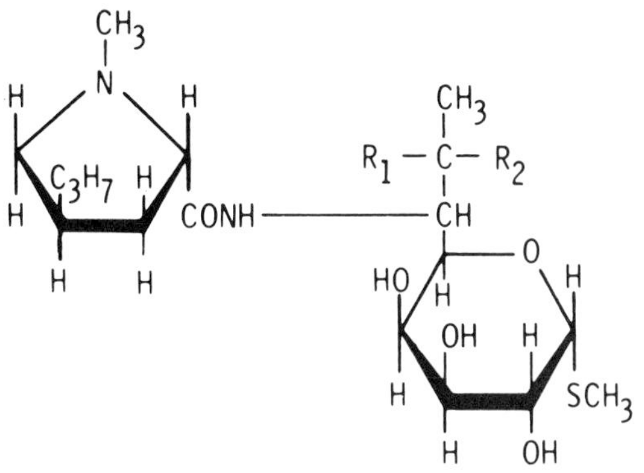

Figure 2.15 Structure of lincomycin (R_1=OH, R_2=H) and clindamycin (R_1=H, R_2=Cl).

of the bacterial 50S ribosomal subunit. Evidence for direct binding of these drugs to 23S RNA in the 50S subunit has been obtained. This leads to the conclusion that these antibiotics (like chloramphenicol) may act either by perturbing an RNA tertiary structure essential for peptidyl transferase activity, or by hampering correct alignment of the peptidyl and aminoacyl substrates at the peptidyl transferase catalytic site.

3.4.6 *Macrolides*

The macrolides comprise a family of antibiotics ranging from erythromycin (discovered in 1952), which has received wide clinical utility, to analogues synthesized within the last few years. Erythromycin (Fig. 2.16) is a 14-membered macrolide consisting of a macrocyclic lactone ring attached to two sugar moieties. Newer macrolides (Figs 2.17–2.19) differ from erythromycin in the size and/or substitution pattern of the lactone ring system and are classified as 14- (Fig. 2.17), 15- (Fig. 2.18) and 16- (Fig. 2.19) membered macrolides. Some of the newer macrolides are now marketed (clarithromycin, azithromycin, midecamycin, rokitamycin, roxithromycin), whereas others are still in development.

These predominantly bacteriostatic antibiotics selectively bind to a single high affinity site on the 50S subunit of the 70S bacterial ribosome but do not bind to mammalian 80S ribosomes. The antimicrobial binding site is located in the peptidyl tRNA binding region of the 50S subunit, causing dissociation of peptidyl-tRNA from ribosomes and hence inhibition of bacterial protein synthesis. Macrolides bind directly to 23S ribosomal RNA in the 2058–2062 nucleotide region of the molecule. However, although the actual macrolide target appears to be located in the 23S RNA, the binding of macrolides to this site is influenced by certain 50S ribosomal proteins, particularly L4.

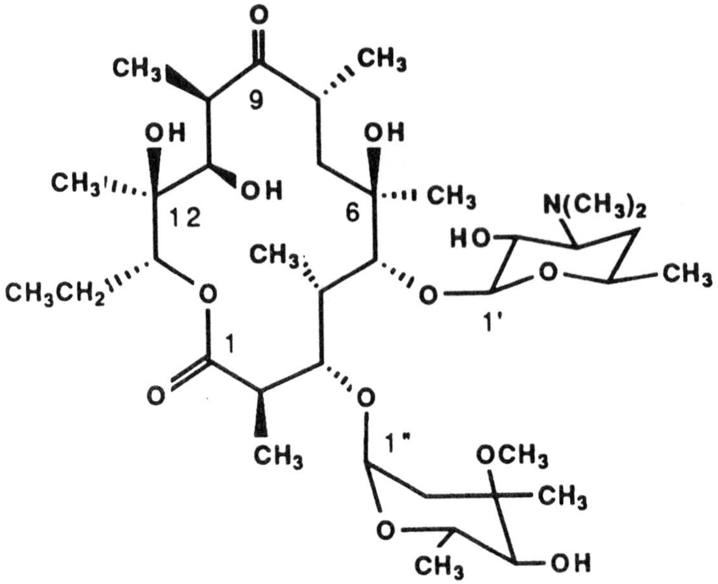

Figure 2.16   Structure of erythromycin (14-membered macrolide).

Although erythromycin is a well-established antibiotic, it has a number of pharmacological deficiencies. These include (a) decomposition under acidic conditions, leading to variable oral bioavailability and the formation of breakdown products causing gastrointestinal intolerance, (b) an elimination half-life which necessitates repeated dosing, and (c) relatively poor tissue and cellular penetration. Compared with erythromycin the newer macrolides display improved acid stability, decreased tendency to cause adverse gastrointestinal side effects, greater and more consistent oral absorption, increased tissue and cellular penetration and prolonged persistence in the body. Furthermore, they can be administered once (e.g. azithromycin) or twice (e.g. clarithromycin) daily, instead of the three or four times for erythromycin.

3.4.7 *Streptogramins*

These antibiotics can be classified into two major groups, A and B. Antibiotics of the A group (e.g. streptogramin A; Fig. 2.20) possess a large non-peptide ring which is polyunsaturated. Members of the B group (e.g. streptogramin B; Fig. 2.20) are cyclic hexadepsipeptides containing unusual amino acids. Generally these antibiotics are bacteriostatic and inhibit protein synthesis directed by 70S ribosomes. Antibiotics of group A distort the ribosomal A site in such a way that both the binding of aminoacyl tRNA and the peptidyl transferase reaction are inhibited. It has been postulated that antibiotics in group B block translocation

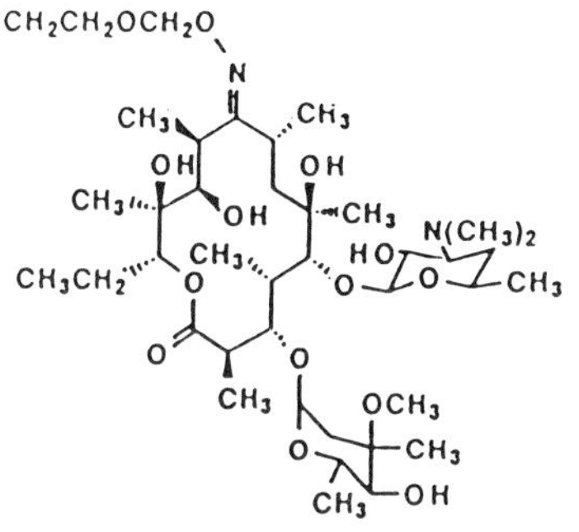

Roxithromycin

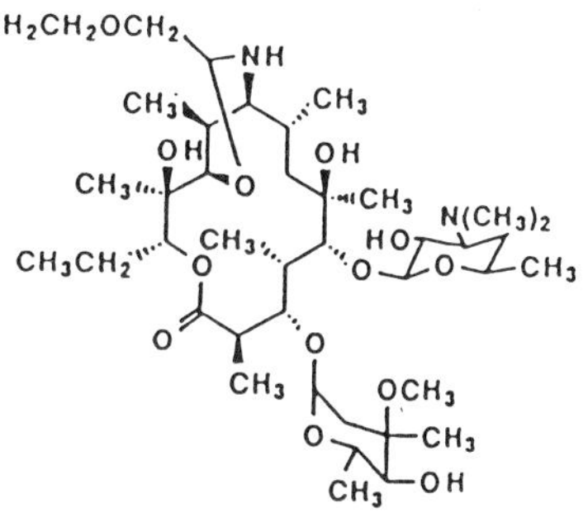

Dirithromycin

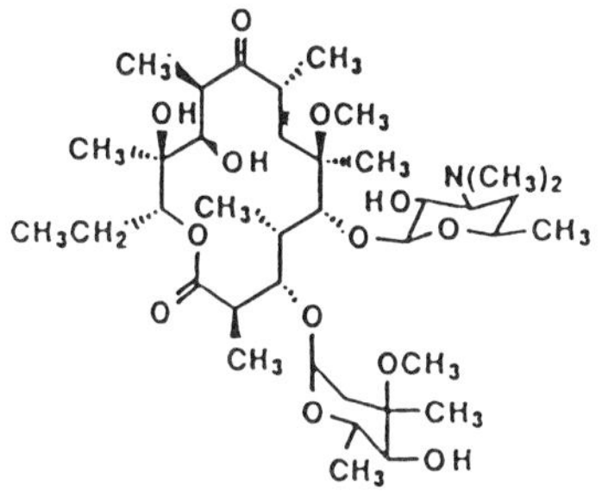

Clarithromycin

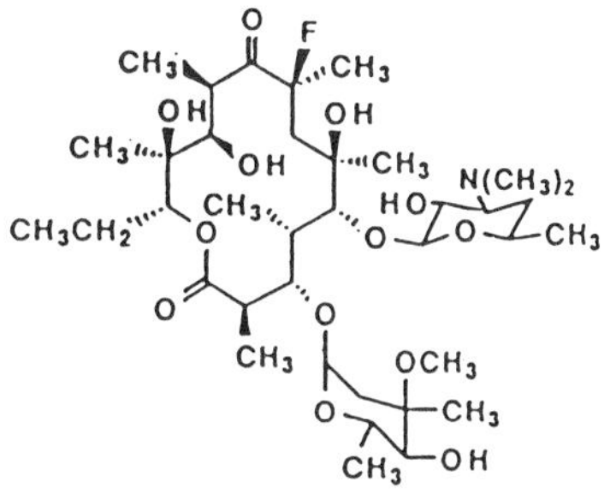

Flurithromycin

Figure 2.17 Structure of newer 14-membered macrolides.

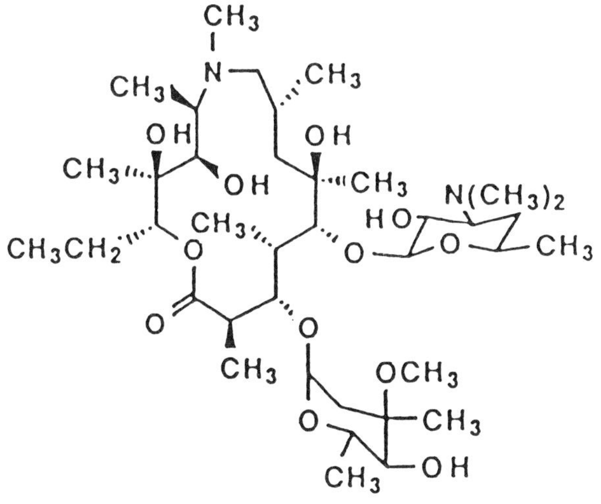

Figure 2.18 Structure of azithromycin (15-membered macrolide).

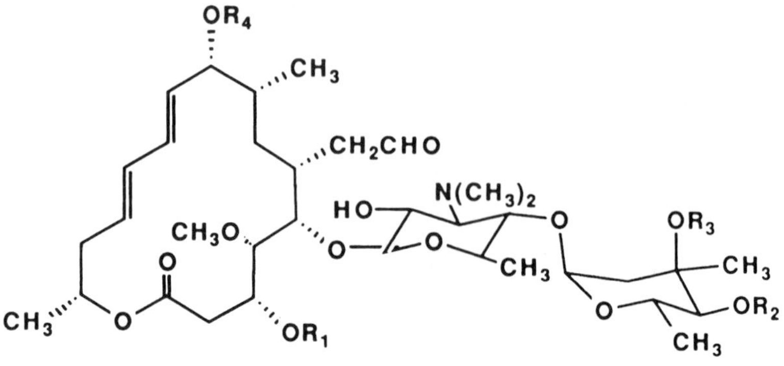

Figure 2.19 Structure of 16-membered macrolides.

	R₁	R₂	R₃	R₄
Rokitamycin	H	Bu	Pr	H
Leucomycin A₅	H	Bu	H	H
Josamycin	Ac	iVal	H	H
Miocamycin	Pr	Pr	Ac	Ac
Midecamycin	Pr	Pr	H	H
Triacetylspiramycin	Ac	Ac	Ac	Forosaminyl
Spiramycin I	H	H	H	Forosaminyl

Ac = Acetyl, Pr = Propionyl, Bu = Butyryl, iVal = isoValeryl

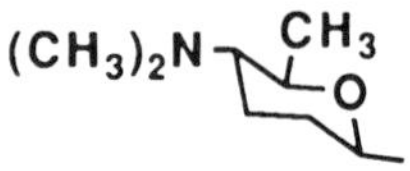

of the growing polypeptide chain from the A site to the P site (although EF-G dependent GTPase activity is unaffected).

Group A and B antibiotics exhibit a marked synergism towards Gram-positive bacteria when both drugs are present in a mixture. This appears to result from an increased affinity of group A antibiotics for the ribosome in the presence of group B antibiotics.

3.4.8 Tetracyclines

The tetracyclines (Fig. 2.21) comprise a group of clinically useful broad-spectrum bacteriostatic antibiotics that inhibit protein synthesis. These drugs prevent protein

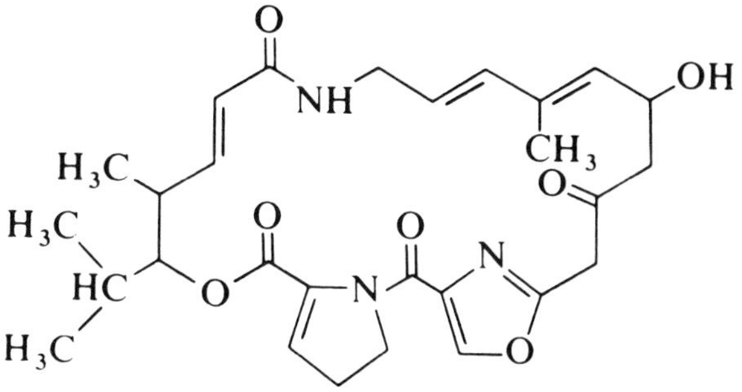

Streptogramin A

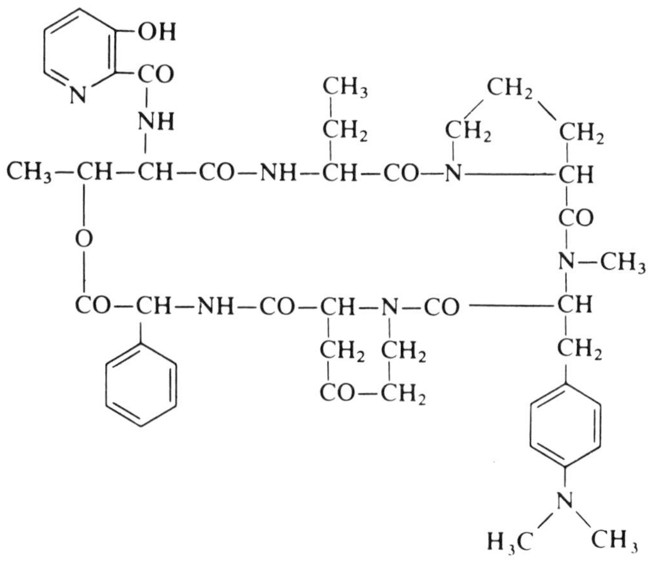

Streptogramin B

Figure 2.20 Structure of streptogramin A and B.

synthesis on both 70S and 80S ribosomes, although 70S ribosomes are more sensitive. Another factor explaining the selective activity of these antibiotics against bacteria arises from their concentration within bacterial but not mammalian cells.

Tetracyclines inhibit the binding of aminoacyl tRNA to the ribosomal acceptor

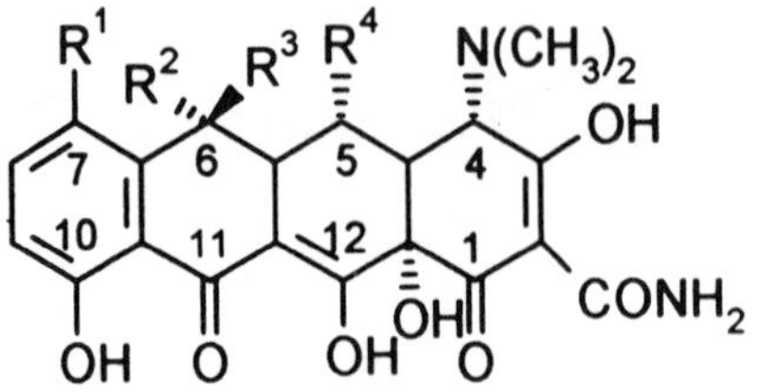

Antibiotic	R^1	R^2	R^3	R^4
Tetracycline	H	CH_3	OH	H
Oxytetracycline	H	CH_3	OH	OH
Chlortetracycline	Cl	CH_3	OH	H
Demethylchlortetracycline	Cl	H	OH	H
Methacycline	H	$= CH_2$		OH
Doxycycline	H	CH_3	H	OH
Minocycline	$-N(CH_3)_2$	H	H	H

Figure 2.21   Structure of tetracycline and some of its analogues.

(A) site by disruption of codon–anticodon interaction between tRNA and mRNA. This inhibitory effect results from the binding of tetracycline to a single site in the 30S ribosomal subunit. This binding site involves a region of 16S ribosomal RNA which contains base A892. However, the anticodon of bound aminoacyl tRNA is spatially proximal to the 16S RNA region containing base number 1400. This suggests that the tertiary folding of 16S ribosomal RNA brings the 892 and 1400 regions into close proximity and that tetracyclines block aminoacyl tRNA binding by interference with the folding of the 892–1400 region after binding of antibiotic to the region containing base number 892. Tetracycline also appears to interact with protein S7 during binding to 16S ribosomal RNA in the 30S particle. However, this protein does not associate with either the 892 or the 1400 base regions (Fig. 2.8). Possibly the binding of tetracycline to 16S RNA leads to gross distortion of ribosome structure so that protein S7 is presented to the 892–1400 RNA domain.

  A number of tetracycline analogues (e.g. chelocardin and 6-thiatetracycline) previously believed to be inhibitors of protein synthesis are now no longer thought to exert their antimicrobial activity by this mechanism. These agents, in contrast to the tetracyclines shown in Fig. 2.21, are bactericidal and cause non-specific damage to the bacterial cytoplasmic membrane. Because of their non-selective properties they cannot be used in systemic treatment of bacterial infections.

4
Antibiotics that inhibit peptidoglycan synthesis

4.1 Introduction

As noted in Chapter 1, nearly all bacteria possess peptidoglycan in their cell walls, but this macromolecule is absent from mammalian cells. Consequently, the development of antibiotics that inhibit peptidoglycan synthesis can provide very useful chemotherapeutic agents. There are indeed a large number of antibiotics that inhibit peptidoglycan synthesis and in recent years much effort has been devoted to the development of new ones.

Peptidoglycan synthesis (Fig. 2.22) takes place in three major stages:

(1) synthesis of precursors in the cytoplasm;
(2) transfer of precursors to a lipid carrier molecule (undecaprenyl phosphate) which transports them across the cytoplasmic membrane;
(3) insertion of glycan units into the cell wall, attachment by transpeptidation and further final maturation steps.

The following section provides examples of antibiotics which inhibit peptidoglycan synthesis by interfering with reactions taking place during one of the stages outlined (Fig. 2.22).

4.2 Stage 1 inhibitors

4.2.1 D-cycloserine

D-cycloserine is an analogue of D-alanine (Fig. 2.23) and blocks peptidoglycan synthesis by competitive inhibition of two enzymes, alanine racemase and D-alanyl-D-alanine synthetase. Therefore, both the formation of D-alanine from L-alanine and the synthesis of the D-alanyl-D-alanine dipeptide prior to its addition to the UDP-MurNAc tripeptide are inhibited (Fig. 2.22).

4.2.2 Fosfomycin

Fosfomycin (phosphonomycin) (Fig. 2.24) inhibits peptidoglycan synthesis by covalently binding to a cysteinyl residue in the enzyme phosphoenolpyruvate:UDP-GlcNAc-3-enolpyruvyltransferase ('pyruvyl transferase') (Fig. 2.22).

4.3 Stage 2 inhibitors

4.3.1 Bacitracin

Bacitracin (Fig. 2.25) complexes with the membrane-bound pyrophosphate form of the undecaprenyl (C55-isoprenyl) lipid carrier molecule that remains after the

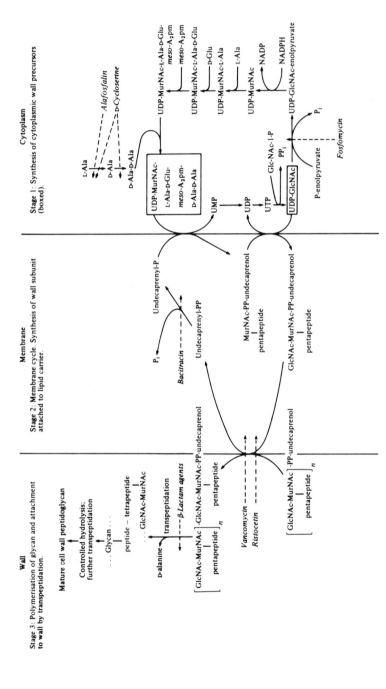

Figure 2.22 Peptidoglycan biosynthesis and the sites of inhibition by antibiotics. Additional amino acids present in the cross-bridge of some bacteria are normally added when the wall subunit is bound to undecaprenylpyrophosphate. This addition has no effect on the mechanism of action of any of the 'cell wall' antibiotics. GlcNAc, *N*-acetylglucosamine; MurNAc, *N*-acetylmuramyl; mesoA$_2$pm, diaminopimelic acid. (Reproduced, with permission, from Reynolds (1985).)

disaccharide–pentapeptide unit has been transferred to the nascent peptidoglycan chain. Binding of bacitracin prevents the enzymic dephosphorylation of the carrier lipid to its monophosphate form, a step which is required for another round of synthesis and transfer of the disaccharide–peptide unit (Fig. 2.22). Inhibition by bacitracin is therefore associated with an interaction between antibiotic and substrate, rather than the antibiotic and the dephosphorylating enzyme.

4.4 Stage 3 inhibitors

4.4.1 Glycopeptide antibiotics

Vancomycin, ristocetin and teicoplanin (teichoplanin) are examples of glycopeptide antibiotics that interfere with glycan unit insertion (Fig. 2.22). Vancomycin (Fig. 2.26(a)) undergoes hydrogen bonding to the acyl-D-alanyl-D-alanine terminus of various peptidoglycan precursors (Fig. 2.26(b)). In particular, it binds to the GlcNAc-MurNAc-pentapeptide-pyrophosphate-undecaprenol precursor and to the growing point of the peptidoglycan, thereby inhibiting the transglycosylation step by which glycan units are polymerized within the peptidoglycan (Fig. 2.22). Strictly speaking the transglycosylase enzyme is not inhibited, but the complex of vancomycin with the peptide prevents the substrate from interacting with the active site of the enzyme. Vancomycin is therefore another example of an antibiotic that combines with a peptidoglycan substrate rather than an enzyme. The mode of action of ristocetin and teicoplanin is similar.

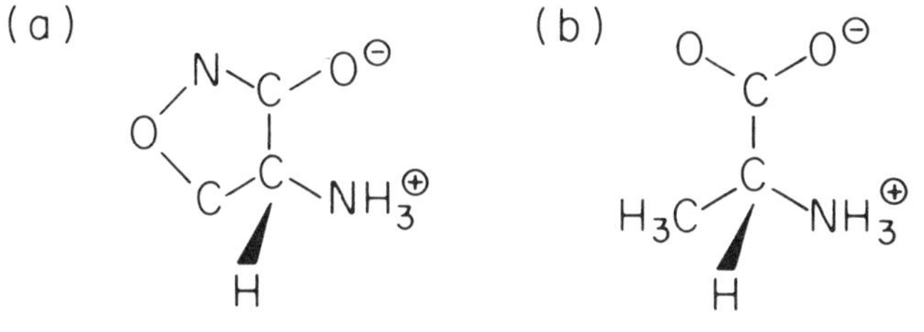

Figure 2.23 Structure of (a) D-cycloserine and (b) D-alanine.

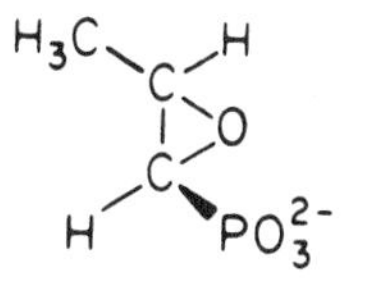

Figure 2.24 Structure of fosfomycin.

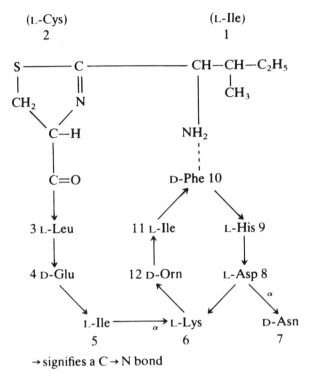

→ signifies a C → N bond

Figure 2.25 Structure of bacitracin.

4.4.2 β-Lactam antibiotics

4.4.2.1 Introduction

Without doubt the β-lactam antibiotics represent the most important group of drugs that inhibit the final stage of peptidoglycan synthesis. During the last decade there has been a dramatic increase in the number of these antibiotics synthesized or discovered and in our understanding of how they act as inhibitors of peptidoglycan synthesis. In view of their importance as clinically useful antibacterial agents, these antibiotics will be considered in detail. Unfortunately it is beyond the scope of this book to consider the clinical applications of this group of antibiotics.

β-Lactams derive their name from the possession of a four-membered cyclic amide ring (Fig. 2.27). Until recently, such antibiotics were defined and classified by a trivial nomenclature, the name of a compound usually relating to the producing organism and a chemical feature of the compound. More recently, they have been categorized by a system based on a defined parent β-lactam skeleton giving ten classes of compound (Fig. 2.27). Thus, the penicillins and

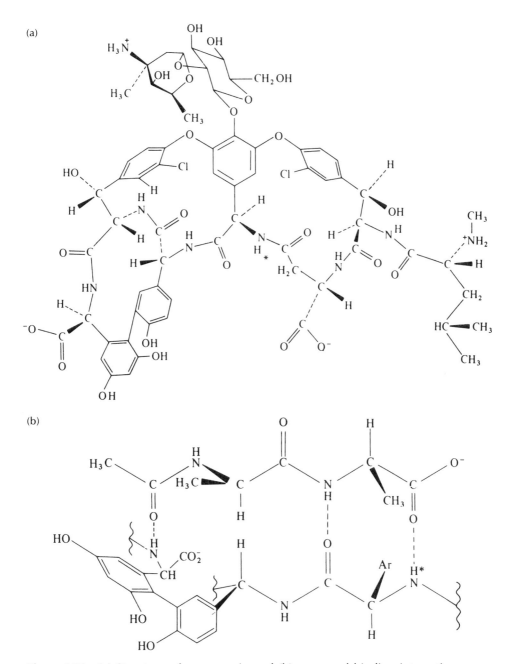

Figure 2.26 (a) Structure of vancomycin and (b) proposed binding interactions between acetyl-D-alanyl-D-alanine and vancomycin. The same hydrogen atom is marked with an asterisk in (a) and (b) to allow the structures to be aligned. (Reproduced, with permission, from Rogers *et al.* (1980).)

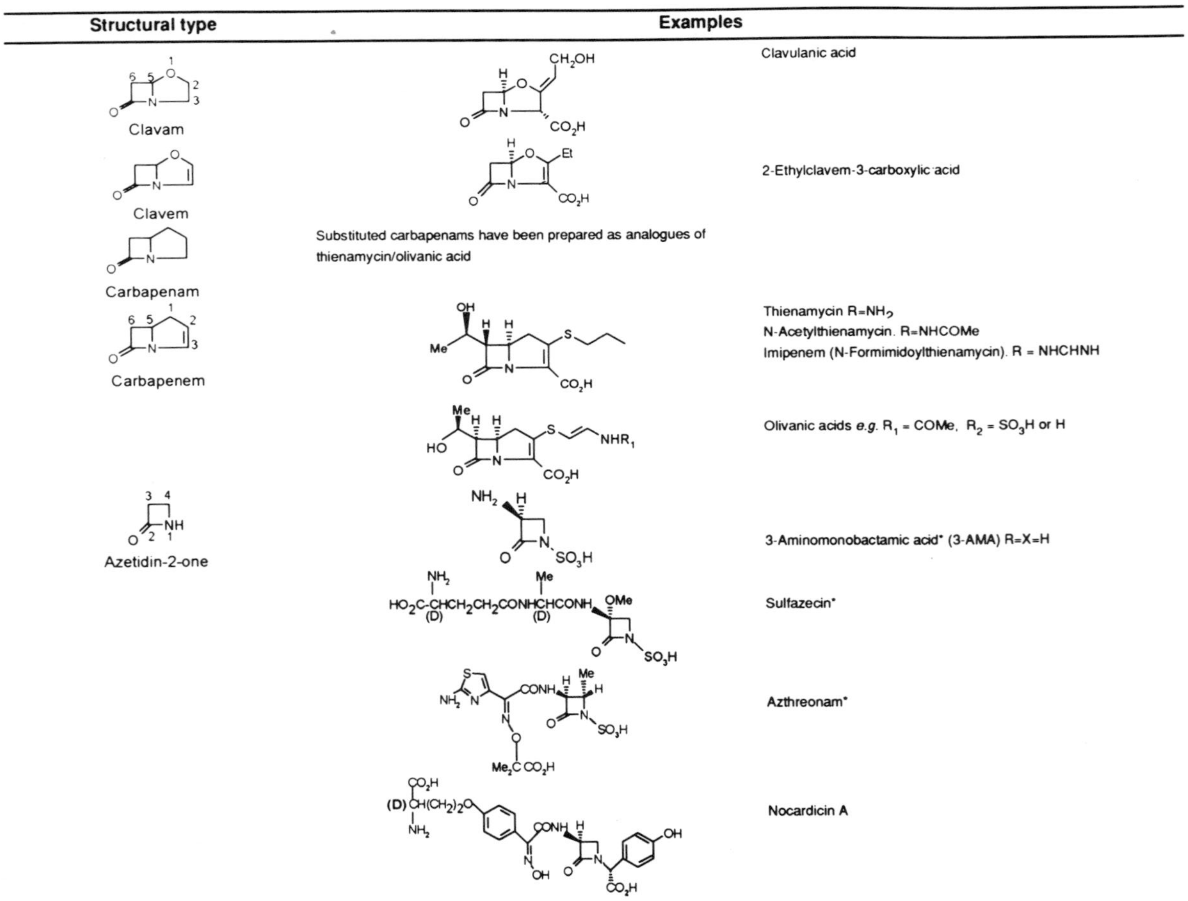

Figure 2.27 Structure of β-lactam antibiotics (*, monobactams). (Based on Brown (1982).)

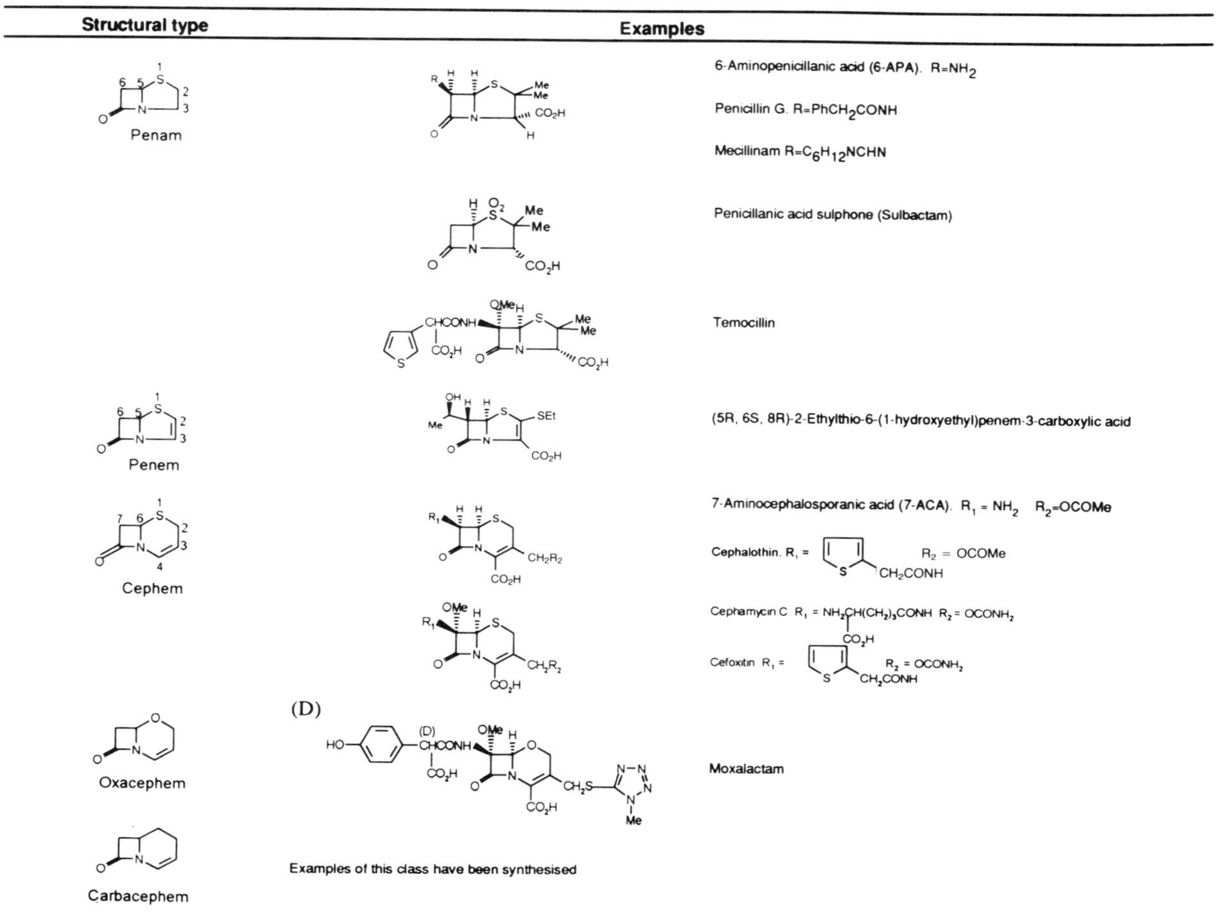

Structural type	Examples

Penam

6-Aminopenicillanic acid (6-APA). R=NH₂

Penicillin G. R=PhCH₂CONH

Mecillinam R=C₆H₁₂NCHN

Penicillanic acid sulphone (Sulbactam)

Temocillin

(5R, 6S, 8R)-2-Ethylthio-6-(1-hydroxyethyl)penem-3-carboxylic acid

Penem

7-Aminocephalosporanic acid (7-ACA). R₁ = NH₂   R₂=OCOMe

Cephalothin. R₁ =   R₂ = OCOMe
                                      CH₂CONH

Cephem

Cephamycin C R₁ = NH₂CH(CH₂)₃CONH R₂ = OCONH₂

Cefoxitin R₁ =   R₂ = OCONH₂
                                      CH₂CONH

Moxalactam

(D)

Examples of this class have been synthesised

Oxacephem

Carbacephem

Figure 2.27 *continued*

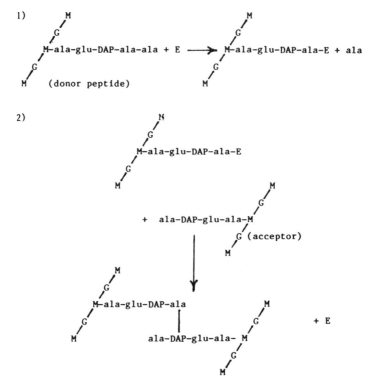

Figure 2.28   The transpeptidation reaction: G, *N*-acetylglucosamine; *N*,*N*-acetylmuramic acid; E, transpeptidase; DAP, diaminopimelic acid. The reaction shown applies to *E. coli*, but it should be remembered that some bacteria contain additional amino acids in the cross-bridge. However, the overall nature of transpeptidation is similar in all bacteria containing peptidoglycan. (1) Formation of enzyme intermediate with release of D-alanine. (2) Transpeptidation reaction with release of enzyme. (Reproduced, with permission, from Park (1987).)

cephalosporins, which are the best known members of the β-lactam antibiotics, are now classified respectively as penams and cephems. Many semisynthetic penam and cephem derivatives have been produced by varying the substituents attached to the β-lactam ring and/or (in the case of the cephems) to the six-membered dihydrothiazine ring (Fig. 2.27).

4.4.2.2 *Early studies (1950–65) on the mode of action of β-lactams*

Early work on the mode of action of penicillin culminated in the theory that its primary target was the transpeptidation reaction that cross-links neighbouring glycan strands (Fig. 2.28). This conclusion was based primarily on studies with intact bacteria treated with benzylpenicillin where it was shown that

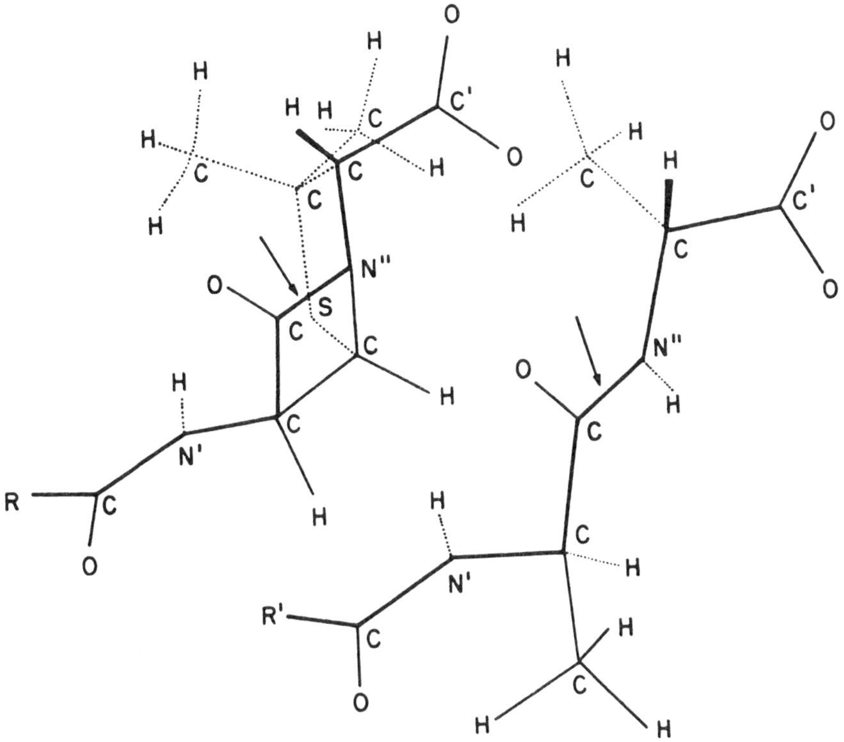

Figure 2.29 Dreiding stereomodels of penicillin (upper left) and of the acyl-D-alanyl-D-alanine end of the nascent peptidoglycan (lower right). Arrows indicate the position of the CO—N bond in the β-lactam ring of penicillin and of the CO—N peptide bond joining the two D-alanine residues. The portion of the penicillin molecule which is believed to resemble the peptide backbone of the acyl-D-ala-D-ala is reproduced in heavy lines. (Reproduced with permission from Tipper, D. J. & Strominger, J. L. (1965) *Proceedings of the National Academy of Sciences (USA)* **54**: 1133 (Fig. 1).)

increased amounts of alanine were present in isolated walls while cross-linkage was decreased. Furthermore, Tipper and Strominger advanced the important hypothesis that penicillin might be a structural analogue of the acyl-D-alanyl-D-alanine portion of the peptide side chain (Fig. 2.29). It was therefore reasonable to suppose that an enzyme catalysing transpeptidation would mistake the antibiotic molecule for the genuine substrate, cleave the β-lactam bond, and, in so doing, be rendered inactive owing to the formation of a stable (covalent) antibiotic–enzyme intermediate. Aspects of this model are indeed still applicable today, although various refinements are necessary in the light of more recent findings.

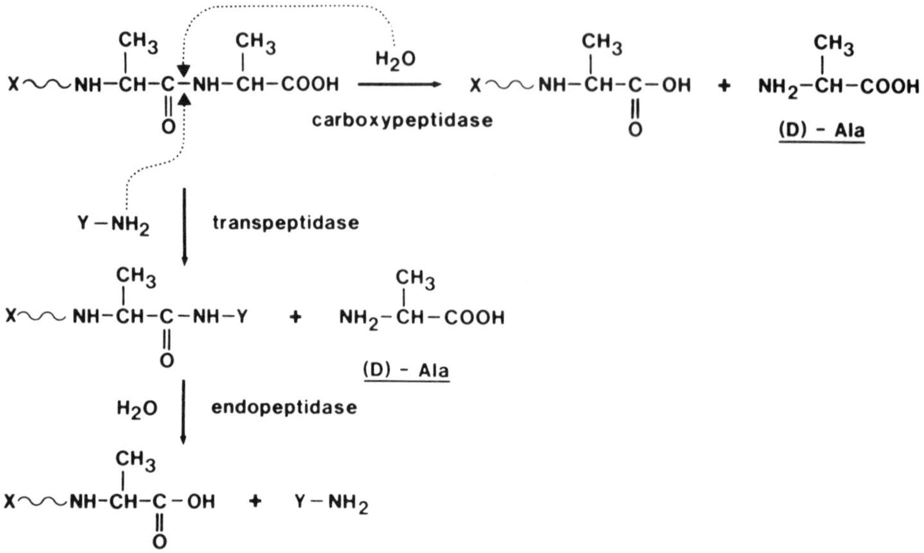

Figure 2.30 Carboxypeptidase, transpeptidase and endopeptidase reactions. All three types of reaction can be catalysed by bacterial penicillin-binding proteins (see text and Table 2.3). Carboxypeptidase reactions are basically similar; in both cases the carbonyl of the penultimate D-alanine is transferred to an exogenous nucleophile. If the latter is water, hydrolysis occurs; if it is an amino group of another peptide, the product is a cross-linked dimer of the two peptides. Endopeptidase activity can hydrolyse such dimers. (Reproduced, with permission, from Tomasz (1983).)

4.4.2.3 *Multiplicity of penicillin-sensitive reactions in bacteria*

Until the 1960s it was assumed that bacteria probably contained only a single type of transpeptidase enzyme and that this represented the unique target for penicillin. However, this simple picture had to be revised following the development of *in vitro* assays of transpeptidation reactions.

The first *in vitro* demonstration of peptidoglycan transpeptidase activity was achieved using *E. coli*. Unexpectedly, it was noted that, in addition to transpeptidation, two further reactions occurred: removal of the carboxyl terminal D-alanine, but without formation of peptide bonds (i.e. a D,D-carboxypeptidase reaction) and cleavage of cross-links between peptide chains (i.e. an endopeptidase reaction) (Fig. 2.30). All three reactions were inhibited by penicillin. Subsequently, similar types of penicillin-sensitive reactions were detected in a variety of other bacteria and in every case the substrate involved was either a D-alanyl–D-alanine bond or a D-alanyl–*meso*-(D)-diaminopimelyl bond. Indeed, it is now apparent that any enzyme which metabolizes a D–D peptide bond is likely to be sensitive to β-lactam antibiotics.

Table 2.3 Properties of the penicillin-binding proteins of *E. coli* K12

PBP	Molecular weight	Molecules/cell	Gene symbol	Proposed function	Examples of antibiotics showed marked affinity
1A	92 000	100	*mrcA (ponA)*	Bifunctional enzymes with transglycosylase and transpeptidase activities. Synthesize peptidoglycan at the growing zones of the side wall.	Benzylpenicillin and most cephalosporins
1Bα	86 500	120	*mrcB (ponB)*		
β	84 000				
γ	81 500				
2	66 000	20	*pbpA*	Bifunctional enzyme with transglycosylase and transpeptidase activity. Initiates peptidoglycan insertion at new growth sites which are then further extended by PBPs 1A, 1B.	Mecillinam, imipenem
3	60 000	50	*ftsI (pbpB, sep)*	Bifunctional enzyme with transglycosylase and transpeptidase activity. Required specifically for formation of the cross-wall at cell division.	Cephalexin and many other cephalosporins, piperacillin, azthreonam
4	49 000	110	*dacB*	D,D-carboxypeptidase and/or D,D-endopeptidase. The first activity may control the extent of peptidoglycan cross-linking by transpeptidases, the second activity causing hydrolysis of cross-links during cell elongation.	Benzylpenicillin, ampicillin, imipenem
5	42 000	1800	*dacA*	D,D-carboxypeptidases that may control the extent of peptidoglycan cross-linking by transpeptidases.	Cefoxitin
6	40 000	600	*dacC*		
7	29 000	?	*pbpG*	Unknown.	Penems

4.4.2.4 *Penicillin-binding proteins*

The identification of more than one penicillin-sensitive reaction in the cell-free peptidoglycan synthetic systems described above implied that several proteins (enzymes) capable of interacting with penicillin (and other β-lactams) might be present in any individual bacterial species. The introduction of radioactive penicillin labelling techniques for the visualization of bacterial proteins that covalently bind penicillin has confirmed this prediction.

Several (usually at least four) penicillin-binding proteins (PBPs) are present in most bacterial species. PBPs are designated numerically, e.g. 1–7 in *E. coli* K12 (Table 2.3). The numerical description of PBPs is strictly a reference to their relative molecular size within the group of PBPs detected in a particular bacterium (PBP1 having the greatest molecular weight). Thus PBP3 of *E. coli* need not have anything in common with PBP3 of *S. aureus*. Nevertheless, within a closely related group of bacteria, such as the Enterobacteriaceae, at least some of the PBPs of comparable molecular size may have similar functions.

PBPs are minor components of the cytoplasmic membrane. For example, in *E. coli* they total about 3000 molecules per cell (Table 2.3), or 1% of total membrane proteins. The likely functions of several PBPs have been established using genetic and biochemical techniques. In view of the information presented in Section 4.4.2.3 it is not surprising to find that PBPs catalyse transpeptidase, carboxypeptidase and endopeptidase reactions. The PBPs of *E. coli* (Table 2.3) represent the most extensively studied set of PBPs. Their functions and the consequences of inhibition by β-lactams are discussed more fully below (Sections 4.4.2.5–4.4.2.10). PBPs can conveniently be considered as two groups, the high molecular weight essential PBPs and the lower molecular weight, generally non-essential, PBPs that appear to play a minor role in peptidoglycan synthesis.

4.4.2.5 *High molecular weight* E. coli *PBPs*

The high molecular weight PBPs (PBPs 1–3) are responsible for net synthesis of peptidoglycan *in vivo*, although their enzymic activities are often difficult to demonstrate *in vitro*. The proteins are products of separate structural genes (Table 2.3), the multiple components of PBP1B arising because alternative translational initiation codons are used within *mrc*B (*pon*B). The gene for each high molecular weight *E. coli* PBP has been sequenced, thereby permitting prediction of the primary amino acid sequences of the corresponding PBPs.

PBPs 1–3 are enzymes which catalyse both the polymerization of the disaccharide units into glycan chains (transglycosylation) and also the cross-linking of their pentapeptide side chains (transpeptidation): they are thus bifunctional peptidoglycan transglycosylases–transpeptidases (Fig. 2.31). The transglycosylation activity of these proteins is not susceptible to β-lactams, unlike the transpeptidase activity (Fig. 2.31). The dual enzymatic activity expressed by these

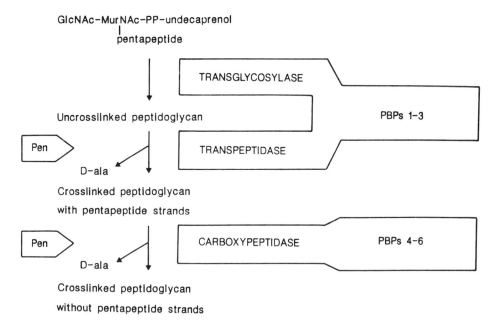

Figure 2.31 Enzymatic formation of cross-linked peptidoglycan in *E. coli* showing the bifunctional activity of PBPs 1–3 as peptidoglycan transglycosylases and penicillin-sensitive transpeptidases. PBPs 4–6 may function as penicillin-sensitive D,D-alanine carboxypeptidases to limit the cross-linking reaction. Pen refers to a penicillin or other β-lactam antibiotic. Note that transglycosylases are insusceptible to β-lactam antibiotics.

PBPs probably results from the presence of two distinct, catalytically active, centres in the same polypeptide, i.e. an amino-terminal domain catalysing the trans-glycosylation reaction and a carboxyl-terminal domain carrying the β-lactam sensitive transpeptidase activity. Presumably the presence of both enzymic activities in the same polypeptide permits close control over the insertion and cross-linking of glycan units into the growing peptidoglycan network.

Inhibition of the transpeptidase activity of the high molecular weight PBPs of *E. coli* by β-lactam antibiotics eventually leads to cell death. Concomitant inhibition of PBPs 1A and 1B leads to rapid cell lysis, inhibition of PBP2 to 'growth' as osmotically stable spherical or ovoid forms and inhibition of PBP3 to filamentation. 'Growth' as spheres following inhibition of PBP2 (e.g. by mecillinam), or as filaments following inhibition of PBP3 (e.g. by cephalexin), can continue for several generations before deformation and collapse (but not necessarily complete lysis) occurs.

4.4.2.6 *Low molecular weight* E. coli *PBPs*

Apart from PBP7, the probable functions of the low molecular weight PBPs (i.e. PBPs 4–6) have been established (Table 2.3). Although PBP4 exhibits D-alanine carboxypeptidase activity *in vitro*, it may also act *in vivo* as an endopeptidase hydrolysing previously formed peptide cross-links in peptidoglycan. The endopeptidase reaction is the reverse of transpeptidation except that the resulting product is a tetrapeptide, not possessing the terminal D-alanine. The endopeptidase activity of PBP4 probably contributes to the remodelling of peptidoglycan necessary for growth and division of the cell. PBPs 5 and 6 catalyse a D-alanine carboxypeptidase reaction (Fig. 2.31). This reaction probably controls the extent of peptidoglycan cross-linking by removing the terminal D-alanine residues from the pentapeptide side chains of nascent peptidoglycan, thereby preventing them from acting as peptide donors in transpeptidation.

Mutants of *E. coli* lacking the enzyme activities of PBP 4 (*dac*B), 5(*dac*A), or 6(*dac*C) and a double mutant (*dac*A, *dac*B) have been isolated. Since these mutants grew normally it has been concluded that neither the carboxypeptidase nor the endopeptidase activities of the respective PBPs were essential for growth, at least under laboratory conditions. However, a role in normal growth for the carboxypeptidase activity provided by these PBPs cannot yet be completely excluded since even the *dac*A, *dac*B double mutant might have sufficient *dac*C-encoded carboxypeptidase activity to maintain growth. The nature of a triple *dac*A,B,C mutant (if it can be isolated) might resolve the question of whether PBP-mediated D-alanine carboxypeptidase activity is required for growth.

Although the enzymatic activity and function of the low molecular weight PBP7 are unknown, its inactivation, particularly by penems (e.g. imipenem) leads to bacterial lysis. However, the steps leading to lysis following inactivation of PBP7 differ from those when PBP1A and 1B are inactivated (see Section 4.5.2).

4.4.2.7 E. coli *PBPs that are killing targets for β-lactams: a summary*

In *E. coli*, PBPs 4, 5 and 6 do not appear to be essential for growth and thus their interaction with β-lactams is not considered to be responsible for the killing action of these antibiotics. The remaining proteins, particularly the high molecular weight PBPs 1A, 1B, 2 and 3, are the primary lethal targets. The binding of a β-lactam, leading to inactivation of transpeptidase activity, is potentially lethal. Rapid lysis (death) results from inactivation of PBPs 1A and 1B, whereas antibiotics showing a preference for PBPs 2 or 3 produce distinct, but transient, morphological changes prior to cell death. Inhibition of bacterial growth by β-lactams (e.g. benzylpenicillin, ampicillin) that have similar affinities for the target proteins is likely to result from the simultaneous inactivation of more than one of the lethal targets. The exact mechanisms leading to cell death are not entirely clear, but this topic is expanded in a later section (Section 4.5).

4.4.2.8 Enzymatic activities of PBPs in other bacteria and identification of β-lactam killing targets

The enzymic activity of PBPs in Gram-negative bacteria other than *E. coli* is not well documented. However, transpeptidase, carboxypeptidase and endopeptidase activities have been ascribed to some PBPs. Only D,D-carboxypeptidase activity has been associated with PBPs purified from Gram-positive bacteria, i.e. natural transpeptidation activity has not been directly demonstrated. Nevertheless, on the basis of findings with *E. coli* and other Gram-negative organisms, it can be assumed that at least some of the PBPs from the Gram-positive bacteria mediate transpeptidation reactions *in vivo* that are susceptible to inhibition by β-lactam antibiotics.

   Although the precise functions of the majority of PBPs found in bacteria other than *E. coli* have not yet been established, a more general approach to the identification of physiologically important PBPs (killing targets) in these organisms has been possible. If the multiple PBPs of bacteria include one or more killing targets for β-lactams, while other PBPs perform less vital activities (e.g. PBPs 4–6 of *E. coli*), it should be possible to identify the former from among all the detectable PBPs by comparing the extent of inhibition of PBPs with the overall susceptibility of the organism as a function of antibiotic concentration. This is based on the principle that PBPs which are saturated at antibiotic concentrations that are either below, or far above, those required to inhibit bacterial growth do not qualify as killing targets. It is beyond the scope of this book to attempt to describe in detail the various conclusions drawn from studies of this type. Nevertheless, it is sufficient to comment that this general approach has identified likely PBP killing targets in *Ps. aeruginosa*, *K. aerogenes*, *Pr. rettgeri*, *E. cloacea*, *H. influenzae* and *B. megaterium*. However, this approach does not yield helpful information with those organisms (e.g. *S. aureus*, *Strep. pneumoniae* and *B. subtilis*) where several, or all, of the PBPs are saturated at similar β-lactam concentrations which are themselves equivalent to the antibiotic concentrations inhibiting growth of the respective organisms.

4.4.2.9 Nature of the substrate and β-lactam binding sites in PBPs

PBPs are enzymes that utilize the D-alanyl-D-alanine moiety of the pentapeptide as a substrate and are believed to form an acyl–enzyme intermediate, with release of the terminal D-alanine during the course of the reaction (Fig. 2.32). The hypothesis of Tipper and Strominger (Section 4.4.2.2) predicts that penicillin and other β-lactams will bind covalently to the same group in the enzymes (PBPs) to which the natural substrate normally binds. Evidence for similar, if not identical, binding sites for substrate and β-lactams has now been obtained, the enzyme active site containing a serine residue through which β-lactams or substrate bind to the enzymes (Fig. 2.32).

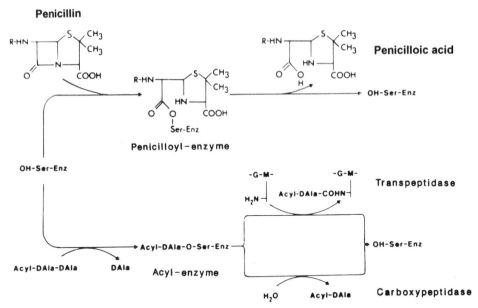

Figure 2.32 Proposed mechanism for the reaction of penicillin-sensitive enzymes with penicillin or acyl-D-Ala-D-Ala. A nucleophile in the enzyme active site (shown as a serine (Ser) residue) reacts with either acyl-D-Ala-D-Ala or penicillin to yield either acyl-D-alanyl-enzyme or penicilloyl-enzyme intermediates. Serine has been established as the residue to which the substrate or inhibitor binds in PBPs 1,2,3,5 and 6 of *E. coli*, PBP 5 of *B. subtilis* and *B. stearothermophilus* and certain carboxypeptidases and transpeptidases from streptomycetes. Subsequent reaction of the acyl-D-alanyl-enzymes with a suitable amino acceptor peptide results in formation of a cross-link and release of the enzyme (transpeptidase). Alternatively, reaction with water results in the release of acyl-D-alanine and enzyme (carboxypeptidase). Although both functions are shown for the same enzyme, individual proteins tend to favour one reaction, i.e. they are D,D-carboxypeptidases with inefficient transpeptidase activity or the reverse may be the case. The penicilloyl-enzyme is more stable than the acyl-D-alanyl-enzyme and consequently the antibiotic residue is not transferred to an amino acceptor. Certain of these complexes do, however, react to release penicillin degradation products (e.g. penicilloic acid) and active enzyme (see Figure 2.33). (Reproduced, with permission, from Lorian (1986).)

The amino acid sequences in the active site regions of several PBPs have been determined. PBPs 1–6 of *E. coli* and PBP 5 of *B. subtilis* contain the active site serine within the sequence Ala/Gly–Ser–X–X–Lys. Thus the sequence Ser–X–X–Lys is conserved in all the PBPs. By themselves these sequencing studies do not establish the three-dimensional architecture of the substrate and inhibitor binding sites. To investigate the contribution of different regions of the polypeptide to the

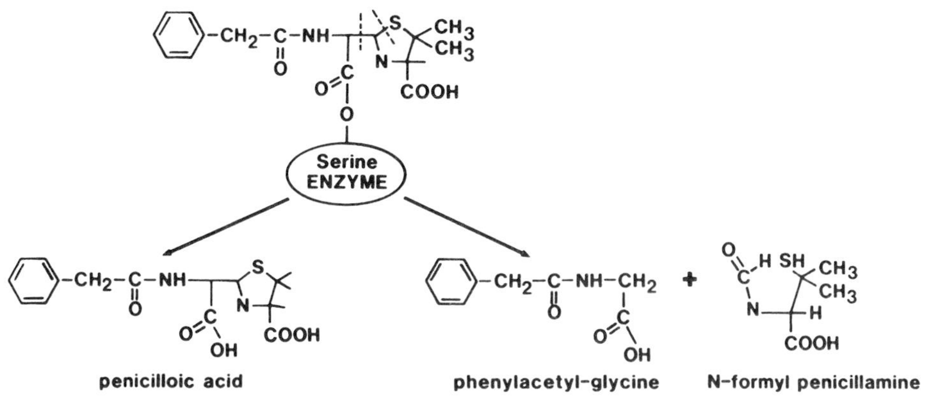

Serine ENZYME

penicilloic acid   phenylacetyl-glycine   N-formyl penicillamine

Figure 2.33   Alternative pathways for the degradation of the β-lactam acyl-enzyme complexes. (Reproduced, with permission, from Tomasz (1983).)

active site it will be necessary to apply X-ray crystallographic techniques to purified PBPs. Such studies are still in their infancy, but it can be assumed that the different affinities displayed by β-lactam antibiotics for the same PBP reflect the three-dimensional shapes of the active site and the drug molecules. Presumably certain pendent groups on the antibiotic molecules can be accommodated by the proteins more easily than others. Although there is considerable evidence for overlapping substrate and β-lactam binding sites in PBPs, enzymological studies suggest that penicillin-sensitive enzymes, in addition to the enzyme active site, may also have other drug recognition sites. Interaction of antibiotic molecules with these sites may influence the reactivity of the enzyme active site.

4.4.2.10   Interaction of β-lactams with PBPs: kinetic studies and fate of the antibiotic molecule

The association (binding and release) of β-lactams with PBPs is represented by the following equation:

$$I + PBP \underset{k_2}{\overset{k_1}{\rightleftharpoons}} IPBP \xrightarrow{k_3} IPBP^* \xrightarrow{k_4} PBP \text{ (active)} + \text{antibiotic (inactive)}$$

where I is the inhibitor (β-lactam), IPBP is the initial non-covalent inhibitor–PBP complex, IPBP* is the inhibitor–PBP complex (demonstrably covalent in most cases), and k_1, k_2, k_3, k_4 are first-order rate constants.

β-Lactams with low rates of acylation ($k_3 < k_2$) or high rates of deacylation (k_4

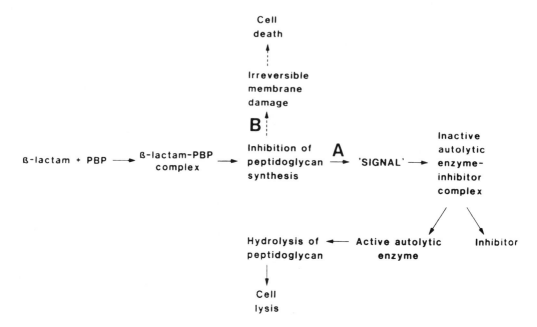

Figure 2.34   Model for the mechanisms by which β-lactam antibiotics kill bacteria by lytic death (route A), or non-lytic death (route B). The nature of the 'signal' resulting from inhibition of peptidoglycan synthesis and leading to lytic death (route A) is unknown. See text for further details. (Reproduced, with modifications, from Lorian (1986).)

high) will be poor inhibitors, in the latter case because the antibiotic is a substrate of the enzyme. However, even in the case of good PBP inhibitors, the penicilloyl complexes undergo deacylation. Decomposition can follow two routes (Fig. 2.33) depending on the PBP and the particular type of β-lactam. The first reaction (formation of a penicilloic acid) is identical to that catalysed by β-lactamases, enzymes distinct from PBPs that mediate bacterial resistance to β-lactams (see Chapter 5).

4.5   Mechanisms by which inhibition of peptidoglycan synthesis leads to bacterial death

4.5.1   Introduction

Exposure of growing bacteria to inhibitors of peptidoglycan synthesis usually leads to cell death. This may result from lytic or non-lytic events (Fig. 2.34). The two types of response are considered more fully in Sections 4.5.2 and 4.5.3.

4.5.2 Lytic death and the role of peptidoglycan degradative enzymes (autolysins)

It has been known for many years that inhibition of further peptidoglycan synthesis can result in the formation of osmotically fragile cells which lyse in the absence of a suitable non-penetrating stabilizer, such as sucrose. Furthermore, the participation of peptidoglycan degradative enzymes in the process had been established by the mid-1950s.

However, the findings summarized above do not explain why cessation of peptidoglycan synthesis can lead to enzymatic degradation of cell walls. The first hypothesis (advanced in the 1960s) considered that the effects of antibiotics such as penicillin resulted primarily from 'unbalanced growth'. Bacterial autolysins, i.e. enzymes hydrolysing bonds in the glycan, or peptide side chains of peptidoglycan (Fig. 2.35), were considered to play an essential role in cell wall synthesis by providing space and acceptor sites for new material to be condensed into the growing wall by peptidoglycan synthetic enzymes. In the presence of penicillin, inhibition of cross-linkage (by transpeptidation) together with continued autolytic activity would, it was proposed, lead to a structurally weakened wall and eventual lysis of the cell because it would no longer be able to withstand the high internal osmotic pressure generated by the cytoplasmic contents. Under such circumstances bacterial lysis would not be due to any specific induction of autolysins, but due to the abrupt arrest of peptidoglycan synthesis leading to an unbalanced state where autolysins continue to cleave peptidoglycan.

The first direct evidence for involvement of autolysins in penicillin-induced lysis of bacteria came from studies with a *Strep. pneumoniae* mutant defective in *N*-acetylmuramyl-L-alanine amidase activity. The parent (wild-type) organism lysed rapidly on treatment with β-lactam antibiotics, but the mutant, although prevented from growing by the drugs, remained viable for much longer periods than the parent strain in the presence of antibiotic. Confirmation of these initial findings has come from further studies on other autolysin-defective bacterial mutants for which the general term 'tolerant' mutant has been coined.

Although autolysins clearly have a role in lytic death, their activity in this process is no longer thought to be related to the 'unbalanced growth' model mentioned above. This modified view has arisen mainly from observations showing that autolysins are not essential enzymes needed for cell wall expansion, but rather are probably involved in degradation of peptidoglycan accompanying cell separation at the end of cell division. Studies with autolysin-defective mutants support this view. For instance, autolysin-deficient mutants of rods or streptococci frequently form long chains of cells and mutant staphylococci have been described that grow as large clumps of cells, suggesting that lowered autolysin activity in each case prevents separation of daughter cells. An attractive theory relating autolysin activity to antibiotic-induced lytic death has been advanced by Tomasz. He speculates that the activity of the autolysins is 'triggered' at the end of the cell cycle by a properly timed and genetically programmed halt in peptidoglycan

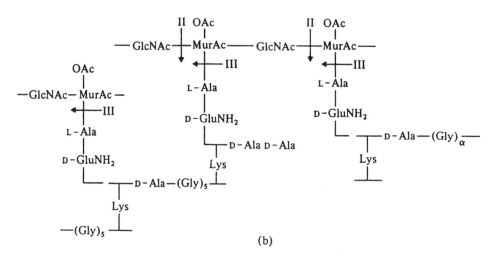

(a)

(b)

Figure 2.35 Bond specificities of three common types of autolytic enzymes. The arrows indicate the bonds hydrolysed by (I) *endo*-muramidase, (II) *endo*-β-N-acetylglucosaminidase and (III) N-acetylmuramyl-L-alanine amidase (amidase). (a) Shows the structure of peptidoglycans present in many bacilli and in all the Gram-negative species examined. (b) Shows the structure of a peptidoglycan with a 'bridge' peptide. The one illustrated is present in *S. aureus*. (Reproduced, with modifications, from Rogers *et al.* (1980).)

synthesis, the whole process permitting controlled separation of daughter cells. Antibiotic- (e.g. penicillin) induced lysis is considered by Tomasz as a premature 'triggering' of terminal events in bacterial cell separation, but differing from the normal physiological process because autolytic activity is not localized, transient or properly timed. The consequences of uncontrolled autolytic activity are lysis and death.

The concept of naturally occurring autolysin inhibitors is also central to Tomasz's theory on lytic death. The activity of autolytic enzymes is proposed to be negatively controlled by one or more natural inhibitors and the bactericidal action of β-lactams (and other inhibitors of peptidoglycan synthesis) is mediated by antibiotic-induced deregulation or 'triggering' of the autolytic system, possibly due to dissociation of autolysin-natural inhibitor complexes (Fig. 2.34). Amphipathic, membrane-associated, substances are implicated as the naturally occurring autolysin inhibitors (regulators), but little is known about the molecular basis of events during the 'triggering' process. Also, it is not known why inhibition of certain essential PBPs, e.g. PBPs 1A and 1B in *E. coli*, leads to very rapid cell lysis, whereas inhibition of other essential PBPs, such as PBP2 of *E. coli*, does not result in rapid 'triggering' of autolytic activity.

A further important point relating to lytic death mechanisms concerns the well-known observation that β-lactams generally do not promote lysis of non-growing bacteria. This phenomenon was first recognized in the 1940s when it was noted that starvation of nutritional auxotrophs protected against the bactericidal effect of penicillin. The exact basis of this phenomenon is still not fully understood, but has been examined to some extent in *E. coli*. When bacteria suffer from nutrient starvation, particularly deprivation of amino acids, the so-called 'stringent response' ensues. This is a regulatory system that suppresses synthesis of certain cellular macromolecules such as stable RNA species, phospholipids and peptidoglycan. The response is mediated, in a complex manner, by the nucleotide guanosine tetraphosphate (ppGpp) which is derived from guanosine pentaphosphate (pppGpp). The latter is synthesized from GTP by a ribosome-associated ATP:GTP 3' pyrophosphotransferase (the product of the *rel*A gene) which is activated during amino acid deprivation. The stringent response inhibits peptidoglycan synthesis at two points: (a) an early step in the synthesis of UDP-MurNAc-pentapeptide and (b) a late step in the polymerization of peptidoglycan catalysed by one or more of the PBPs. The combination of these events presumably prevents the unnecessary accumulation of peptidoglycan intermediates when growth is arrested by amino acid deprivation. The mechanism by which the stringent control system regulates peptidoglycan synthesis is not yet fully understood. However, preliminary evidence suggests that inhibition of peptidoglycan synthesis is a consequence of inhibition of phospholipid synthesis by ppGpp.

On the basis of these and other findings a speculative model has been proposed to explain why most β-lactams are only able to promote lysis of growing *E. coli* (Fig. 2.36). Although β-lactams are able to bind to PBPs that are not actively engaged in peptidoglycan synthesis, such interactions fail to activate the 'trigger'

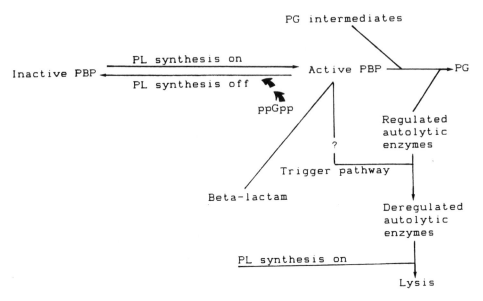

Figure 2.36 Model for regulation of peptidoglycan synthesis and antibiotic-induced lysis: PG, peptidoglycan; PBP, penicillin-binding protein; ppGpp, guanosine tetraphosphate; PL, phospholipid. (From Ishiguro & Kusser (1988), with modifications.)

pathway leading to activation of autolysins. In contrast, binding of β-lactams to PBPs (particularly PBPs 1A and 1B) that are actively engaged in peptidoglycan synthesis leads to activation of autolytic enzymes and cell death. When considering this model it should be remembered that certain β-lactams (e.g. imipenem) promote lysis of non-growing *E. coli* by interaction with PBP 7 (Section 4.4.2.6). Possibly the activity of PBP 7 is not subject to stringent control and remains permanently 'active' even though net peptidoglycan synthesis may have stopped. Alternatively, PBP 7 may be coupled to a different type of 'triggering' pathway from that of PBPs 1A and 1B.

4.5.3 *Non-lytic death*

Although β-lactam antibiotics frequently cause cell lysis, they are able to kill some types of bacteria by a non-lytic process. Death without lysis usually occurs in bacteria that do not possess detectable autolytic activity. McDowell and Lemanski (1988) reported that penicillin-induced death of a group A streptococcus was associated with hydrolysis and loss of RNA from the cell, changes that may arise from irreversible, penicillin-mediated, membrane damage.

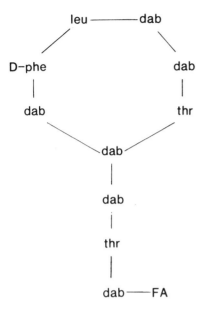

Figure 2.37 Generalized structure of the polymyxins. For polymyxin B the fatty acyl (FA) residue is 6-methyloctanoic acid. dab, ʟ-diaminobutyric acid.

5
Antibiotics that inhibit membrane integrity

5.1 Polymyxins

The polymyxins (e.g. polymyxin B, Fig. 2.37) are a group of cyclic, polycationic, peptides with a fatty acid chain attached to the peptide through an amide linkage. The bactericidal activity of these compounds results from their interaction with the bacterial cytoplasmic membrane causing gross disorganization of its structure. Membranes containing the phospholipid phosphatidylethanolamine are particularly sensitive to polymyxins which explains why Gram-negative bacteria are more susceptible to polymyxins than Gram-positive organisms, because membranes of the latter generally do not contain phosphatidylethanolamine.

Polymyxins have only a minor place in medicine because they also have affinity for mammalian membranes. However, they appear to bind less readily to mammalian membranes than to bacterial membranes. The basis for this discrimination may relate to the presence of cholesterol in mammalian membranes.

5.2 Magainins

Recently, a number of endogenous host defence peptides with antimicrobial activity have been identified in mammals, invertebrates and amphibians. Those from amphibians have been termed magainins and are peptides containing 21–23 residues. These naturally occurring products have relatively poor antibacterial potencies and a limited spectrum of activity. To improve peptide activity and antibacterial spectrum, synthetic analogues have been designed involving selected amino acid substitutions and deletions, repeats of small peptides and protection of sites likely to be susceptible to enzymatic attack. Currently a number of such peptides, e.g. MSI-78, are under development as topical anti-infective agents with potential dermatological, ophthalmic and periodontal applications.

Magainins are bactericidal and bind to the bacterial cytoplasmic membrane forming transmembrane helical channels that dissipate the membrane potential ($\Delta\psi$). The reason that magainins such as MSI-78 exhibit selective antibacterial activity is not fully understood, but may relate to the presence of cholesterol in mammalian membranes which inhibits the membrane insertion event.

6
Antimycobacterial drugs

6.1 Introduction

Recently considerable interest has focused on the chemotherapy of mycobacterial infections due to the resurgence of diseases caused by mycobacteria. Principal mycobacterial infections against which antibacterial agents are employed include tuberculosis (*M. tuberculosis*), leprosy (*M. leprae*) and a collection of diseases (lymphadenitis, pulmonary, cutaneous and disseminated infections) caused by the so-called non-tuberculous or 'atypical' mycobacteria (principally the *M. avium* complex, *M. kansassi*, *M. chelonae*, *M. marinum*, *M. fortuitum* and *M. ulcerans*). Some of the agents employed against these organisms have already been described, e.g. rifampicin, streptomycin and cycloserine. These will not be considered further in this section as it is assumed that their modes of action against mycobacteria are identical to those elucidated in other bacteria. Furthermore, other agents, such as the fluoroquinolones and the newer macrolides that show considerable potential for the treatment of certain mycobacterial diseases, but are not yet approved for such applications, will not be discussed again here. It is important to note that the antibiotics mentioned above, together with the specific antimycobacterial agents described below, are invariably used as components of multidrug treatment regimens, an approach designed to avoid the selection of resistant mutants during monotherapy. Poor patient compliance with such multiple drug regimens is one factor that has contributed to the emergence of multiple-drug-resistant strains of *M. tuberculosis* (see Chapter 8).

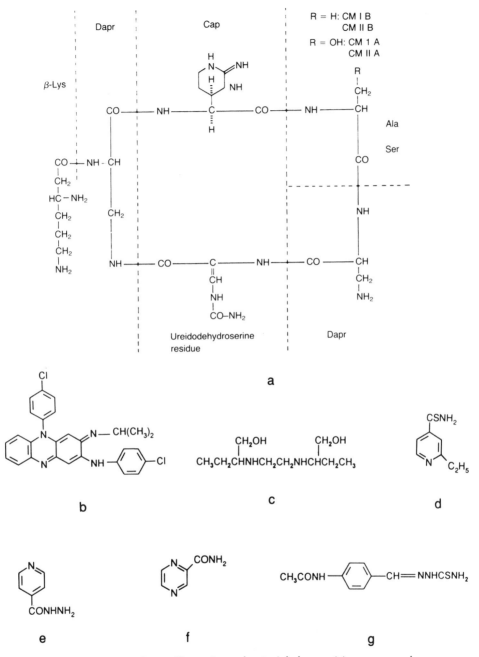

Figure 2.38   Structures of specific antimycobacterial drugs: (a) capreomycin complex (CM) components (β-lys, lysine; Dapr, α,β-diaminopropionic acid; Cap, capreomycidine (α-(2-iminohexahydro-4-pyrimidyl) glycine)); (b) clofazimine; (c) ethambutol; (d) ethionamide; (e) isoniazid; (f) pyrazinamide; (g) thiacetazone.

6.2 Capreomycin

Streptomyces capreolus produces a mixture of antibiotics, known as the capreomycin (CM) complex. CM contains four very similar macrocyclic polypeptides termed CMIA, CMIB, CMIIA and CMIIB (Fig. 2.38). The principal component of CM is CMIB. CMIA differs from the main component CMIB by possession of a serine residue in place of alanine. CMIIA and CMIIB correspond in their ring skeleton to CMIA and CMIB but differ from the latter by the absence of the β-lysine side chain (Fig. 2.38). CM is a so-called 'second-line' antituberculosis agent that is employed when resistance or adverse side effects to the preferred 'first-line' agents occur. The CM components inhibit protein synthesis in *M. tuberculosis*, but the exact mechanism of action is unknown.

6.3 Clofazimine

Clofazimine (Fig. 2.38), a substituted phenazine dye derived from phenylenediamine, is one of the most important components of multidrug treatment regimens for *M. leprae*. Apart from its use in leprosy, clofazimine has also been used in combination with other drugs for treatment of disseminated infections caused by the *M. avium* complex in patients who have acquired immunodeficiency syndrome (AIDS). In addition to its antimycobacterial activity, clofazimine is also active against some other Gram-positive bacteria, but it is not used to treat infections caused by these organisms. Clofazimine binds directly to DNA and inhibits transcription.

6.4 Ethambutol

Ethambutol (Fig. 2.38) is a synthetic compound of the ethylenediamine series. It is one of the 'first-line' antituberculosis agents, but it is also used in the therapy of infections caused by nontuberculous mycobacteria. The primary mode of action of ethambutol appears to be inhibition of mycobacterial arabinogalactan synthesis (Chapter 1). However, the precise step inhibited has not yet been elucidated.

6.5 Ethionamide

Ethionamide (Fig. 2.38) is a synthetic derivative of isonicotinic acid. It is one of the 'second-line' antituberculosis agents and is also used in multiple drug regimens for the treatment of pulmonary infections caused by the *M. avium* complex. Mycolic acid biosynthesis (Chapter 1) is the primary target for inhibition by ethionamide. Although the precise enzymatic step inhibited is not yet known, the protein InhA, which appears to be involved in mycolic acid biosynthesis, is a likely target.

6.6 Isoniazid

Isoniazid (Fig. 2.38), a structural analogue of ethionamide, is an important 'first-line' antituberculosis agent also used in the therapy of infections caused by non-tuberculous mycobacteria. The mode of action of isoniazid has not been fully established but appears to involve conversion (activation) to one or more metabolically active inhibitors within the mycobacterial cell. In *M. tuberculosis* it has been found that expression of the gene *katG*, which encodes an enzyme with catalase and peroxidase activities, is particularly important in conferring an isoniazid-sensitive phenotype. Therefore the catalase–peroxidase enzyme may have a direct role in the biotransformation of isoniazid to one or more inhibitory molecules. The exact target with which activated isoniazid molecules interact has not yet been established, but appears to involve one or more steps in mycolic acid biosynthesis (Chapter 1). One of the targets may be the protein InhA.

6.7 Pyrazinamide

Pyrazinamide (pyrazine-2-carboxylic acid amide) (Fig. 2.38) is a synthetic compound derived from nicotinic acid which has useful antibacterial activity only against *M. tuberculosis*. It is a member of the 'first-line' group of antituberculosis drugs. Pyrazinamide itself may be converted to pyrazinoic acid within the cell by nicotinamidase, an enzyme involved in the production of nicotinic acid from nicotinamide. However, the mode of action of pyrazinoic acid is unknown.

6.8 Thiacetazone

Thiacetazone (Fig. 2.38) is used, usually in combination with isoniazid, as an antituberculosis agent in many developing countries. Its mode of action is unknown.

7
Uptake of antibiotics by bacteria

7.1 Introduction

It is clear that many clinically useful antibiotics have target sites that are located either within the bacterial cell (e.g. inhibitors of protein, DNA and RNA synthesis), or within the cytoplasmic membrane (e.g. β-lactam antibiotics). Therefore, in order to reach these targets, the antibiotic molecules may have to cross either one or two membranes depending on whether the organism is Gram negative and therefore surrounded by both an outer and inner (cytoplasmic) membrane (Figs 1.1 and 1.2), or Gram positive and therefore surrounded only by a cytoplasmic membrane (Figs 1.1 and 1.3).

As noted in Chapter 1, although mycobacteria are Gram-positive organisms, features of their cell envelope bear resemblance to the Gram-negative outer membrane. Uptake of antimycobacterial agents will therefore be considered separately (Section 7.6). Further information in the present section and in Sections 7.2–7.5 deals with the entry of antibiotics into non-mycobacterial species.

Passage of antibiotics across the outer membrane of Gram-negative bacteria can occur by passive diffusion, self-promoted uptake or facilitated diffusion. Passive, or simple, diffusion of antibiotics across the outer membrane occurs primarily through the water-filled pores (porins: see Chapter 1) and is influenced by the molecular size, charge and lipophilic properties of the permeating molecule. Molecules able to diffuse most rapidly through porin channels are, in general, soluble in water and have molecular weights of less than about 600 to gain access to the transmembrane pores. Most porins show little chemical selectivity for permeating solutes, but can either be cation or anion selective. For example, the cation-selective OmpF channel in *E. coli* favours diffusion of zwitterionic over anionic antibiotics, whereas for the anion-selective PhoE channel this situation is reversed. Self-promoted uptake of antibiotics across the outer membrane of Gram-negative organisms is not well understood and is restricted to polycationic antibiotics such as the aminoglycosides and polymyxins (see below). Self-promoted uptake involves destabilization and disorganization of the outer membrane as a result of displacement of divalent cations by these antibiotics. Facilitated diffusion involves uptake through a channel or carrier which is specific for a given substrate owing to possession of a specific binding site. Until recently it had been assumed that the outer membrane is essentially impermeable to hydrophobic molecules. However, the outer membrane bilayer does allow the penetration of such molecules, although the rate is 50–100 times slower than that through phospholipid-containing bilayers. Nevertheless, decreased permeation of hydrophobic molecules through the outer membrane is responsible for the intrinsic resistance of Gram-negative bacteria to certain antibiotics, whereby the outer membrane 'shields' intracellular targets from antibiotic action: see Chapter 5. This also applies to hydrophilic antibiotics that may simply be too large to gain entry to the porin channels.

Transfer of antibiotics across the bacterial cytoplasmic membrane results from either passive diffusion or active transport of the drug molecules. Active transport involves specific carrier proteins that are coupled to an energy source. When metabolic energy is available antibiotics can be accumulated within the cell against a concentration gradient. The energy for transport may derive from ATP or the proton-motive force (PMF). ATP-coupled transport is referred to as primary transport, whereas PMF-dependent processes are described as secondary systems. Active transport of antibiotics into bacteria usually results from 'illicit' transport, i.e. the antibiotic bears sufficient structural resemblance to a naturally occurring molecule to be able to utilize the normal transport carrier.

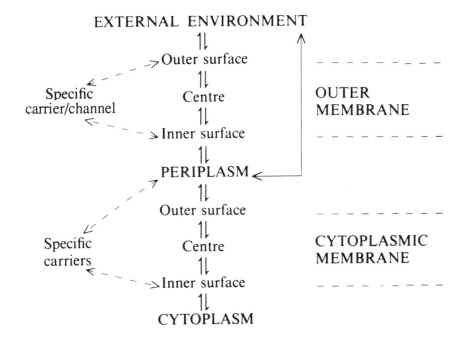

Figure 2.39 Model depicting the routes of entry of antibiotics across the Gram-negative bacterial cell envelope: ←--→, involvement of specific carrier proteins; ⇌, passive diffusion and partitioning which can involve 'self-promoted' transfer (see text); ←→, passive diffusion through non-specific hydrophilic pores. (Reproduced, with permission, from Chopra & Ball (1982).)

Figs 2.39 and 2.40 present models depicting the routes of entry of antibiotics into Gram-negative and Gram-positive cells and the following sections consider in detail the uptake of those antibiotics whose mode of action has been described in earlier sections of this chapter. The antibiotics are grouped into the same major divisions used previously.

7.2 Inhibitors of nucleic acid synthesis

7.2.1 Introduction

Of those antibiotics described in Section 2, information on transport mechanisms is only available for the quinolones. Since the target (DNA gyrase) of these antibiotics is located intracellularly, they must be able to cross both outer and cytoplasmic bacterial membranes.

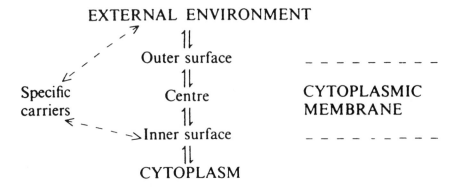

Figure 2.40 Model depicting the routes of entry of antibiotics across the cytoplasmic membrane of Gram-positive bacteria: ←→, involvement of specific carrier proteins; ⇌, passive diffusion and partitioning. (Reproduced, with permission, from Chopra & Ball (1982).)

7.2.2 *Uptake of quinolones*

Most quinolones are low molecular weight (<400 Da) hydrophilic molecules that are predicted to cross bacterial outer membranes through porin channels. In *E. coli* and *Salm. typhimurium* direct evidence for involvement of the OmpF porin in quinolone uptake has been obtained. Preferential use of OmpF over other porins relates to the formation of quinolone–magnesium chelates favouring use of the cation-selective OmpF channel.

The mechanism of uptake of quinolones across the bacterial cytoplasmic has been controversial. Initial evidence favoured the involvement of an active transport process coupled to the PMF, but a consensus is now emerging that uptake is a simple diffusion process dictated by the pH gradient across the cytoplasmic membrane.

7.3 Inhibitors of protein synthesis

7.3.1 *Introduction*

Of those protein synthesis inhibitors considered in Section 3.4, information on transport is available for mupirocin, the AGAC group, chloramphenicol and tetracyclines.

7.3.2 *Mupirocin*

The hydrophobic nature of this antibiotic suggests that it will not easily penetrate the outer membrane of most Gram-negative bacteria. This is consistent with the observation that mupirocin has poor activity against *E. coli* and high activity against deep rough mutants of *Salm. typhimurium*, but is about 500-fold more active against *S. aureus* than *E. coli*. Thus, although the *E. coli* outer membrane 'shields' the inner membrane from the antibiotic, it is able to cross the cytoplasmic membrane of Gram-positive bacteria. Transport of mupirocin into *B. subtilis* and *S. aureus* is energy independent but temperature dependent. These features suggest non-carrier-mediated passive diffusion across the cytoplasmic membrane, an uptake mechanism that is consistent with the hydrophobic nature of the antibiotic.

7.3.3 Aminoglycoside–aminocyclitol antibiotics

Since the primary site of action of AGACs is the bacterial ribosome, these drugs will need to cross both outer and cytoplasmic membranes before reaching their target.

AGAC passage across the outer membrane employs an unusual non-porin pathway. In both *E. coli* and *Ps. aeruginosa*, AGAC antibiotics promote their own uptake across the outer membrane. Self-promoted uptake involves the displacement of divalent cations from lipopolysaccharide by the polycationic aminoglycosides. This interferes with cross-bridging between neighbouring lipopolysaccharide molecules which leads to outer membrane destabilization and enhancement of antibiotic uptake.

Uptake of AGAC antibiotics across the bacterial cytoplasmic membrane is essential for antibacterial activity and is similar in Gram-positive and Gram-negative bacteria. It displays unusual energy-dependent characteristics with a dual requirement for the membrane potential component of the PMF and for a functioning electron transport chain. The former is probably the driving force for uptake of AGAC antibiotics across the cytoplasmic membrane, the electron transport requirement possibly reflecting a role for respiratory quinones as carriers. However, there is no direct proof of a role for quinones or other membrane components as carriers for AGAC antibiotics.

7.3.4 Chloramphenicol

Since the target of this antibiotic is intracellular, the drug must therefore be able to cross bacterial outer and cytoplasmic membranes. The antibiotic crosses the outer membrane by passive diffusion through transmembrane porins and crosses the cytoplasmic membrane probably by using two (as yet unidentified) active transport systems. Studies in *E. coli* on the nature of energy coupling for chloramphenicol transport suggest the involvement of both primary and secondary transport processes for drug uptake.

7.3.5 Tetracyclines

Since tetracyclines act intracellularly they must cross both outer and cytoplasmic membranes. Although a variety of tetracycline analogues exists (Fig. 2.21),

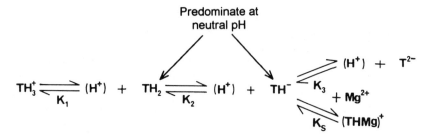

Figure 2.41 Dissociation scheme for tetracycline. Tetracycline is an acid which has three protonation sites with pK values of 3.3 (pK_1), 7.7 (pK_2) and 9.7 (pK_3) which are assigned to the tricarbonylmethane group (C1 through C3 region, Fig. 2.21), the phenolic β-diketone system (C10 through C12 region, Fig. 2.21), and the dimethylamino group (C4 substituent, Fig. 2.21). The anion (TH$^-$) chelates Mg^{2+} to form the coordination complex (THMg)$^+$. The forms that cross the bacterial cytoplasmic membrane (TH$_2$) and diffuse through *E. coli* OmpF porins (THMg)$^+$ are indicated.

detailed studies on the transport of these antibiotics have been confined mostly to tetracycline itself. Furthermore, attention has been primarily focused on the basis of uptake into *E. coli*.

In order to consider tetracycline uptake an overview of the protonation and chelation behaviour of tetracycline is necessary. Tetracycline is an acid which can ionize in an aqueous solution (Fig. 2.41). It has three protonation sites with pK values of 3.3, 7.7 and 9.7 (see legend for Fig. 2.41). At neutral pH the forms TH$_2$ and TH$^-$ predominate with the anion chelating magnesium in the medium to form the cationic chelate THMg$^+$. Diffusion, in particular by the THMg$^+$ species, occurs through the cation-selective OmpF porin channel thereby delivering tetracycline to the periplasm. In the periplasm, conversion to TH$_2$ occurs and it is this uncharged tetracycline species that crosses the cytoplasmic membrane. The apparent energy-dependent accumulation of tetracycline represents distribution of this uncharged species across the membrane in response to the pH gradient component of the PMF. There is no evidence for involvement of a carrier protein in uptake. Since the cytoplasmic pH (approximately 7.8) is higher than the external pH (approximately 6.1) the uncharged tetracycline species dissociates into anion (TH$^-$) and proton (H$^+$) on entering the cell. This dissociation is further facilitated by the formation of magnesium–tetracycline chelates in the cytoplasm, resulting in intracellular accumulation of antibiotic. Fig. 2.42 presents a model for the uptake of tetracycline across the cytoplasmic membrane and its accumulation in bacteria. The form THMG$^+$ is the active tetracycline species that binds to the ribosome to inhibit protein synthesis.

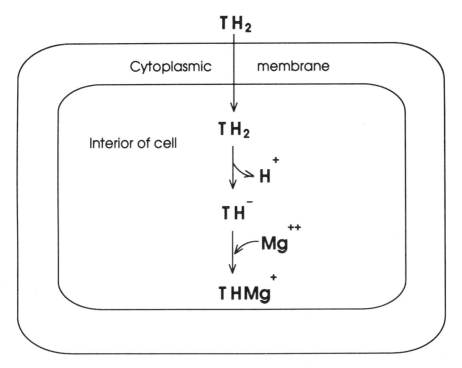

Figure 2.42 Proposed mechanism for tetracycline uptake across the bacterial cytoplasmic membrane.

7.4 Antibiotics that inhibit peptidoglycan synthesis

7.4.1 D-cycloserine

Since the D-cycloserine target enzymes (alanine racemase and D-alanyl-D-alanine synthetase) are intracellular, the drug must be able to cross both outer and cytoplasmic bacterial membranes.

Little is known about uptake of the antibiotic across the bacterial outer membrane, but it is assumed to diffuse passively through porin channels. The nature of D-cycloserine transport across the *E. coli* cytoplasmic membrane is well defined. The antibiotic is accumulated by the D-alanine transport system which is coupled to the PMF. The ability of D-cycloserine to utilize the D-alanine transport system reflects the structural similarity between the two molecules (Fig. 2.23).

7.4.2 Fosfomycin

Since fosfomycin (phosphonomycin: Fig. 2.43) inhibits a cytoplasmic target enzyme, the antibiotic must be able to cross bacterial outer and cytoplasmic

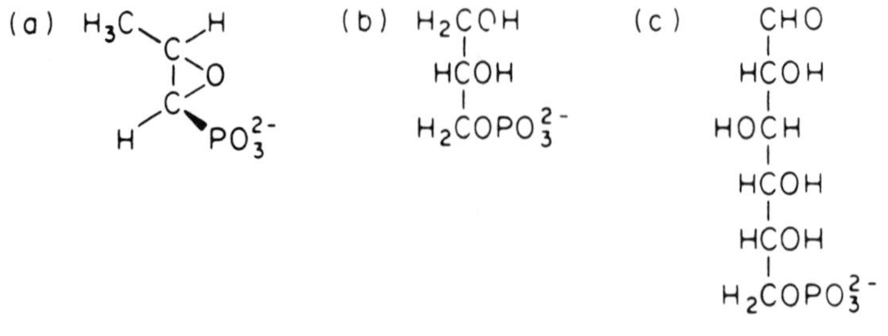

(a) H_3C — $\overset{H}{\underset{\displaystyle \overset{|}{C}}{C}}$ — O ... $\overset{\displaystyle}{\underset{PO_3^{2-}}{C}}$ H

(b) H_2COH
$HCOH$
$H_2COPO_3^{2-}$

(c) CHO
$HCOH$
$HOCH$
$HCOH$
$HCOH$
$H_2COPO_3^{2-}$

Figure 2.43 Structures of (a) fosfomycin, (b) glycerol-3-phosphate and (c) glucose-6-phosphate.

membranes. In *E. coli*, passage across the outer membrane is mediated by the glpT protein which may act as a specific channel both for fosfomycin entry and the naturally occurring molecule sn-glycerol-3-phosphate (Fig. 2.43). Transport across the cytoplasmic membrane can be mediated by either the sn-glycerol-3-phosphate or the hexose phosphate transport systems reflecting the structural similarity between the antibiotic and the naturally occurring molecules (Fig. 2.43). Both these transport systems are coupled to the PMF.

7.4.3 Bacitracin A and glycopeptide antibiotics

These antibiotics all comprise large molecules (bacitracin 1411 Da; vancomycin, ristocetin and teicoplanin about 3300 Da) that are too large to cross Gram-negative outer membranes. Hence these antibiotics exhibit poor antibacterial activity towards Gram-negative organisms. Their ability to inhibit targets in Gram-positive bacteria does not depend on transport into the cell since the targets are exposed at the cell surface.

7.4.4 β-Lactams

As already discussed (Section 4.4.2) inhibition of bacterial growth by β-lactam antibiotics is a complex process which involves the binding of drug molecules to PBPs that are located on the surface of bacterial cytoplasmic membranes. Therefore, in Gram-negative organisms these antibiotics must cross the bacterial outer membrane to exert their inhibitory effects.

The majority of β-lactams cross the outer membrane by passive diffusion through porin channels. In *E. coli*, this primarily involves the OmpF and OmpC porins. The rate of influx of β-lactams through the porins is influenced by a number of factors that include drug hydrophobicity, size and net charge. In general, increases in hydrophobicity, size or net negative charge tend to decrease the rate of permeation of β-lactams through porin channels.

Imipenem represents one class of β-lactam agent that differs from the majority of β-lactam antibiotics described above. Imipenem (molecular weight 299) permeates poorly through the OmpF and OmpC porin channels that can accommodate other β-lactams of higher molecular weight. In *Ps. aeruginosa* imipenem uses an alternative, specific porin, OmpD, which may have a counterpart in other Gram-negative organisms.

7.5 Antibiotics that inhibit membrane integrity

7.5.1 *Introduction*

Although magainins possess activity against Gram-negative bacteria and therefore presumably gain access across the outer membrane, the mechanism involved is unknown. However, some information on polymyxin uptake is available (Section 7.5.2).

7.5.2 *Polymyxins*

As already noted (Section 5.1) the bactericidal activity of these compounds results primarily from their interaction with the bacterial cytoplasmic membrane causing gross disorganization of its structure. Therefore, in order to reach their target site in Gram-negative organisms, polymyxins need to cross the bacterial outer membrane. This is achieved primarily by self-promoted uptake of polymyxins across the outer membrane whereby divalent cations are displaced leading to membrane destabilization and further insertion of antibiotic molecules into the outer membrane bilayer.

7.6 Antimycobacterial drugs

As noted in Chapter 1, an understanding of the molecular organization of the mycobacterial cell envelope is just beginning to emerge. Consequently little is known about the uptake of specific antibiotics into mycobacteria. However, by analogy with the Gram-negative outer membrane, two general routes of uptake probably exist for passage of molecules across the outer regions of the mycobacterial cell envelope. One route probably involves passive diffusion of hydrophilic molecules through the recently identified mycobacterial porins (see Chapter 1) and the second route, for hydrophobic molecules, passive diffusion following dissolution into the lipid-containing regions of the envelope. Since many of the agents effective against mycobacteria are hydrophobic, it is likely that the lipid penetration route is the more important uptake pathway for antimycobacterial drugs. This view is further supported by the following:

(a) chemically synthesized analogues of isoniazid and kanomycin that are more hydrophobic than their parent molecules exhibit enhanced antimycobacterial activity;

(b) many hydrophilic molecules penetrate the mycobacterial cell envelope very poorly, e.g. β-lactam antibiotics penetrate *Mycobacterium chelonae* 1000 times more slowly than *E. coli*.

The low permeability to relatively hydrophilic molecules such as β-lactam antibiotics undoubtedly contributes to the intrinsic resistance to this class of antibiotic displayed by the mycobacteria.

8
Conclusions

A very large number of antibiotics (about 6000) have now been identified and this chapter has focused on the mode of action of the most important antibacterial antibiotics. The molecular basis by which these compounds prevent bacterial growth has been considered in detail, but it is beyond the scope of this book to describe their specific clinical uses. Readers interested in this important aspect of antibiotic usage can refer to the specific texts on the subject cited in the reference list at the end of this chapter. However, it should be remembered that the presence of antibiotic-resistant organisms, particularly in the hospital environment, may influence the choice of antibiotic used for a particular therapeutic purpose. The subject of antibiotic resistance is considered in detail in Chapter 5.

Further reading

Books

(a) *With an emphasis on the mode of action of antibiotics*

Franklin, T. J. & Snow, G. A. (1989). *Biochemistry of Antimicrobial Action*. Fourth edition. Chapman & Hall, London.

Gale, E. F., Cundliffe, E., Reynolds, P. E., Richmond, M. H. & Waring, M. J. (1981). *The Molecular Basis of Antibiotic Action*. John Wiley & Sons, London.

Hooper, D. C. & Wolfson, J. S. (eds) (1993). *Quinolone Antimicrobial Agents*. Second edition. American Society for Microbiology, Washington, DC.

Lorian, V. (1986). *Antibiotics in Laboratory Medicine*. Second edition. Williams and Wilkins, Baltimore.

Rogers, H. J., Perkins, H. R. & Ward, J. B. (1980). *Microbial Cell Walls and Membranes*. Chapman & Hall, London.

(b) *With an emphasis on the clinical application of antibiotics*

Gorbach, A., Bartlett, J. G. & Blacklow, N. R. (1992). *Infectious Diseases*. W. B. Saunders, Philadelphia.

Kuckers, A. & McBennett, N. (1987). *The Use of Antibiotics*. Fourth edition. William Heinemann, London.

Lambert, H. P. & O'Grady, F. W. (1992). *Antibiotic and Chemotherapy*. Sixth edition. Churchill Livingstone, Edinburgh.

Review articles

Anonymous (1990). Diagnosis and treatment of disease caused by nontuberculous mycobacteria. *American Review of Respiratory Diseases* **142**: 940–953.

Brisson-Noel, A., Trieu-Cuot, P. & Courvalin, P. (1988). Mechanism of action of spiramycin and other macrolides. *Journal of Antimicrobial Chemotherapy* **22** (Suppl. B): 13–23.

Brown, A. G. (1982). Beta-lactam nomenclature. *Journal of Antimicrobial Chemotherapy* **10**: 365–368.

Brown, G. M. & Williamson, J. M. (1987). Biosynthesis of folic acid, riboflavin, thiamine and pantothenic acid. In *Escherichia coli and Salmonella typhimurium*. Cellular and Molecular Biology, Volume 1 (ed. F. C. Neidhardt) pp. 521–538. American Society for Microbiology, Washington, DC.

Cairns, D., Hay, J. & Seal, D. V. (1993). The new macrolides: expanding the frontiers of antimicrobial chemotherapy. *Pharmaceutical Journal* **251**: 317–320.

Casewell, M. W. & Hill, R. L. R. (1987). Mupirocin ('pseudomonic acid')—a promising new topical antimicrobial agent. *Journal of Antimicrobial Chemotherapy* **19**: 1–5.

Cashel, M. & Rudd, K. E. (1987). The stringent response. In *Escherichia coli and Salmonella typhimurium*. Cellular and Molecular Biology, Volume 2 (ed. F. C. Neidhardt) pp. 1410–1438. American Society for Microbiology, Washington, DC.

Chopra, I. (1985). Mode of action of the tetracyclines and the nature of bacterial resistance to them. In *The Tetracyclines*. Handbook of Experimental Pharmacology, Volume 78 (eds J. J. Hlavka & J. H. Boothe) pp. 317–392. Springer-Verlag, Berlin.

Chopra, I. (1989). Transport of antibiotics into bacteria. *Annual Reports in Medicinal Chemistry* **24**: 139–146.

Chopra, I. (1993). The magainins: antimicrobial peptides with potential for topical application. *Journal of Antimicrobial Chemotherapy* **32**: 351–353.

Chopra, I. (1995). Tetracycline uptake and efflux in bacteria. In *Drug Transport in Antimicrobial and Anticancer Chemotherapy* (ed. N. H. Georgopapadakou) pp. 221–243. Marcel Dekker, New York.

Chopra, I. & Ball, P. R. (1982). Transport of antibiotics into bacteria. *Advances in Microbial Physiology* **23**: 183–240.

Chopra, I., Hawkey, P. M. & Hinton, M. (1992). Tetracyclines: molecular and clinical aspects. *Journal of Antimicrobial Chemotherapy* **29**: 245–277.

Cundliffe, E. (1987). On the nature of antibiotic binding sites in ribosomes. *Biochimie* **69**: 863–869.

Davis, B. D. (1988). The lethal action of aminoglycosides. *Journal of Antimicrobial Chemotherapy* **22**: 1–3.

Doyle, R. J. & Koch, A. L. (1987). The functions of autolysins in the growth and division of *Bacillus subtilis*. *CRC Critical Reviews in Microbiology* **15**: 169–222.

Hancock, R. E. W. & Bellido, F. (1992). Antibiotic uptake: unusual results for unusual molecules. *Journal of Antimicrobial Chemotherapy* **29**: 235–239.

Hershey, J. W. B. (1987). Protein synthesis. In *Escherichia coli and Salmonella typhimurium*. Cellular and Molecular Biology, Volume 1 (ed. F. C. Neidhardt) pp. 613–647. American Society for Microbiology, Washington, DC.

Ishiguro, E. E. & Kusser, W. (1988). Regulation of peptidoglycan biosynthesis and antibiotic-induced autolysis in nongrowing *Escherichia coli*: a preliminary model. In *Antibiotic Inhibition of Bacterial Cell Surface Assembly and Function* (eds P. Actor, L. Daneo-Moore, M. L. Higgins, M. R. J. Salton & G. D. Shockman) pp. 189–194. American Society for Microbiology, Washington, DC.

Kirst, H. A. & Sides, G. D. (1989). New directions for macrolide antibiotics: structural modifications and *in vitro* activity. *Antimicrobial Agents and Chemotherapy* **33**: 1413–1418.

Kirst, H. A. & Sides, G. D. (1989). New directions for macrolide antibiotics: pharmacokinetics and clinical efficacy. *Antimicrobial Agents and Chemotherapy* **33**: 1419–1422.

Maxwell, A. (1992). The molecular basis of quinolone action. *Journal of Antimicrobial Chemotherapy* **30**: 409–414.

Moazed, D. & Noller, H. F. (1987). Interaction of antibiotics with functional sites in 16S ribosomal RNA. *Nature (London)* **327**: 389–394.

Nagarajan, R. (1991). Antibacterial activities and modes of action of vancomycin and related glycopeptides. *Antimicrobial Agents and Chemotherapy* **35**: 605–609.

Nikaido, H. & Thanassi, D. G. (1993). Penetration of lipophilic agents with multiple protonation sites into bacterial cells: tetracyclines and fluoroquinolones as examples. *Antimicrobial Agents and Chemotherapy* **37**: 1393–1399.

Nikaido, H. & Vaara, T. (1986). Molecular basis of bacterial outer membrane permeability. *Microbiological Reviews* **49**: 1–32.

Noller, H. F. & Nomura, M. (1987). Ribosomes. In *Escherichia coli and Salmonella typhimurium*. Cellular and Molecular Biology, Volume 2 (ed. F. C. Neidhardt) pp. 104–125. American Society for Microbiology, Washington, DC.

Noller, H. F., Stern, S., Moazed, D., Powers, T., Svensson, P. & Changchien, L.-M. (1987). Studies on the architecture and function of 16S rRNA. *Cold Spring Harbor Symposia on Quantitative Biology* **52**: 695–707.

Park, J. T. (1987). Murein synthesis. In *Escherichia coli and Salmonella typhimurium*. Cellular and Molecular Biology, Volume 1 (ed. F. C. Neidhardt) pp. 663–671. American Society for Microbiology, Washington, DC.

Piddock, L. J. V. (1991). Mechanism of quinolone uptake into bacterial cells. *Journal of Antimicrobial Chemotherapy* **27**: 399–403.

Reynolds, P. E. (1985). Inhibitors of bacterial cell wall synthesis. In *The Scientific Basis of Antimicrobial Chemotherapy*, 38th Symposium of the Society for General Microbiology (eds D. Greenwood & F. O'Grady) pp. 13–40. Cambridge University Press, Cambridge.

Rosen, B. P. & Kashket, E. R. (1978). Energetics of active transport. In *Bacterial Transport* (ed. B. P. Rosen) pp. 559–620. Marcel Dekker, New York, Basel.

Russell, A. D. (1988). Design of antimicrobial chemotherapeutic agents. In *Introduction to the Principles of Drug Design* (ed. H. J. Smith) pp. 265–308. Wright, London.

Shockman, G. D., Daneo-Moore, L., McDowell, T. D. & Wong, W. (1981). Function and structure of the cell wall—its importance in the life and death of bacteria. In *Beta-lactam Antibiotics, Mode of Action, New Developments and Future Prospects* (eds M. R. J. Salton & G. D. Shockman) pp. 31–65. Academic Press, New York.

Spratt, B. G. (1983). Penicillin binding proteins and the future of β-lactam antibiotics. *Journal of General Microbiology* **129**: 1247–1260.

Storm, D. R., Rosenthal, K. S. & Swanson, P. E. (1977). Polymyxin and related peptide antibiotics. *Annual Review of Biochemistry* **46**: 723–763.

Tomasz, A. (1983). Mode of action of β-lactam antibiotics—a microbiologist's view. In *Antibiotics Containing the beta-Lactam Structure*. Handbook of Experimental Pharmacology, Volume 67 (eds A. L. Demain and N. A. Solomon) pp. 15–97. Springer-Verlag, Berlin.

Walsh, C. T. (1989). Enzymes in the D-alanine branch of bacterial cell wall peptidoglycan assembly. *Journal of Biological Chemistry* **264**: 2393–2396.

Woese, C. R., Gutell, R., Gupta, R. & Noller, H. F. (1983). Detailed analysis of the higher-order structure of 16S-like ribosomal ribonucleic acids. *Microbiological Reviews* **47**: 621–669.

Wolinski, E. (1992). Antimycobacterial drugs. In *Infectious Diseases* (eds A. Gorbach, J. G. Bartlett & N. R. Blacklow) pp. 313–319. W. B. Saunders, Philadelphia.

Zhang, Y. & Young, D. B. (1993). Molecular mechanisms of isoniazid: a drug at the front line of tuberculosis control. *Trends in Microbiology* **1**: 109–113.

Research papers

Banerjee, A., Dubnau, E., Quemard, A., Balasabramanian, V., Um, K. S., Wilson, T., Collins, D., de Lisle, G. & Jacobs, W. R. (1994). *inhA*, a gene encoding a target for isoniazid and ethionamide in *Mycobacterium tuberculosis*. *Science* **263**: 227–230.

Douthwaite, S. (1992). Interaction of the antibiotics clindamycin and lincomycin with *Escherichia coli* 23S ribosomal RNA. *Nucleic Acids Research* **20**: 1417–1420.

Kirano, K. & Tomasz, A. (1979). Triggering of autolytic cell wall degradation in *Escherichia coli* by beta-lactam antibiotics. *Antimicrobial Agents and Chemotherapy* **16**: 838–848.

McDowell, T. D. & Lemanski, C. L. (1988). Absence of autolytic activity (peptidoglycan nicking) in penicillin-induced nonlytic death in group A streptococcus. *Journal of Bacteriology* **170**: 1783–1788.

Quemard, A., Laneelle, G. & Lacave, C. (1992). Mycolic acid synthesis: a target for ethionamide in mycobacteria? *Antimicrobial Agents and Chemotherapy* **36**: 1316–1321.

Takayama, K. & Kilburn, J. O. (1989). Inhibition of synthesis of arabinogalactan by ethumbutol in *Mycobacterium smegmatis*. *Antimicrobial Agents and Chemotherapy* **33**: 1493–1499.

Tuomanen, E. & Schwartz. J. (1987). Penicillin-binding protein 7 and its relationship to lysis of nongrowing *Escherichia coli*. *Journal of Bacteriology* **169**: 4912–4915.

CHAPTER THREE

Antiseptics, disinfectants and preservatives: their properties, mechanisms of action and uptake into bacteria

1
Introduction

Biocides have been used for many centuries. The ancient Egyptian art of mummification relied in part on the use of balsams which contained natural preservatives. The preservation of food by salting or mixing with natural spices has also been known since ancient times. Various agents (wine, vinegar, honey, mercuric chloride) found use as wound dressings. In the nineteenth century, antiseptic surgery was introduced and disinfectant usage expanded considerably to control the spread of infection in hospitals. An important landmark was reached in 1897 when Kronig and Paul, with help from Ikeda, introduced their famous work on the dynamics of disinfection, the principles of which still form the basis of our present knowledge.

Currently, antimicrobial compounds (other than antibiotics) are used for their antiseptic, disinfectant or preservative activity. These terms were defined in Chapter 1 (Section 1) and so suffice to state here that disinfectants are normally used on inanimate objects (although it is permissible to use the term 'disinfection of the skin', for example pre-operatively), antiseptics may be applied to living tissues and preservatives are incorporated into various types of food, pharmaceutical and cosmetic products to prevent contamination or spoilage. The broad term 'biocide' is used to describe agents with these properties.

Individual infectious agents differ considerably in their response to biocides (Table 3.1). Probably the most resistant of all are 'slow viruses', known as prions. Amongst the bacteria, bacterial spores are invariably the least sensitive, followed by acid-fast bacteria, then Gram-negative organisms and finally the most sensitive, Gram-positive non-sporing, non-acid-fast bacteria such as staphylococci.

The initial reaction between an antibacterial agent and a bacterial cell involves binding to the cell surface. Changes to the outer layers may then occur to allow agents to penetrate the cell to reach their primary site of action at the cytoplasmic membrane or within the cytoplasm. The effect of the primary target site may lead to additional, secondary, changes elsewhere in the organism. Such secondary

96

Table 3.1 Relative sensitivity[a] of microorganisms to disinfectants and other biocides

Type of microorganism[b]	Sensitivity to biocides	Comment
Viruses	Non-enveloped more resistant than enveloped Most resistant: prions ('slow viruses')	Picornaviruses and parvoviruses may show resistance just below acid-fast bacteria
Bacteria	Non-sporing bacteria are most susceptible Acid-fast bacteria are more resistant Bacterial spores are more resistant	*Ps. aeruginosa* may show high resistance, e.g. to QACs Probably associated with waxy 'overcoat' Less so than prions
Fungi	Fungal spores may be resistant	Rather less so than acid-fast bacteria
Parasites	Coccidia may be highly resistant	Similar to bacterial spores

[a]Mechanisms of bacterial resistance to biocides are considered in Chapters 6 and 7.
[b]See also Section 3.
QACs, quaternary ammonium compounds.

alterations may also contribute to the bacteriostatic or bactericidal activity of the biocide. For these reasons, it may not always be easy to define the mode of action of a biocide.

This chapter considers the properties and mechanisms of antibacterial action of a range of antiseptics, disinfectants and preservatives, and of the possible ways in which they enter bacterial cells. It is first necessary, however, to describe those factors that influence their activity, since some of these are important in assessing the mechanism of action of a biocide.

2
Factors influencing activity

The antimicrobial activity of biocides depends markedly on several factors, the most important of which will be considered briefly here. These are time of exposure, concentration, temperature, pH, the presence of organic matter and the type of microorganism.

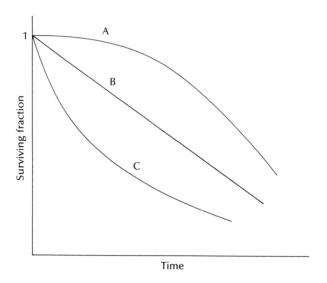

Figure 3.1   Different types of response of microorganisms to a biocide: A, initial shoulder followed by exponential death; B, exponential death; C, initial exponential death followed by tailing off.

2.1 Time of exposure

Contrary to popular advertising, the death of microorganisms exposed to a biocide is not an instantaneous event, but takes place over a period of time (Fig. 3.1). Depending on the nature of the biocide and its concentration, a series of death curves of different shapes may be produced. However, such data provide little information about killing mechanisms at the molecular level.

2.2 Concentration

When concentration rises (e.g. D to H, Fig. 3.2) the rate of bacterial inactivation increases. However, the effect of concentration varies from biocide to biocide. When the logarithm of the time needed to kill a specified number of cells is plotted against the logarithm of the concentration, a straight line is produced, the slope (η) of which (Fig. 3.3) is known as the concentration exponent or dilution coefficient.

This is a measure of the effect of concentration (or dilution) on antibacterial activity. The value of η can also be deduced from the equation

$$C^{\eta}t = \text{constant} \tag{1}$$

or

$$C_1^{\eta}t_1 = C_2^{\eta}t_2 \tag{2}$$

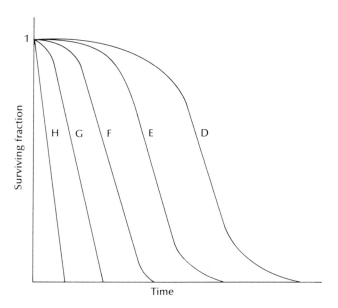

Figure 3.2 Effect of concentration of biocide on rates of microbial death: D, lowest concentration through intermediate concentrations (E–G) to H, highest concentration.

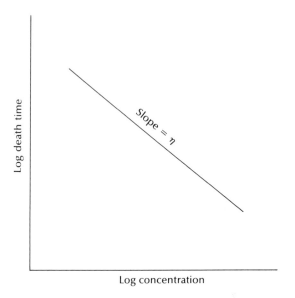

Figure 3.3 Plot of logarithm of concentration against logarithm of time for each concentration to bring about a specified degree of microbial inactivation: slope of line is η.

Table 3.2 The possible relationship between η values and mechanism of action of antibacterial agents

Group	Antibacterial agent[a]	Mechanism of action[a]
A ($\eta < 1$–2)	Hydrogen peroxide	—SH reactor
	Mercury compounds	—SH reactors
	Chlorhexidine	Membrane disrupter
	QACs	Membrane disrupter
	Formaldehyde	Interacts with protein
	Glutaraldehyde	—NH$_2$ groups and nucleic acids
	Acridines	Intercalating agents
	Iodine	—SH reactor (oxidation)
	Chlorine	—SH reactor (oxidation)
B ($\eta = 2$–4)	Parabens ⎫	See Table 3.5 for specific details
	Sorbic acid ⎭	
	Benzoic acid	
C ($\eta > 4$)	Aliphatic alcohols ⎫	
	Phenolics	Membrane disrupters
	Benzyl alcohol ⎬	
	Phenylethanol ⎭	

[a]Other reactions have also been proposed for some biocides, e.g. hydrogen peroxide, iodine and chlorine: see Sections 5 and 6.

in which t_1 and t_2 are the times required to kill a specified number of cells after exposure to concentrations C_1 and C_2 respectively.

Antibacterial agents with high η values lose their activity rapidly on dilution, whereas those with low η values retain much of their original activity. The η value for a particular compound is probably related to its mechanism of action and accordingly biocides have been classified into three general categories, A, B and C (Table 3.2).

2.3 Temperature

The antibacterial activity of most chemicals increases when the temperature is raised. This can be expressed in mathematical terms by determining the times (t_1 and t_2) necessary to kill a particular suspension at temperatures T_1 and T_2 respectively, from which the temperature coefficient (θ) can be calculated, namely

$$\theta^{T_2 - T_1} = t_1/t_2 \qquad (3)$$

θ refers to the effect of temperature per 1 °C rise and nearly always has a value between 1 and 1.5. It is more usual to specify the θ^{10} value (also known as Q_{10}

by analogy with enzymatic reactions) which is the change in activity per 10 °C rise in temperature. Examples of Q_{10} values are as follows: phenols and cresols, 3–5; formaldehyde, 1.5; aliphatic alcohols, 30–50. Antibacterial agents that are not sporicidal at ambient temperatures, e.g. phenols, become so at elevated temperatures.

2.4 pH

The activity of many antibacterial compounds is influenced quite markedly by changes in pH. Examples include phenols (Section 5.1.1.1), organic acids (Section 5.3.1.1), glutaraldehyde (Section 4.1), quaternary ammonium compounds (QACs) and chlorhexidine (Sections 5.1.1.2 and 5.1.1.3) and various halogens (Sections 6.6 and 6.7.1).

Reasons for this change of activity are twofold.

(a) There may be an effect on the molecule, e.g. an increase in pH increases the dissociation of organic acids, the undissociated form making the greatest contribution to killing (see Fig. 3.4). Hypochlorous acid (HOCl) and diatomic iodine (I_2) contribute most to the activity of hypochlorites and iodine formulations, respectively, and occur at highest levels at acid pH. Glutaraldehyde combines most strongly with amino and sulphydryl groups in proteins at alkaline pH, where it is consequently most active.
(b) There is an alteration in the bacterial cell surface: as pH rises, the cell surface becomes more negatively charged. Cationic-type bactericides such as the quaternaries, chlorhexidine and diamidines (e.g. pentamidine, propamidine) which react with negatively charged groups thus become more effective bactericides at increased pH.

2.5 Organic matter

Organic matter may occur in several forms, especially as blood or serum, faeces, dirt, milkstone, etc. Antibacterial agents, e.g. chlorine-releasing compounds, that are highly reactive chemically thus tend to lose activity rapidly and to a considerable extent in the presence of organic matter, with which they combine strongly.

3

General classification of biocides

Three different levels of biocidal activity, encompassing fungi and viruses as well as bacteria, have been recognized:

(i) high level—with action against bacterial spores (although prolonged periods of time may be necessary if large numbers of bacterial spores are present),

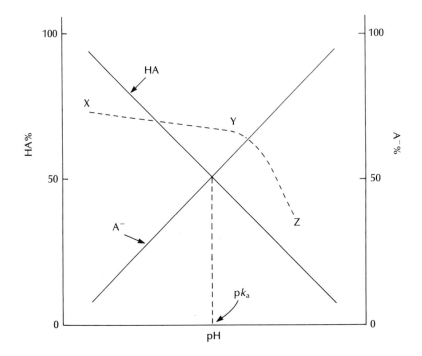

Figure 3.4 Relationship between pH and the ionization and bactericidal activity of an acid, HA. Bactericidal activity is shown by the broken line XYZ, in which maximum activity is demonstrated at X with a slight decrease at Y and a considerable drop in efficacy at Z.

non-sporulating bacteria, fungi and lipid enveloped and non-lipid-enveloped viruses;
(ii) intermediate level—with action against mycobacteria and other non-sporulating bacteria, fungi, non-lipid viruses (although virucidal activity may be limited) and lipid viruses;
(iii) low level—with action against non-sporulating bacteria (except mycobacteria) and some fungi and viruses.

On the basis of this classification, glutaraldehyde (Section 4.1) is a high-level biocide, whereas chlorhexidine and the QACs (Sections 5.1.1.3 and 5.1.1.2, respectively) are low-level biocides.

The variation in response of different bacteria to biocides is a manifestation, at least in part, of the nature of the organisms in question. Chapter 1 described the chemical composition and structure of cell walls of non-sporulating bacteria, including mycobacteria, and of the spore coats and cortex of bacterial spores. These clearly have an important role to play in the uptake of biocides by bacterial cells.

3.1 Bacterial spores

Of the different types of bacteria, bacterial spores are generally the least sensitive to biocides. Many biocides are sporistatic, not sporicidal, even at high concentrations, although a sporicidal effect may be achieved at elevated temperatures. Sensitivity and resistance of spores to biocides are considered in detail in Chapters 4 and 7.

3.2 Mycobacteria

There is increasing concern about the re-emergence of tuberculosis and the development in AIDS patients of this and other mycobacterial infections (Chapter 1, Section 2.2.4). The mycobacteria consist of a diverse group of acid-fast bacteria (AFB), the best-known of which are *Mycobacterium tuberculosis* and *M. leproe*. Assuming greater importance is *M. avium intracellulare* (MAI), part of the MAIS group (*M. avium–M. intracellulare*), because of its association with AIDS patients, and *M. chelonei*, which is sometimes isolated from endoscopes (Chapter 6, Section 2.7).

As a group, the mycobacteria are more sensitive than bacterial spores, but are invariably more resistant than other non-sporulating bacteria. Mycobactericidal agents are considered to be amphoteric (ampholytic) surfactants, ethylene oxide gas, halogens, alcohols, phenolic compounds, especially cresol–soap formulations, and usually aldehydes such as glutaraldehyde and formaldehyde. The uptake of biocides into mycobacteria has, however, been little studied. Possible mechanisms of mycobacterial resistance to biocides are discussed in Chapter 6.

3.3 Cocci

Gram-positive cocci such as staphylococci and streptococci are usually more sensitive to biocides than are Gram-negative bacteria. Methicillin-resistant *S. aureus* (MRSA) may be less sensitive than methicillin-sensitive (MSSA) strains, as discussed in Chapter 6, but enterocci, even antibiotic-resistant strains, are not particularly resistant to biocides.

3.4 Gram-negative rods

Generally, Gram-negative rods are less susceptible to many biocides than are Gram-positive cocci. This reduced biocidal activity is most marked with *Pseudomonas aeruginosa*, *Ps. cepacia*, *Proteus* spp. and *Providencia stuartii* (Chapter 6).

4

Properties and mechanisms of action of agents interacting with outer cellular components

A variety of antiseptics and disinfectants interact with outer cellular components, although viability is not always affected. These agents are considered in greater detail in the following sections. The reader should also refer to Figs 1.2, 1.3 and 1.9 for a detailed picture of the structure and chemical composition of the outer cell layers.

4.1 Glutaraldehyde

Glutaraldehyde is a saturated 5-carbon dialdehyde that, at alkaline pH, possesses high microbicidal activity (bacteria and their spores, fungi, viruses). In its simplest form, it exists as a monomeric dialdehyde, $CHO \cdot (CH_2)_3 \cdot CHO$, but can also occur as a dimer, trimer or polymer. Studies are continuing in an attempt to obtain a full understanding of its chemical structure. The monomer is the most active species. Despite its potential toxicity to medical staff, glutaraldehyde remains an invaluable compound for high-level disinfection purposes in endoscopy units. Acid solutions are stable, but 'activated' solutions (alkalinized) are potent biocides but retain activity for only about two weeks, although some 'long-acting' solutions are available.

Glutaraldehyde interacts predominantly with amino groups in proteins and enzymes. One of the most important factors affecting activity is pH: as the external pH rises, the number of reactive sites on the cell to which the aldehyde binds increases. The enhanced activity at alkaline pH is associated with changes in the bacterial cell surface rather than the glutaraldehyde molecule, because activity against bacteria is demonstrated within minutes (non-sporulating organisms) whereas chemical instability becomes apparent over a period of days.

Because of its interaction with amino groups, glutaraldehyde binds to important components in bacterial cell envelopes, e.g. proteins, peptide chains in peptidoglycan and the teichoic acids in the cell walls of Gram-positive bacteria. Evidence for these interactions is as follows.

(i) Peptidoglycan isolated from *B. subtilis* and treated with glutaraldehyde is less sensitive than the untreated polymer to lysozyme. The aldehyde reacts with 30–50% of the ε-NH_2 groups probably causing two tripeptide side chains to be joined when free groups are available (Fig. 3.5).

(ii) Ester-linked D-alanine residues in *B. subtilis* wall teichoic acids react with glutaraldehyde.

(iii) Pretreatment of wall peptidoglycan in *S. aureus* decreases peptidoglycan breakdown on subsequent exposure to lysotaphin, an antistaphylococcal enzyme with murein hydrolase activity.

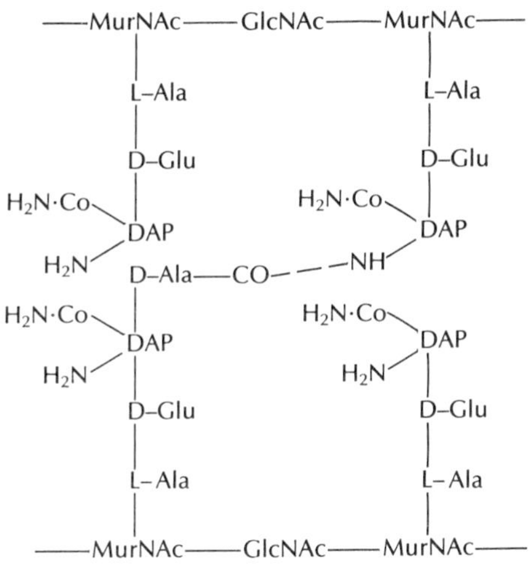

```
——MurNAc———GlcNAc———MurNAc——
       |                    |
     L–Ala                L–Ala
       |                    |
     D–Glu                D–Glu
 H₂N·Co    |        H₂N·Co    |
       ＼DAP              ＼DAP
 H₂N／  |          H₂N／
       D–Ala——CO———— —NH
 H₂N·Co    |        H₂N·Co
       ＼DAP              ＼DAP
 H₂N／  |          H₂N／  |
       D–Glu                D–Glu
       |                    |
     L–Ala                L–Ala
       |                    |
  ——MurNAc———GlcNAc———MurNAc——
```

Figure 3.5 Peptide side chains in *Bacillus subtilis* peptidoglycan showing availability of amino groups for interaction with glutaraldehyde.

In Gram-negative bacteria, glutaraldehyde interacts principally with outer components of the cells, notably lipoprotein.

The high degree of cross-linking produced at the cell surface means that the bacterial cell is unable to undertake most, if not all, of its essential functions. The question must be asked whether this cross-linking is sufficient to explain its lethal effect, because the dialdehyde also binds strongly to the cytoplasmic membrane. Thus, glutaraldehyde-treated mureinoplasts (which have peptidoglycan as the outer layer) exhibit a decrease in transport capacity and *B. megaterium* protoplasts and *E. coli* spheroplasts treated with glutaraldehyde resist lysis when transferred to a medium of low osmotic pressure. Furthermore, release of certain membrane-bound enzymes is prevented by glutaraldehyde treatment. Glutaraldehyde is thus a highly reactive molecule and an effective biocide. In intact cells, however, it is likely that its effect at the cell surface is an important aspect of its mechanism of action.

4.2 Permeabilizers

A permeabilizer is a chemical that increases the permeability of the outer membrane of Gram-negative bacteria. Included in this definition are ethylenediamine tetraacetic acid (EDTA), polycations, lactoferrin and transferrin, polyphosphates and certain acids. Clearly, there is potential in developing biocide formulations containing an appropriate permeabilizer in order to enhance, or to increase, the spectrum of activity of an antibacterial agent. Formulations are already available in which increased activity of (a) chloroxylenol and (b) a QAC against *Ps. aeruginosa* has been achieved.

EDTA shows significant activity against *Ps. aeruginosa* and lesser activity against other Gram-negative bacteria. The integrity of the outer leaflet of the outer membrane is maintained by hydrophobic LPS–LPS and LPS–protein interactions and the presence of divalent cations, notably Mg^{2+}, is essential for stabilizing the strong negative charges of the core oligosaccharide chain of the LPS molecules. EDTA binds these cations, thereby releasing up to about 50% of the LPS molecules, and causing non-polar phospholipids associated with the inner membrane to be exposed at the cell surface so that hydrophobic molecules can now enter the cell. In this way, EDTA achieves a non-specific increase in cell permeability. Polycations such as polylysine (lysine$_{20}$) also induce LPS release, as do the iron-binding proteins lactoferrin and transferrin (Table 3.3).

Lactoferricin B is a peptide produced by gastric pepsin digestion of bovine lactoferrin. Lactoferricin B is a much more potent antibacterial agent than lactoferrin and binds rapidly to the bacterial cell surface. Its activity and binding are reduced in the presence of divalent cations. It damages the bacterial outer membrane, although its major site of action is on the cytoplasmic membrane.

Citric acid, gluconic acid and malonic acid (all used at alkaline pH) also act as permeabilizers. These act as chelating agents and their activity is quenched by the addition of divalent cations. Like EDTA, they induce the release of alkaline phosphatase from ·*Ps. aeruginosa* and their action as permeabilizing agents must be linked to their effects on outer membrane permeability in Gram-negative bacteria.

The role of a compound as a permeabilizer can be readily measured, for example

(i) by determining whether cells become sensitive to lysozyme-induced lysis (Fig. 3.6(a))—Gram-negative bacteria are normally not permeated by the enzyme unless the outer membrane is altered,

(ii) by assessing whether cells become sensitive to the growth-inhibitory effects of a hydrophobic antibiotic, such as novobiocin (Fig. 3.6(b)), and

(iii) by measuring the extent of the binding of fluorescent *N*-phenylnaphthylamine (NPN) to membranes of target cells (Fig. 3.6(c)).

The examples provided in Fig. 3.6 are diagrammatic representations of published data and give evidence of the rapid effect of permeabilizers on the outer membranes of Gram-negative cells.

4.3 Other agents

The enzyme lysozyme digests peptidoglycan by cleaving β, 1–4 links. Hypochlorites induce lysis of Gram-positive bacteria, ostensibly by an effect on the cell wall, but have other effects on bacterial cells; in particular they act as oxidizing agents, reacting with −SH groups (Section 6.7.1). High concentrations of the anionic surfactant sodium lauryl sulphate lyse isolated outer membranes of Gram-negative

Table 3.3 Permeabilizing agents

Type of agent	Specific example(s)	Mechanism(s) of action
Chelator	EDTA and similar agents	*Ps. aeruginosa*: leakage; lysis (prevented in equiosmotic sucrose); removal of some Mg^{2+} and release of some LPS Resistant pseudomonads: no leakage, lysis or release of Mg^{2+} or LPS Coliforms: leakage; no lysis. Some release of Mg^{2+} and LPS
	Citric acid, gluconic acid, malonic acid (all at alkaline pH)	*Ps. aeruginosa*: becomes sensitive to lysozyme-induced lysis
	Polyphosphates (sodium hexametaphosphate)	*Ps. aeruginosa* and *E. coli*: rendered sensitive to lysozyme-induced lysis and to hydrophobic drugs
Polycations	Poly-L-lysine (PLL) (lys)$_{20}$	Displacement of Mg^{2+} and consequent release of some LPS. Cells become sensitive to hydrophobic drugs
	Spermidine, diaminoacetone, N-(2-pyrimidinyl)-piperazine	
Iron-binding proteins	Lactoferrin, transferrin, lactoferricin B	All act as chelators, with LPS loss

bacteria, probably by affecting the protein components of the outer membrane, but this agent also acts on the inner membrane (Section 5.1.1.2).

The so-called 'membrane-active' agents (Section 5) such as the biguanides, QACs and diamidines (see Fig. 3.10(f): e.g. dibromopropamidine) can also damage the cell wall or outer membrane. Dibromopropamidine isethionate causes severe damage to the outer membrane of Gram-negative bacteria, and promotes the increased uptake of a second, unrelated, compound. It has been proposed (see Section 8) that these cationic agents are able to promote their own uptake into Gram-negative cells by damaging the outer membrane so that they are able to reach their major target sites at the cytoplasmic membrane and deeper within the cell, e.g. nucleic acids and proteins (see also Section 6).

5

Properties and mechanisms of action of membrane-active agents

The term 'membrane-active agent' is, rather loosely, used to describe an antimicrobial agent that damages the inner (cytoplasmic, plasma) membrane.

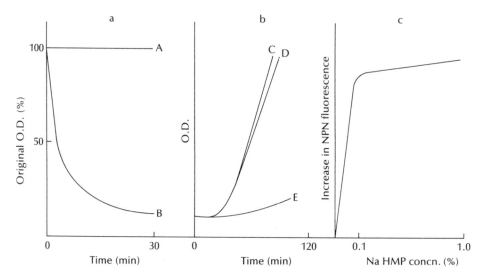

Figure 3.6 Measurement of permeabilizer activity by (a) lytic method, (b) growth inhibition procedure, (c) binding of a fluorescent probe to membranes. (a) A, tris buffer (alkaline pH).+ lysozyme; B, tris buffer (alkaline pH) + lysozyme + permeabilizer. (b) C, growth ± permeabilizer; D, growth + novobiocin (hydrophobic antibiotic); E, growth + permeabilizer + novobiocin. (c) NaHMP (sodium hexametaphosphate) drastically increases binding of NPH (*N*-phenylnaphthylamine) to membranes of target cells.

Several such compounds are known, and include polymyxins (Chapter 2), phenols, parabens, biguanides, QACs and alcohols (see below). These differ quite markedly in chemical structure and it is therefore unlikely that they have exactly the same effect on the cytoplasmic membrane. Perturbation of homeostatic mechanisms in microorganisms can also be achieved by physical processes such as mild heat shock. Only chemically induced damage to homeostasis will be considered here, but it must be pointed out that greater cellular damage will usually be achieved by chemicals used at elevated temperatures.

The cytoplasmic membrane (also known as the inner membrane in Gram-negative bacteria) is composed essentially of lipids and protein. Some details were given in Chapter 1 (Figs 1.2 and 1.3). A more detailed description is the Singer–Nicholson model (Fig. 3.7), in which the membrane is conceived as a fluid mosaic model in which globular proteins are embedded in a phospholipid matrix or bilayer. The membrane is semipermeable, controls the presence of solutes into and out of the cytoplasm and is associated with several important enzymes. As such, it is a prime target for the action of many biocides. Damage to the membrane can take several forms: leakage of intracellular constituents (Fig 3.8), total disruption causing cell lysis (Table 3.4), dissipation of the proton-motive force

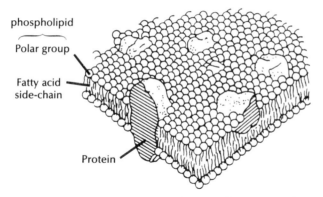

phospholipid

Polar group

Fatty acid
side-chain

Protein

Figure 3.7 The proposed structure of the cytoplasmic membrane:
Singer–Nicholson fluid mosaic model.

(PMF) (Section 5.3) and inhibition of membrane-associated enzyme activity
(Section 5.4).

5.1 Leakage of intracellular constituents

Damage to the cytoplasmic membrane is usually manifested by the release of
intracellular constituents (Fig. 3.8). The first index of membrane injury is
potassium (K^+) leakage, followed by inorganic phosphates (Pi), pool amino acids
and material absorbing at 260 nm (rather non-specific since it could indicate RNA
or DNA or even, to some extent, protein material). More specific information can
be obtained by examining leakage of RNA, DNA and protein. Alternatively, the
cells can be preloaded with a radioactive compound, e.g. $^{42}K^+$, $^{86}Rb^+$ or
^{32}P-phosphate, and the leakage from treated cells measured by liquid scintillation
counting. The QAC cetrimide induces more rapid leakage from Gram-positive
than Gram-negative bacteria, the latter being less susceptible because the outer
membrane presents a barrier to the agent (see Chapter 6).

Leakage is best considered as a measure of the generalized loss of function of
the cytoplasmic membrane as a permeability barrier. The rate and extent of leakage
may depend on the concentration of the inhibitor and the time and temperature
of exposure. Leakage may be related to bacteriostasis but not necessarily to cell
death. For example, the activity of phenoxyethanol has been determined against
E. coli at 35 °C and 10 °C. The resulting temperature coefficient (Q_{25}) values
showed a 38-fold reduction in bactericidal activity but only a twofold reduction
in leakage of intracellular constituents. In contrast, there is a direct relationship
between membrane damage and cell death in *E. coli* treated with a polymeric
biguanide since Q_{10} values of about 2 were produced for both bactericidal activity
and loss of intracellular substances. In studying the mechanism of action of a

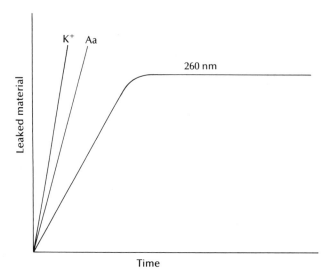

Figure 3.8 Rate of leakage of intracellular materials from bacteria exposed to a membrane-active agent: Aa, amino acids; 260 nm, 260 nm-absorbing material.

biocide, it is thus important to correlate biochemical and other changes with growth-inhibitory and lethal concentrations.

5.1.1 Nature and mechanisms of agents inducing leakage

Several chemically unrelated biocides damage the bacterial cytoplasmic membrane, inducing leakage of intracellular constituents. They include phenolics, biguanides, quaternary ammonium compounds (QACs) and alcohols.

5.1.1.1 Phenols and cresols

Phenols and cresols are widely used as general disinfectants and as preservatives, but must not be employed when food may become exposed to them. The tar obtained as a by-product in the destructive distillation of coal is the source of most of the phenols (tar acids) used to produce disinfectants. Typically, coal tar contains the following fractions (boiling range in parentheses): phenol (182 °C), cresols (189–205 °C), xylenols (210–230 °C) and high-boiling tar acids (230–310 °C).

Cresols consist of 2- (*ortho*-), 3- (*meta*-) and 4- (*para*-) cresol, the xylenols of six isomeric dimethylphenols and ethylphenols. Cresols and xylenols are available commercially as a combined fraction (cresylic acid) and the high boiling tar acids constitute the higher alkyl homologues of phenol, which form the basis of what are known as the Black fluids and White fluids. Examples of chemical structures are provided in Fig. 3.9. As the fractions are ascended, water solubility decreases

Table 3.4 Membrane-active agents and permeability of *Bacillus megaterium* (strain KM) protoplasts (see also Section 5.2)

Antibacterial agent[a]	Protoplast inducer[b]	Protoplast permeable to	Protoplast impermeable to
None (control)	Lys Pen	$NH_4^+CH_3COO^-$	Sucrose K^+Cl^- $Na^+NO_3^-$
TCC	Lys Pen	Sucrose NH_4^+ $NO_3^-CH_3COO^-Cl^-$	Na^+K^+
CHA or CPC	Lys Pen	Sucrose $NH_4^+K^+$ $Na^+CH_3COO^-Cl^-NO_3^-$	None found

[a]TCC, trichlorocarbanilide; CHA, chlorhexidine diacetate; CPC, cetylpyridinium chloride.
[b]Lys, lysozyme; Pen, benzylpenicillin.

and bactericidal activity increases but so, unfortunately, does inactivation by organic matter.

Phenol itself may also be manufactured by a synthetic process and other synthetic (non-coal-tar) phenolics include 2-phenylphenol, 4-hexylresorcinol, chlorocresol (4-chloro-3-methylphenol) and chloroxylenol (4-chloro-3,5-dimethyl-phenol), all of which are used as antibacterial agents.

Structure–activity relationships in the phenol series demonstrate that

(a) *para* (4) substitution of an alkyl chain of up to 6 carbon atoms in length (straight rather than branched chain substituents) increases antibacterial activity,

(b) halogenation increases activity, and further still if this is at the *para* (4) position, and an alkyl group is introduced at the *ortho* (2) site, both in relation to the phenol group, and

(c) nitration increases activity but also increases systemic toxicity.

Phenols are predominantly membrane-active agents, but will also cause intracellular coagulation of cytoplasmic constituents. They are sometimes considered merely as protein precipitants, but this term masks the more subtle effects they have on bacterial cells.

Phenols, cresols and their chlorinated derivatives induce leakage of intracellular materials from bacteria. Penetration into the lipid-rich interior of the cytoplasmic membrane is an important step in the activity of 4-*n*-alkylphenols. Phenolic compounds which were at one time employed in antiseptic soaps and shampoos included hexachlorophane (Fig. 3.9) and tetrachlorosalicylanilide (TCS). These are now considered to be toxic. High (bactericidal) concentrations of these and the less toxic fentichlor induce leakage of intracellular constituents, but low concentrations have more specific effects as described in Sections 5.3.1.4 (TCS,

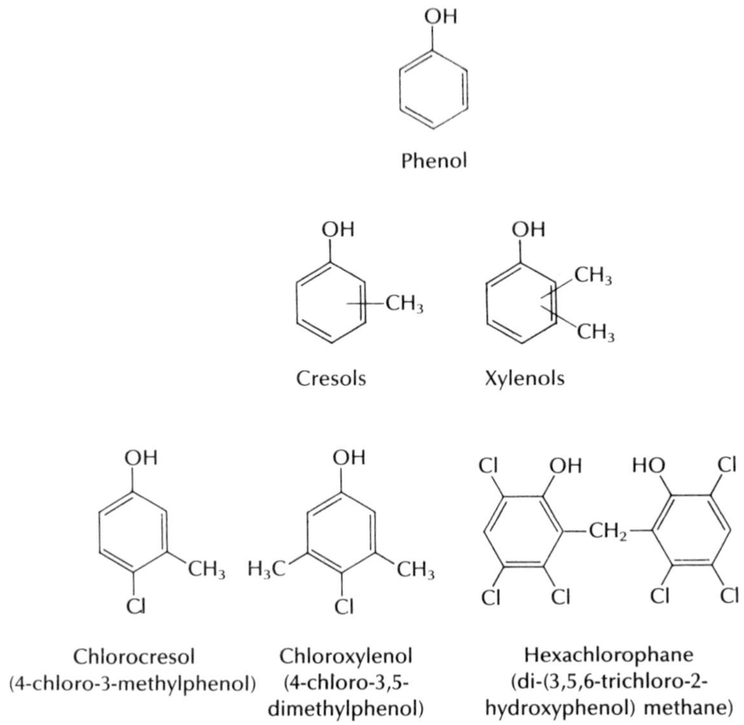

Phenol

Cresols

Xylenols

Chlorocresol
(4-chloro-3-methylphenol)

Chloroxylenol
(4-chloro-3,5-
dimethylphenol)

Hexachlorophane
(di-(3,5,6-trichloro-2-
hydroxyphenol) methane)

Figure 3.9   Some phenols and cresols.

fentichlor) and 5.4.1.1 (hexachlorophane). Phenol itself induces the release of ^{14}C-glutamate from *E. coli*, but leakage occurs without a drop in viable numbers and thus precedes death. Phenol damages the permeability barrier, permitting the rapid diffusion of low-molecular-weight substances from the metabolic pool, but cells may be able to recover rapidly following its removal.

5.1.1.2   Surface-active agents (surfactants)

Surface-active agents contain two structural regions, a hydrocarbon, water-repellent (hydrophobic) group and the other a water-attracting (hydrophilic or polar) group. Depending on the basis of the charge or absence of ionization of the hydrophilic group, surface-active agents are classified into the following four groups of compounds: cationic, anionic, amphoteric and non-ionic.

(1) *Cationic agents.* Primarily these are represented by the QACs (Fig. 3.10(a)), which are organically substituted ammonium compounds in which the nitrogen atom has a valency of 5, and four of the substituted radicals (R^1–R^4) are alkyl or heterocyclic radicals and the fifth (X^-) is a small anion. The sum of the carbon atoms in the four R groups is >10. In those QACs with potent

antimicrobial activity, at least one of the R groups has a chain length in the range C_8–C_{18}. The QACs are active against Gram-positive bacteria (but not spores) and less so against Gram-negative organisms, especially *Ps. aeruginosa*. Activity is markedly reduced in the presence of organic matter. The QACs are membrane-active agents, inducing a generalized increase in permeability (Table 3.5).

The QACs induce leakage of intracellular constituents from treated bacteria, which is indicative of membrane damage. The release of nitrogenous and phosphorus-containing substances was described by Hotchkiss in 1944, and Salton in 1951 demonstrated that the QAC cetrimide induced a more rapid rate of leakage from Gram-positive than Gram-negative cells. K^+ ions are released first, followed by PO_4^{3-} and then by 260 nm absorbing material, indicative of larger molecular weight compounds: see Fig. 3.8.

Low, bacteriostatic, concentrations of cetrimide are claimed to have an effect on the PMF (Section 5.3.1.4). The effects of QACs on bacterial protoplasts are described in Section 5.2.1.

(2) *Anionic agents.* These are compounds which, in aqueous solution, dissociate into a large complex anion responsible for the surface activity and a smaller cation. Examples are the alkali metal and metal soaps and lauryl ether sulphates (e.g. sodium lauryl (dodecyl) sulphate). Generally, they have strong detergent but weak antimicrobial properties, although high concentrations will induce lysis of Gram-negative bacteria (Section 4.3). Fatty acids are active against Gram-positive but not Gram-negative bacteria.

Anionic surfactants such as sodium lauryl sulphate (SLS) disrupt permeability barriers, inducing the leakage of intracellular constituents. They also cause protoplast lysis (Section 5.2.1) and produce a general denaturation of cell proteins. High concentrations (2%) of SLS dissolve cell walls of *E. coli*.

(3) *Amphoteric (ampholytic) agents.* Amphoteric agents are compounds of mixed anionic–cationic character, and combine the detergent properties of anionic surfactants with the bactericidal properties of cationic surfactants. Examples include dodecyl-di(aminoethyl)-glycine and dodecyl-β-alanine.

Amphoteric surfactants cause the leakage of intracellular constituents from bacteria, but their precise mechanism of action is unknown.

(4) *Non-ionic agents.* These consist of a hydrocarbon chain attached to a non-polar water-attracting group, which is usually a chain of ethylene oxide units, e.g. cetomacrogols and sorbitan derivatives such as the polysorbates (Tweens). Low concentrations affect the permeability of the outer parts of the envelopes of Gram-negative cells whereas high concentrations overcome the activity of QACs, parabens and phenols.

5.1.1.3 *Biguanides and polymeric biguanides*

Chlorhexidine (Fig. 3.10(b)) is a member of a family of N^1,N^5-substituted biguanides, and is available as dihydrochloride, diacetate (acetate) and gluconate

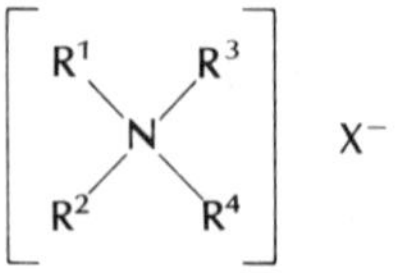

$$\left[\begin{array}{ccc} R^1 & & R^3 \\ & N & \\ R^2 & & R^4 \end{array} \right] \quad X^- \quad \text{General structure}$$

(a)

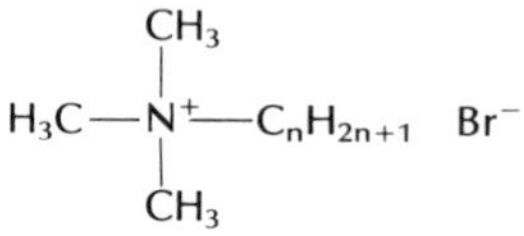

$$H_3C-\overset{\overset{\displaystyle CH_3}{|}}{\underset{\underset{\displaystyle CH_3}{|}}{N^+}}-C_nH_{2n+1} \quad Br^-$$

(n = 12, 14 or 16)
Cetrimide

(a mixture of dodecyl-, tetradecyl-and
hexadecyl-trimethylammonium bromide)

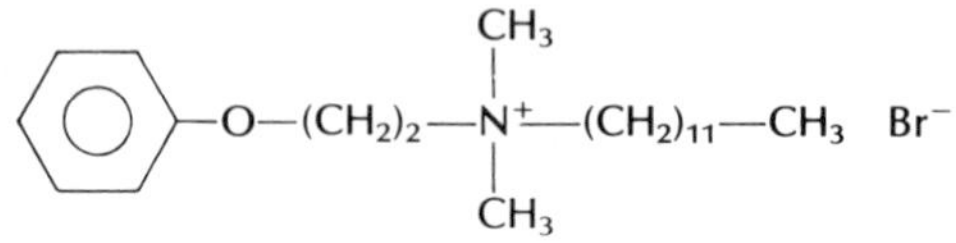

Domiphen bromide
(dodecyldimethyl-2-phenoxyethyl-
ammonium bromide)

$$\bigcirc\!\!-O-(CH_2)_2-\overset{\overset{\displaystyle CH_3}{|}}{\underset{\underset{\displaystyle CH_3}{|}}{N^+}}-(CH_2)_{11}-CH_3 \quad Br^-$$

$$\bigcirc\!\!-CH_2-\overset{\overset{\displaystyle CH_3}{|}}{\underset{\underset{\displaystyle CH_3}{|}}{N^+}}-C_nH_{2n+1} \quad Cl^-$$

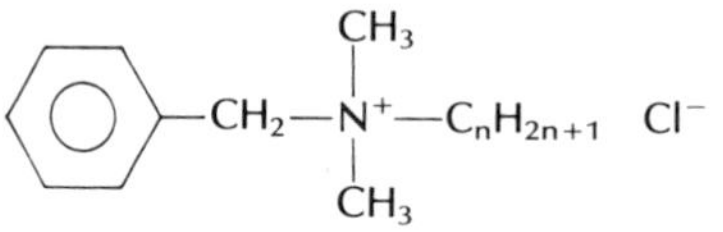

(n = 8 to 18)
Benzalkonium chloride

(a mixture of alkyldimethylbenzyl-
ammonium chlorides)

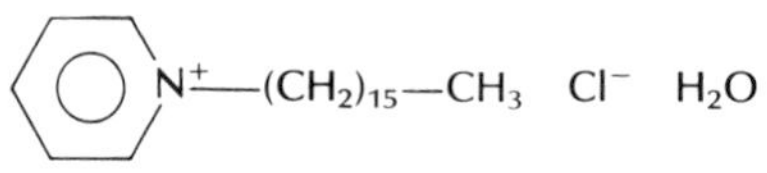

$$\bigcirc\!\!-N^+\!\!-(CH_2)_{15}-CH_3 \quad Cl^- \quad H_2O$$

Cetylpyridinium chloride
(1-hexadecylpyridinium chloride)

(b)

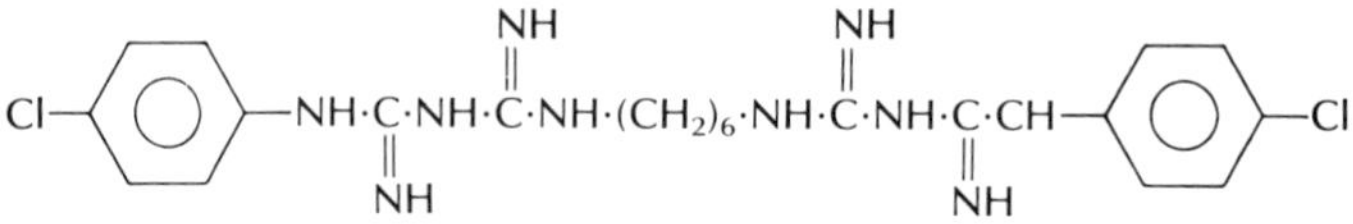

$$Cl\!-\!\!\bigcirc\!\!-NH\cdot C\cdot NH\cdot C\cdot NH\cdot(CH_2)_6\cdot NH\cdot C\cdot NH\cdot C\cdot CH\!-\!\!\bigcirc\!\!-Cl$$

with NH above and NH below the C groups

(c)

$$H_3C\cdot(H_2C)_3\cdot C\cdot H_2C\cdot NH-C\cdot NH\cdot C\cdot NH\cdot(CH_2)_6\cdot NH\cdot C\cdot NH\cdot C\cdot NH\cdot CH_2\cdot C\cdot(CH_2)_3CH_3$$

with H, CH₂, CH₃ and NH substituents

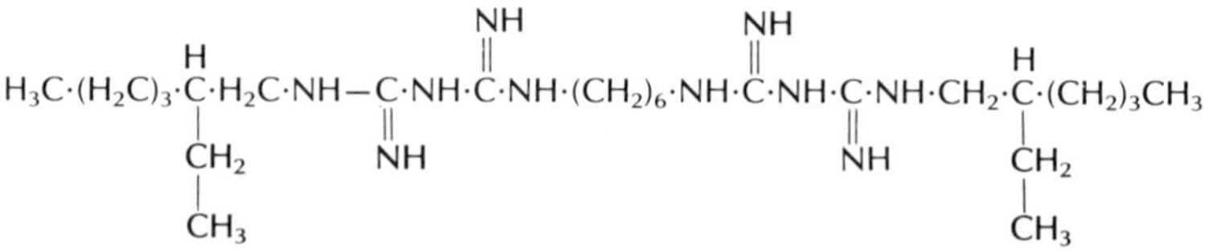

Figure 3.10 (a) General structure of quaternary ammonium compounds (QACs) and some examples; (b) chlorhexidine; (c) alexidine; (d) polyhexamethylene biguanide (PHMB); (e) bronopol; (f) some diamidines (propamidine, dibromopropamidine).

(d), (e), (f) Propamidine, Dibromopropamidine

Figure 3.10 *continued*

salts. It is active against both Gram-positive and Gram-negative bacteria, but is not sporicidal and is not lethal to acid-fast bacteria (mycobacteria). Most Gram-positive bacteria are inhibited at a chlorhexidine concentration of 1 mg/l and many Gram negatives at 2–2.5 mg/l; however, *Ps. aeruginosa* may require higher concentrations (20–>50 mg/l) and *Proteus* spp. and *Providencia* spp. are usually insensitive. Activity is reduced in the presence of serum, blood, pus and other organic matter, and, because of its cationic nature, in the presence of soaps and other anionic compounds, and also by non-ionic surfactants (such as the polysorbates) and phospholipids.

Chlorhexidine is predominantly a membrane-active agent, but it has several effects on susceptible bacteria which contribute to its overall bactericidal efficacy (Table 3.5). The biguanide has a biphasic effect on membrane permeability (Fig. 3.11): an initial high rate of leakage of intracellular constituents occurs as the concentration of chlorhexidine increases, but, at higher biocide concentrations, coagulation or precipitation of the cytosol occurs so that leakage is progressively decreased. It must be emphasized that there is no obvious relationship between the quantity of cell constituents released and the drop in viability.

Alexidine (Fig. 3.10(c)) possesses ethylhexyl end groups and thus differs from chlorhexidine (Fig. 3.10(b)). Alexidine is more rapidly bactericidal than chlorhexidine and produces a significantly faster alteration in bacterial permeability. Studies with mixed lipid and pure phospholipid vesicles demonstrate that alexidine and Vantocil produce lipid phase separation and domain formation (Fig. 3.12).

Vantocil is a heterodisperse mixture of polyhexamethylene biguanides (PHMB,

Table 3.5　Summary of effects of membrane-active agents

Antibacterial agent(s)	Effect(s) on bacterial cell	Mechanism of action
Phenols	Leakage; protein denaturation	Generalized membrane damage
QACs	Leakage; protoplast lysis; discharge of pH component of Δp in PMF	Generalized membrane damage
Chlorhexidine	Leakage; protoplast lysis; high concentrations interact with cytoplasmic constituents	Concentration-dependent effects: membrane integrity affected (low), protoplasm congealed (high)
PHMB	Impairment of outer membrane; leakage resulting from cytoplasmic membrane damage	Phase separation and domain formation of acidic phospholipids of cytoplasmic membrane
Alexidine	Leakage (more rapidly than chlorhexidine); spheroplast lysis	More rapid perturbation of membrane integrity than chlorhexidine; causes phase separation and domain formation of membrane lipids
Hexachlorophane	Leakage; protoplast lysis; respiration inhibited	Inhibits membrane-bound electron transport chain
Phenoxyethanol	Leakage; low concentrations stimulate total oxygen uptake and uncouple oxidative phosphorylation; H^+ translocation	Proton-conducting uncoupler
Sorbic acid	Transport inhibition (conflicting data reported); inhibition of ΔpH across membrane	Transport inhibitor (effect on PMF); another unidentified mechanism?
Parabens	Leakage; transport inhibition; selective inhibition of ΔpH across membrane	Concentration-dependent effects; transport inhibited (low), membrane integrity affected (high)

Fig. 3.10(d) in which $n = 2$–30, with a mean of 5.5) with a molecular weight of approximately 3000. It is active against Gram-positive and Gram-negative bacteria (*Ps. aeruginosa* and *P. vulgaris* are less sensitive) but is not sporicidal. Because of the residual positive charges on the polymer, it is precipitated from aqueous solutions by anionic compounds which include soaps and detergents based on alkyl

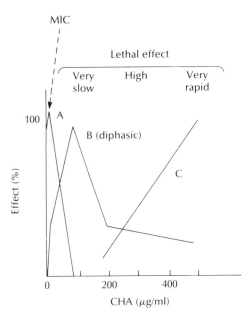

Figure 3.11 Effect of chlorhexidine diacetate (CHA) on *E. coli*: effects on viability, triphenyltetrazolium chloride (TTC) reduction (A), leakage of intracellular constituents (B) and intracellular coagulation and precipitation of nucleic acids and proteins (C). MIC, minimum inhibitory concentration. (Based on Longworth (1971).)

sulphates. PHMB is a membrane-active agent which also impairs the integrity of the outer membrane of Gram-negative bacteria. Activity of PHMB increases, on a weight basis, with increasing levels of polymerization; this is linked to enhanced membrane perturbation.

Although such membrane-active agents perturb homeostasis, the manner in which they interact with the membrane itself is not always clear. QACs and chlorhexidine combine with membrane phospholipids and thereby bring about disruption of the membrane. Anionic agents, unlike cationic ones, interact with the protein moiety of the membrane which is thus completely disrupted. PHMB causes domain formation of the acidic phospholipids of the cytoplasmic membrane. Permeability changes ensue and there is believed to be an altered function of some membrane-associated enzymes. The proposed sequence of events during its interaction with the cell envelope of *E. coli* is as follows (see Fig. 3.12).

(1) There is rapid attraction towards the negatively charged bacterial cell surface with specific and strong adsorption to phosphate-containing compounds.
(2) The integrity of the outer membrane is impaired and PHMB is attracted towards the inner membrane.
(3) Binding to phospholipids occurs followed by an increase in inner membrane permeability involving K^+ loss and accompanied by bacteriostasis.

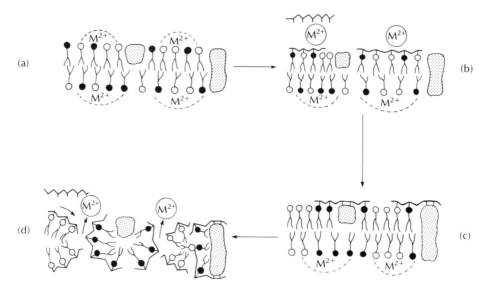

Figure 3.12   Proposed mechanism of action of PHMB: (a) cytoplasmic membrane conforming to fluid mosaic model (Singer–Nicholson) and stabilized by metallic cations; (b) surface cations displaced by PHMB, which binds to phospholipids causing changes in packing; (c) phospholipid phase separation induced, with K^+ efflux and loss of enzyme function (bacteriostatic effect); (d) aggregation of destabilized zones, complete loss of membrane function (bactericidal effect). (Based on P. Broxton *et al.* (1984) *Journal of Applied Bacteriology* **57**: 115–124.) PHMB, ⋀⋀⋀ ; M^{2+}, divalent cation; ⋏ acidic phospholipid; ⋏ neutral phospholipid.

(4) Complete loss of membrane function, and precipitation of intracellular constituents, leading to a bactericidal effect.

Increased molecular size of PHMB increases the magnitude of the domain so that membrane perturbation is enhanced. Alexidine can also cause lipid phase separation and domain formation, whereas chlorhexidine does not produce this effect. The nature of the end group in the biguanide molecule (ethylhexyl in alexidine, chlorophenol in chlorhexidine) might thus influence its ability to produce lipid domains in the cytoplasmic membrane.

5.1.1.4 Alcohols

Several alcohols are rapidly bactericidal even to acid-fast bacteria. However, they are not sporicidal. Some important alcohols are as follows.

(a) Ethanol (ethyl alcohol, C_2H_5OH) is active only in the presence of water.
(b) Methanol (methyl alcohol, CH_3OH) has poor activity but has been claimed to potentiate the sporicidal activity of hypochlorites (Chapter 7).

(c) Isopropanol (propan-2-ol, isopropyl alcohol, $(CH_3)_2CHOH$) is a more effective bactericide than ethanol.

(d) Phenylethanol (phenylethyl alcohol, $C_6H_5 \cdot CH_2 \cdot CH_2OH$) has selective activity against Gram-negative bacteria.

(e) Phenoxyethanol ($C_6H_5 \cdot O \cdot CH_2 \cdot CH_2OH$) possesses significant activity against *Ps. aeruginosa* but is less active against other Gram-negative organisms and Gram-positive bacteria.

(f) Bronopol (2-bromo-2-nitropran-1,3-diol; Fig. 3.10(e)) is an aliphatic halogenonitro compound which possesses a broad antibacterial spectrum including *Ps. aeruginosa* but is not sporicidal. Its activity is reduced in the presence of 10% serum and especially by sulphydryl compounds (Section 5.4.1.2). Bronopol oxidizes thiol groups to disulphides, an action that is reversed by sulphydryl compounds (Fig. 3.21(a)).

Ethanol and isopropanol are membrane disrupters. Phenylethanol and phenoxyethanol also induce generalized loss of cytoplasmic membrane function, but both have other, more specific, effects (see, for example, the discussion on phenoxyethanol in Section 5.3.1.4).

Ethanol causes a rapid release of intracellular constituents from bacteria, and disorganization of the membrane probably results from penetration of the solvents into the hydrocarbon interior of the cytoplasmic membrane. Ethanol has pleiotropic effects on bacteria. Inhibition of DNA, RNA, protein and peptidoglycan synthesis in *E. coli* are secondary effects that follow membrane damage. Other responses, which include inhibition of enzymes involved in glycolysis, fatty acid and phospholipid synthesis, and effects on membrane permeability and solute uptake, all result directly from an ethanol-induced disruption of membrane structure and function.

5.1.1.5 Other biocides

Other agents such as organic acids and esters may also induce leakage of intracellular constituents. In addition, they dissipate the PMF and will thus be considered elsewhere (Section 5.3).

5.2 Membrane disruption: agents causing lysis of wall-deficient forms

Although an antibacterial agent may cause extensive cytoplasmic membrane damage, this will not necessarily result in cell lysis. However, bacterial cells without cell walls (protoplasts) or with modified cell envelopes (spheroplasts) will lyse after exposure to a biocide that causes gross membrane damage.

Protoplasts and spheroplasts are osmotically fragile forms that lyse when transferred from a non-penetrating medium of high osmotic pressure, e.g. 0.5 M sucrose, to water or to a solute which readily penetrates the cytoplasmic membrane. For example, the membrane of *B. megaterium* protoplasts is naturally permeable to glycerol, NH_4^+ and acetate (CH_3COO^-) ions; however, protoplasts are stable in, for example, ammonium chloride because the membrane is impermeable to chloride (Cl^-) ions. Protoplast stability thus occurs in the presence of

(a) a membrane-permeable and a membrane-impermeable ion pair, where the non-permeant ion prevents entry of the permeable species, e.g. acetate, or
(b) two membrane-impermeable ions.

Therefore, the effects of antibacterial agents on protoplasts (or spheroplasts) suspended in sucrose or other solutes can be used to obtain information about their mechanism of action, e.g. by examining biocide-induced lysis in solutions of acetate salts (caesium, Cs; sodium, Na; lithium, Li) data about membrane permeability towards these cations can be obtained (Table 3.4).

5.2.1 *Nature and mechanisms of agents inducing major membrane disruption*

Low concentrations of chlorhexidine and QACs cause lysis of spheroplasts and protoplasts suspended in sucrose, but at higher concentrations lysis is reduced because of intracellular precipitation or coagulation (Fig. 3.13). Parallels have been noted between bactericidal action against whole cells and lytic activity on protoplasts of *M. lysodeikticus* of detergents containing a dodecyl chain ($C_{12}H_{25}$) attached to a charged group. The order of activity was

$$C_{12}H_{25}-NH_3^+ > NMe_3^+ > -SO_4^- > -SO_3^-$$

Cationic agents (QACs) react with phospholipid components (Fig. 3.7) in the cytoplasmic membrane, thereby producing distortion of the membrane and protoplast lysis under osmotic stress. Isolated membranes do not undergo disaggregation on exposure to QACs because membrane distortion is not sufficiently drastic. Anionic surfactants, in contrast, interact with the protein components (Fig. 3.7) of cytoplasmic membranes; these proteins are solubilized, so that anionic detergents will lyse protoplasts and disaggregate isolated membranes (in the absence of osmotic stress).

Alcohols also will induce protoplast lysis. Alcohols having equal thermodynamic activities, i.e. effective as opposed to actual concentrations, produce equal degrees of lysis of *M. lysodeikticus* protoplasts, and the amount of damage that they produce is probably related to their concentrations in the lipid phase.

Useful information about the selectivity of membrane action can be obtained by studying the effects of biocides on protoplasts or spheroplasts suspended in various solutes (Table 3.4).

Trichlorocarbanilide induces lysis in ammonium chloride because it increases Cl^- permeability whereas tetrachlorosalicylanilide induces lysis in ammonium nitrate by increasing NO_3^- permeability (Table 3.4). However, QACs and

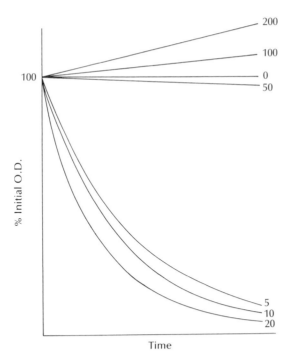

Figure 3.13 Lysis of protoplasts of *Bacillus megaterium* by chlorhexidine (the numerals on the curves have units of μg/ml). Note that, at concentrations above 50 μg/ml, lysis is prevented because of intracellular precipitation.

chlorhexidine produce lysis of protoplasts suspended in various solutes because they effect a generalized, rather than specific, membrane damage. The effects and conclusions are summarized in Table 3.5.

Chlorhexidine-induced rate of lysis of spheroplasts in acetate salts is inversely proportional to the hydrated ionic radii of the cations, i.e. greatest in Cs (atomic weight 132.9) and least in Li (atomic weight 6.94).

5.3 Dissipation of proton-motive force

As pointed out in Chapter 1, Mitchell's chemiosmotic theory envisages a mechanism whereby active transport, oxidative phosphorylation and adenosine triphosphate (ATP) synthesis in chloroplasts, mitochondria and bacteria, as well as bacterial flagellar movement, can be explained. These are powered by a PMF generated by ATP hydrolysis of metabolic oxidoreductions (Fig. 3.14). The PMF is expressed as a gradient across the cytoplasmic membrane and in bacteria is demonstrated with the interior of the cell alkaline and negatively charged in relation to the external environment. Another pertinent aspect of Mitchell's theory is that the cytoplasmic membrane must be non-conducting and not readily permeable to protons and other ions.

As described in Chapter 1, the theory may be expressed mathematically as follows:

$$\Delta p = \Delta \psi - Z \Delta pH$$

in which Δp is the PMF, ψ the membrane electrical potential, ΔpH the transmembrane pH gradient, and Z a constant ($2.303RT/F$) with a value of 61 at $37\,°C$. Z is a factor converting pH values to millivolts.

The electron transport chain is fixed in a definite direction in the membrane. In consequence, the protons generated during the oxidation of substrate (SH$_2 \to$ S, Fig. 3.14), leading eventually to the reduction of oxygen, are transported from the interior of the cell outwards. The fact that a PMF is also generated by ATPase hydrolysis of ATP explains the existence of a PMF in anaerobic bacteria and in facultative organisms metabolizing anaerobically.

Some antibacterial agents interfere with oxidative phosphorylation by stimulating oxygen uptake whilst inhibiting phosphorylation. These are called uncouplers or uncoupling agents.

5.3.1 *Nature and mechanisms of agents dissipating the PMF*

5.3.1.1 *Organic acids and esters*

Saturated straight-chain monocarboxylic acids are classified into the following groups, the acids being listed by their common name (systematic name in parentheses):

(1) short-chain fatty acids (C_1–C_6), e.g. formic (methanoic), acetic (ethanoic) and propionic (propanoic) acids;
(2) medium-chain fatty acids (C_7–C_{10}), e.g. caprylic (octanoic) and capric (decanoic) acids;
(3) long-chain fatty acids (C_{12}–C_{18}), e.g. lactic (dodecanoic), myristic (tetradecanoic), palmitic (hexadecanoic) and stearic (oxtadecanoic) acids.

Common derivatives of these straight-chain monocarboxylic acids include unsaturated, e.g. sorbic (2,4-hexadienoic acid Fig. 3.15), hydroxylic, e.g. citric, lactic and phenolic, e.g. benzoic (Fig. 3.15), salicylic, acids.

Several acids (a few inorganic and some aromatic and aliphatic) are used as preservatives in food and/or pharmaceutical products, whereas others, e.g. salicyclic and undecylenic, are sometimes incorporated into products used for the topical treatment of fungal skin infections. Acids used as food preservatives include acetic, sorbic, propionic, dehydroacetic and benzoic acids. Pharmaceutically, sorbic and benzoic acids are sometimes employed as preservatives, as are the esters, considered below, of *para-* (4-) hydroxybenzoic acid (Fig. 3.15). Acetic and propionic acids are better known as acidulants (Section 5.3.1.2).

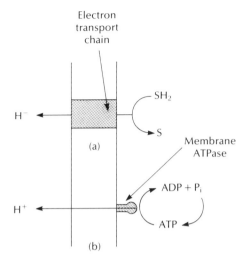

Figure 3.14 Mitchell's chemiosmotic theory. Generation of PMF by (a) electron transport chain and (b) hydrolysis of adenosine triphosphate (ATP). $SH_2 \rightarrow S$: oxidation of substrate. (For further information on ATPase, see Fig. 3.23.)

Organic acids are often termed fatty, lipophilic, weak or carboxylic acids. They are weakly acid, because they do not readily donate H^+ in aqueous solution, but the salts (Na, K) dissociate completely. For microorganisms, organic acids act either as a source of carbon and energy or as inhibitory agents. This apparent contradiction depends on

(i) the concentration of the acid and the pH,
(ii) its ability to enter the microbial cell, and
(iii) the capacity of the microbe to metabolize it.

Environmental pH is one of the major factors affecting the activity of organic acids, activity decreasing as the pH rises (Fig. 3.4). In aqueous solutions of mineral acids, but not of weaker organic acids, complete ionization occurs. The latter type will contain three components and these can be considered as being an acid of symbol HA and the ionized components A^- and H^+. The ionization constant, K_a, of the acid is represented by

$$K_a = [A^-][H^+]/[HA]$$

and the pK_a value (the pH at which 50% ionization occurs) varies with different acids, e.g. benzoic acid 4.2, sorbic acid 4.8. At pH values greater than pK_a, antibacterial activity decreases rapidly, permitting the conclusion that the undissociated moiety (HA) makes the greatest contribution to inhibitory activity (Fig. 3.4). In fact, it had often been assumed that HA was totally responsible for the antimicrobial effect of organic acids. This, however, did not consider the behaviour of an acid inside the microbial cell. Over an external pH range of 5.5–9, the pH

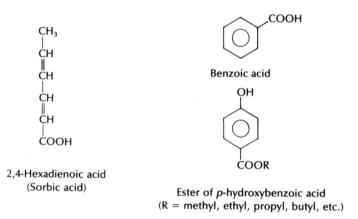

Figure 3.15   Some organic acids and esters of *p*- (4-) hydroxybenzoic acid.

value (pH$_i$) of the bacterial cytoplasm is strictly regulated, so that when molecules of an organic acid have entered a cell they will dissociate almost entirely. This hypothesis itself assumes, of course, that dissociation in the cytosol can be equated to that in aqueous solutions. However, it is now believed that both the proton and anion contribute to the growth-inhibitory effect.

The most important esters of organic acids are those of *para*- (4-) hydroxybenzoic acid (Fig. 3.15). These, known as the parabens, consist usually of the methyl, ethyl, propyl, butyl and sometimes benzyl esters. Their activity is less susceptible to changes in pH and they are employed as pharmaceutical, cosmetic and food preservatives.

Studies with pharmaceutical and food preservatives have demonstrated that lipophilic acids (e.g. propionic, sorbic, benzoic, 4-hydroxybenzoic) and the parabens inhibit the active uptake of some amino and oxo acids in *E. coli* and *B. subtilis*. Despite the long history of these agents as food and pharmaceutical preservatives, their exact mode of action continues to be the subject of debate. Sorbic acid affects the PMF in *E. coli* and accelerates the movement of H$^+$ ions from low pH media into the cytoplasm (see Fig. 3.16). Acidification of the cytoplasm to about pH 6 is sufficient to prevent growth. In the light of current knowledge, it may be rather tentatively concluded that sorbic acid dissipates ΔpH across the membrane and inhibits solute transport. The membrane potential ($\Delta\psi$) is reduced but to a much smaller extent than ΔpH (Fig. 3.16).

The cytoplasmic membrane is thus a prime target site for organic acids.

5.3.1.2   *Organic acids used as acidulants*

In addition to deliberate usage as preservatives (e.g. benzoic and sorbic acids, Section 5.3.1.1), organic acids can also be employed as acidulants, i.e. to lower

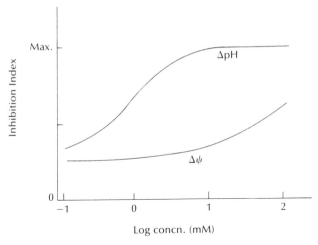

Figure 3.16 Effect of sorbic acid on ΔpH and Δψ in *E. coli* membrane vesicles. (Based on T. Eklund (1985) *Journal of General Microbiology* **131**: 73–76.)

artificially the pH of foods. Such acids include acetic, citric and lactic acids, which may also possess antimicrobial activity. Microbial growth is usually limited at lower pH and this approach can be complemented by adding lower concentrations of organic acid preservatives. Low pH can also potentiate the activity of bicarbonates, nitrites (Chapter 4) and sulphites (Section 5.5.1). Strong inorganic acids will also lower the external pH; however, these are non-permeant and hence do not affect the internal pH(cytoplasmic, pH_i) to the same extent as permeant weak, lipophilic acids.

A low pK_a value is not the only significant feature of acidulants. Thus,

(i) sorbate and acetate have similar pK_a values, but the former is a much more potent antibacterial agent,
(ii) organic acids used as preservatives are more potent inhibitors of bacterial growth than are other weak acids of similar pH, and
(iii) weak organic acid preservatives are more effective inhibitors of pH homeostasis than are other acids of similar structure.

The mechanism of action of organic acid preservatives and acidulants cannot thus be explained solely by an alteration of pH_i. Acetic acid interacts with the cytoplasmic membrane to neutralize the electrochemical potential (PMF); it also lowers pH_i and may cause denaturation of proteins. Propionic acid produces a general inhibition caused by acidification of the bacterial cytoplasm and, more importantly, a specific inhibition of an, as yet, unidentified function.

Incubation of bacterial cells at low pH may also damage the outer membrane, as evidenced by the increased sensitivity to bile salts in *E. coli*.

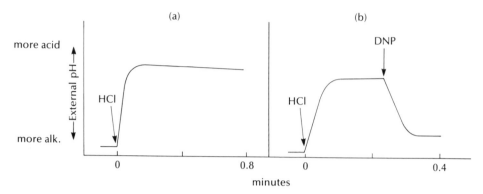

Figure 3.17 Effect of dinitrophenol (DNP, 5×10^5 M) on proton flux in the obligate anaerobe *Chlostridium perfringens*. (a) Control, cells exposed only to hydrochloric acid (external pH falls). (b) Cells exposed to hydrochloric acid and then to DNP. DNP causes an instantaneous influx of protons (seen as a sudden rise in external pH) and a complete discharge of the proton gradient. (Based on D. C. Daltrey & W. B. Hugo (1974) *Microbios* **11**: 131–146.)

5.3.1.3 Dinitrophenol

2,4-Dinitrophenol (DNP) inhibits ATP synthesis while stimulating respiration, i.e. it acts as an uncoupler of oxidative phosphorylation. DNP is a weak lipophilic acid which 'short circuits' the membrane, thereby causing a backflow of protons across the cytoplasmic membrane into the cell with the consequent collapse of Δp, the PMF (Fig. 3.17). The cellular activities powered by the PMF are inhibited. Provided that substrate accumulation was not dependent on proton-driven active transport, cellular respiration (oxygen uptake) would continue whereas ATP synthesis, which is dependent on the PMF, would cease. Thus, the phenomenon of the uncoupling of oxidative phosphorylation can now be explained at the molecular level.

5.3.1.4 Other agents

Low concentrations of phenoxyethanol induce proton translocation in *E. coli* but higher concentrations produce gross membrane damage (Fig. 3.18). Fentichlor and TCS inhibit energy-dependent uptake of amino acids and glucose into cellular material. TCS also discharges the membrane potential component ($\Delta\psi$) in *Enterococcus faecalis*. The QAC cetrimide has been claimed to discharge the pH component of Δp in *S. aureus* at concentrations that inhibit bacterial growth.

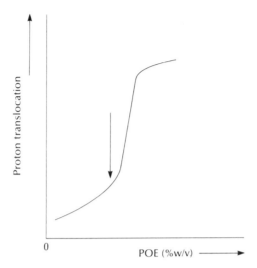

Figure 3.18 Rate of phenoxyethanol (POE)-induced proton translocation in *E. coli*: relationship between POE concentration and its effect on gross membrane damage (arrow indicates POE concentration causing gross membrane damage). (Based on P. Gilbert, E. G. Beveridge & P. B. Crone (1977) *Microbios* **19**: 17–26.)

5.4 Inhibition of membrane enzymes

The cytoplasmic membrane contains phospholipids and proteins. Many of the proteins are enzymes, e.g. those associated with the electron transport chain that use the electrochemical potential of protons to power the complex active transport system (Section 5.3). One antibacterial agent, hexachlorophane, specifically affects the electron transport chain and other biocides interact with thiol groups in membrane enzymes. Nevertheless, it is now generally accepted that enzyme inactivation is unlikely to be a primary mechanism of action since it is only one of many effects that biocides have on a bacterial cell.

5.4.1 *Nature and mechanisms of agents inhibiting membrane enzyme activity*

Several biocides interact with and inhibit membrane enzyme activity. In some rare instances, this effect is sufficient to explain the mechanism of action of the antibacterial compound, but in others the inhibition is only one out of many inhibited sites, as pointed out above.

5.4.1.1 *Hexachlorophane*

The phenolic agent hexachlorophane (hexachlorophene, HCP) induces the leakage of intracellular material from *B. megaterium*. The threshold concentration of HCP

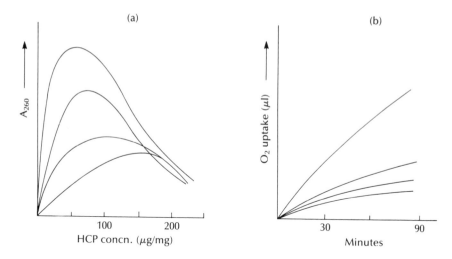

Figure 3.19 Mode of action of hexachlorophane (HCP) on *B. megaterium*. (a) HCP-induced leakage of 260 nm-absorbing material after (top to bottom) 300, 180, 60 and 30 min. (b) Effect on endogenous respiration of HCP concentrations (top to bottom) of 0, 2.5 and 8 μg/mg (8 μg/mg is also the minimum lethal dose). Note that the greatest amount of leakage (A_{260}) occurs at concentrations much higher than 8 μg/mg. (Figures redrawn from the data of (a) H. L. Joswick *et al.* (1971) *Journal of Bacteriology* **109**: 492–500 and (b) J. J. Frederick *et al.* (1974) *Antimicrobial Agents and Chemotherapy* **6**: 712–721.)

for bactericidal activity is 10 μg/mg cell dry weight, yet peak leakage occurs at concentrations >50 μg/mg and cytological changes above 30 μg/ug. Furthermore, HCP is bactericidal at 0 °C despite causing little leakage at this temperature. The primary effect of HCP is to inhibit the membrane-bound part of the electron transport chain (Fig. 3.19(b)) and the other effects noted above are thus secondary ones occurring only at high HCP concentrations (Fig. 3.19(a)).

5.4.1.2 *Agents interacting with thiol groups*

Some inhibitors interact with the thiol groups found in enzymic and structural protein (and this thus includes interaction with cytoplasmic membrane constituents). The thiol groups derived from cysteine residues are vital for the activity of many enzymes. Reaction with, or oxidation of, these essential groups produces cell inhibition or cell inactivation, but it is possible to reverse this by adding a thiol-containing compound, such as thioglycollic acid or cysteine.

Interaction of a mercury compound with enzyme or protein thiol groups and its reversal by means of a sulphydryl (thiol-containing) compound are depicted in Fig. 3.20. Other metals such as silver and copper and the element arsenic react

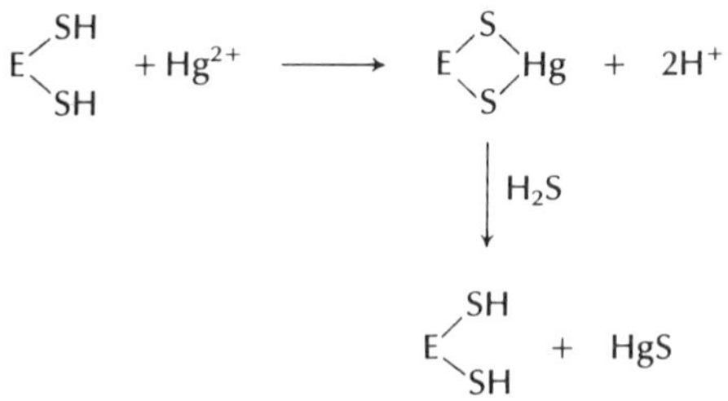

$$E\!<^{SH}_{SH} + Hg^{2+} \longrightarrow E\!<^{S}_{S}\!\!>Hg + 2H^+$$

$$\downarrow H_2S$$

$$E\!<^{SH}_{SH} + HgS$$

Figure 3.20 Effect of mercury compound on enzyme (E) —SH groups and reversal by thiol-containing compounds.

similarly. Bronopol (Section 5.1.1.4) oxidizes thiol groups to disulphides, and this action may also be reversed by sulphydryl compounds (see Fig. 3.21(a)).

The isothiazolones (Fig. 3.22(a)–(c)) are widely used as preservatives. Three members have been comprehensively studied in recent years: 1,2-benzisothiazol-3-one (BIT), 5-chloro-*N*-methylisothiazol-3-one (CMIT) and *N*-methylisothiazol-3-one (MIT).

At growth-inhibitory concentrations, BIT has little effect on membrane integrity of *S. aureus* but a significant effect on active transport and oxidation of glucose. Very marked losses of activity of isolated thiol-containing enzymes ATPase and glyceraldehyde-3-phosphate dehydrogenase (which participates in the pathway of glucose oxidation) occur, but BIT has no action on a non-thiol-containing enzyme, asparaginase. These results clearly suggest that the mechanism of action of BIT is associated with its interaction with —SH groups.

Thiol-containing compounds, such as cysteine and glutathione, rapidly quench the activity of BIT, CMIT and MIT against *E. coli*. Non-thiol amino acids, valine and histidine, also quench the activity of CMIT, which might thus react with amines as well as with essential thiol groups. Unlike the other two isothiazolones, CMIT is able to induce frame-shift and base-pair substitution mutations in the Ames mutagenicity test. Furthermore, CMIT induces morphological changes in treated cells suggestive of an additional effect on DNA synthesis.

BIT is believed to react with glutathione (GSH) to produce the initial by-product depicted in Fig. 3.22(d), further interaction causing the release of oxidized thiol dimers to give a reduced, ring-opened form of BIT (Fig. 3.22(e)) and eventually BIT dimers. CMIT is considered to react differently, with the formation of a mixed disulphide (Fig. 3.22(f)) and the release of a mercaptoacrylamide (Fig. 3.22(g)) which is unstable and tautomerizes to give a thioacetyl chloride (Fig. 3.21(h)), which is highly reactive.

5.4.1.3 *Other agents*

Chlorhexidine has been claimed to be a specific inhibitor of membrane-bound adenosine triphosphatase (ATPase). Enzymes coupling the diffusion of protons

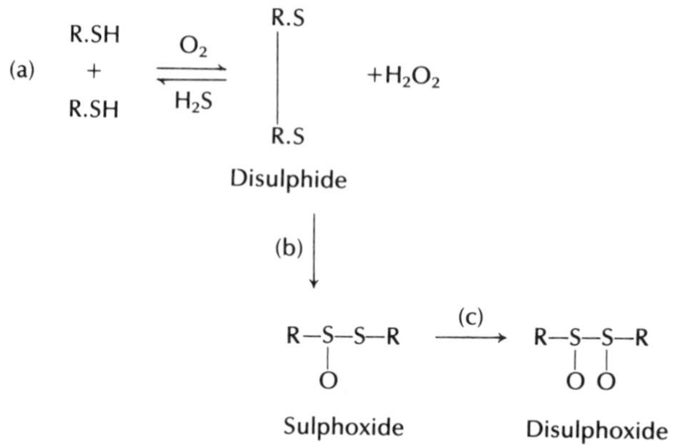

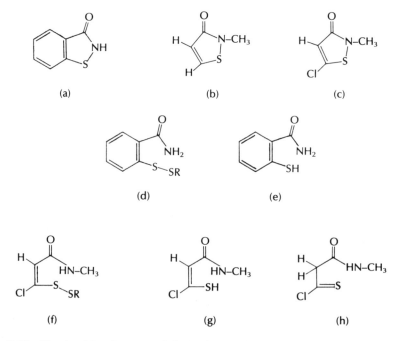

(a)

R.SH
+ $\xrightleftharpoons[H_2S]{O_2}$
R.SH

R.S
|
|
R.S

+H$_2$O$_2$

Disulphide

(b) |

R—S—S—R $\xrightarrow{(c)}$ R—S—S—R
     | | |
     O   O O

Sulphoxide   Disulphoxide

Figure 3.21 Oxidation of thiol groups to (a) disulphides (and possible reversal), (b) sulphoxides and (c) disulphoxides.

(a)

(b)

(c)

(d)

(e)

(f)

(g)

(h)

Figure 3.22 The isothiazolones and their chemical reactivity: (a) benzisothiazolone (BIT); (b) methylisothiazolone (MIT); (c) chloro-*N*-methylisothiazolone (CMIT). Interaction of BIT with glutathione (GSH) produces (d) the initial by-product. (e) A reduced ring-open form of BIT and (not shown) BIT dimers. Interaction of CMIT with cysteine (RSH) produces (f) a mixed disulphide, with the release of (g) a mercaptoacrylamide which yields (h) a thioacetyl chloride.

MEMBRANE

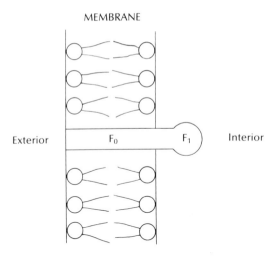

Exterior F_0 F_1 Interior

Figure 3.23 Adenosine triphosphatase (ATPase): F_0, membrane-bound (integral, pore-forming unit); F_1, soluble, catalytic unit; ⊃◯, phospholipid.

back through the membrane to ATP synthesis are globular bodies protruding from the membrane surface (Fig. 3.23). The protruding knob (F_1) is a soluble protein attached to the membrane through another set of proteins (F_0) embedded in the membrane. F_1 is readily removed, F_0 only when the membrane is destroyed. Some *E. coli* mutants have been isolated that lack ATPase activity because of a defective F_1 although F_0 is unaffected, and the permeability of the cytoplasmic membrane of these mutants to protons is greatly enhanced. N,N^1-dicyclohexylcarbodiimide (DCCD) and the antifungal compound oligomycin act at the F_0 site, but membrane-bound ATPase is probably not the primary target of chlorhexidine action, since activity is inhibited only at high biguanide concentrations.

5.5 Nature and mechanisms of agents possibly affecting membrane activity

5.5.1 Sulphites

The main compound used to generate sulphur dioxide and related anions for use as preservatives in foods and beverages is sodium metabisulphite (sodium disulphite, $Na_2S_2O_5$). Other compounds include sodium sulphite (Na_2SO_3) and bisulphite (sodium hydrogen sulphite, $NaHSO_3$) and the corresponding potassium salts. Sodium metabisulphite is also an important pharmaceutical antioxidant.

There are three species in which sulphites can exist in solution:

(a) $SO_2 \cdot H_2O$, which predominates at very low pH (0–2);

(b) as the bisulphite ion, HSO_3^-, which predominates at higher pH (3–6 approximately);

(c) as the sulphite ion (SO_3^{2-}), which predominates at alkaline pH.

The antimicrobial action of sulphites is greatest at low pH values, and it is likely that only molecular SO_2 can pass across the bacterial cytoplasmic membrane.

Interaction of sulphites with outer bacterial cell layers has not been described. In yeasts, sulphites appear to cross the membrane by passive rather than active transport and it is possible that they interact with the lipid and especially the protein component of the cytoplasmic membrane. Similar effects might occur in bacteria.

5.6 Mechanisms of action of membrane-active agents: summary

As noted above, biocides can damage the bacterial cytoplasmic membrane by various mechanisms. A summary is provided in Table 3.5. It must be emphasized that a distinction has often been drawn between the effects of low and high concentrations of a biocide. Low concentrations, usually associated with bacteriostasis, often produce far more subtle damage than the gross damage produced by lethal concentrations. For example, low (bacteriostatic) concentrations of chlorhexidine induce K^+ loss, whereas progressively higher concentrations increase both the extent of the membrane damage and the size of the permeable species, i.e. $Cs^+ > Na^+ > Li^+$ (Section 5.2.1).

6
Agents interacting with cytoplasmic constituents: properties and mechanism of action

Several biocides interact with cytoplasmic constituents. With some agents, noticeable interaction occurs only at high concentrations. For example, at high concentrations the biguanide chlorhexidine causes intracellular coagulation or precipitation of proteins and nucleic acids. Undoubtedly these effects play at least some role in the bactericidal action of the agents. Other biocides alkylate proteins, and still others cross-link proteins, so that it is difficult to pinpoint an exact target site in the cell. Bearing this limitation in mind, the interaction of various antibacterial agents with cytoplasmic components will now be considered in more detail.

6.1 Nature and mechanisms of alkylating agents

Alkylation is defined as the conversion

$$H-X \rightarrow R-X$$

in which R is an alkyl group. The biological activity of the alkylating agents is indicated by reaction with nucleophilic groups.

Some vapour phase disinfectants act as alkylating agents. Ethylene oxide ($CH_2 \cdot CH_2 \cdot O$), propylene oxide ($CH_2 \cdot CH \cdot O \cdot CH_3$) and β-propiolactone are bactericidal and sporicidal, although activity may be slow and may depend on factors such as gaseous concentration, time of exposure, temperature and especially relative humidity.

Ethylene oxide combines with the amino, carboxyl, sulphydryl and hydroxyl groups in bacterial protein, as depicted in Fig. 3.24. It also interacts with nucleic acids with a principal site of interaction at N-7 of guanine moieties in DNA to produce 7-(2'-hydroxyethyl) guanine (Fig. 3.25), the second most reactive site being at N-3 of adenine moieties. The other alkylating agents react similarly with proteins and DNA.

6.2 Nature and mechanisms of cross-linking agents

Formaldehyde is used as a disinfectant in both the liquid (e.g. formalin) and the vapour phases. It is microbicidal with lethal activity against bacteria and their spores. It is an extremely reactive chemical and combines with protein, RNA and DNA, interaction with the latter probably explaining its mutagenic activity. It interacts with protein to give intermolecular cross-links, but also acts as an alkylating agent (see above) by virtue of its interaction with $-NH_2$, $-COOH$, $-SH$ and $-OH$ groups.

Interaction of glutaraldehyde with proteins involves a reaction between the dialdehyde and the α-amino groups of amino acids, the rate of reaction being pH dependent and increasing considerably over the pH range 4–9.

6.3 Nature and mechanisms of intercalating agents

Antibacterial dyes include the triphenylmethane group (e.g. crystal violet) and the acridines. The acridines are weakly active against Gram-positive and Gram-negative bacteria but are not sporicidal. They are more effective at alkaline pH and compete with H^+ ions for anionic sites on the cell surface. Activity increases with the degree of acridine ionization but this must be cationic in nature, i.e. acridine derivatives that are ionized to form anions or zwitterions are only poorly antibacterial in comparison with those that form cations.

The acridine series of antibacterial dyes illustrate how small changes in the chemical structure of the molecule greatly alter the biological activity. Acridines combine with several sites on or in the bacterial cell, the most important of which is DNA. The attachment results from intercalation of an acridine molecule between two layers of base pairs in such a way that the primary amino groups are held in ionic linkage by two phosphoric acid residues of the DNA spiral with

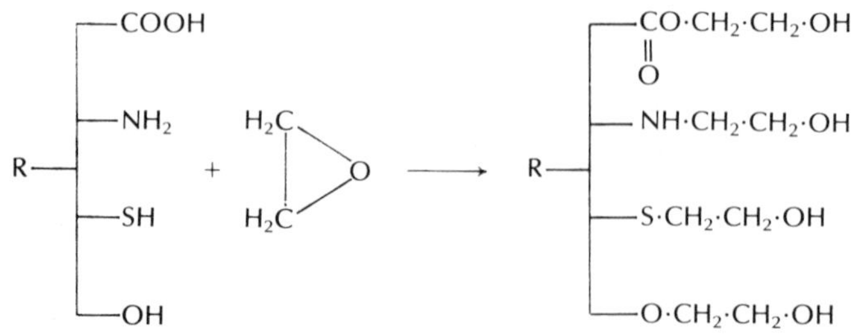

Figure 3.24 Interaction of ethylene oxide with protein groups.

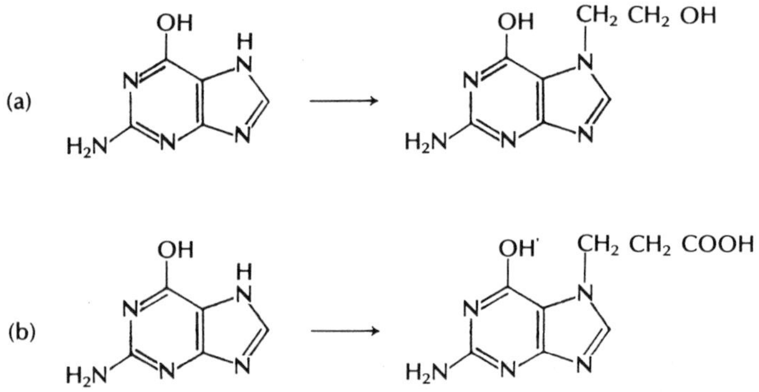

Figure 3.25 Interaction with guanine of (a) ethylene oxide and (b) β-propiolactone.

the flat skeleton of the acridine ring (Fig. 3.26(a)) resting on the purine and pyrimidine molecules to which it is held by van der Waals forces (Fig. 3.26(c); cf. normal DNA in Fig. 3.26(b)).

6.4 Nature and mechanisms of other nucleic-acid-binding agents

The triphenylmethane dyes are more active against Gram-positive than Gram-negative bacteria but are not sporicidal. They react with acid groups, in particular nucleic acids, within the cell. Intercalation is not involved and the interaction is probably of a non-specific nature.

The isethionate salts of pentamidine, propamidine and their dibromo derivatives (Fig. 3.10(f)) are occasionally used as biocides. They are cationic, are more active at alkaline than at acid pH and are considerably more effective against Gram-positive than Gram-negative organisms. Their precise mechanism of action has not been elucidated: they are nucleic-acid-binding (NAB) agents, but inhibit protein synthesis more effectively than RNA or DNA synthesis. Other NAB agents include

(a)

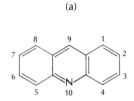

ACRIDINE
(International Union of Chemistry numbering)

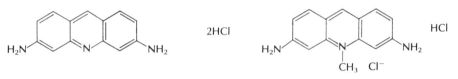

2HCl

HCl

3,6, Diaminoacridine dihydrochloride

3,6-Diamino-10-methylacridinium
chloride hydrochloride

Acriflavine

HCl,H₂O

H₂SO₄, 2H₂O

9-Aminoacridine hydrochloride
(Aminacrine hydrochloride)

3,6-Diaminoacridine hemisulphate
(Proflavine)

(b)   (c)

Figure 3.26   (a) Chemical structure of acridines. Secondary structures of (b) normal
DNA and (c) of DNA containing intercalated proflavine molecules.

the QACs and chlorhexidine, but they act in this manner only at high concentrations.

6.5 Nature and mechanisms of ribosome-binding agents

Sulphydryl reagents dissociate 70S ribosomes into 30S and 50S subunits, the effect being dependent on concentration, time of contact and especially of temperature. The effect may be reversed by β-mercaptoethanol. Hydrogen peroxide also dissociates 70S ribosomes into their ribosomal units, and this effect can be reversed by Mg^{2+} ions.

6.6 Nature and mechanisms of agents that interact with cytoplasmic protein

Several biocides at high concentrations, e.g. chlorhexidine, QACs and phenolics, cause cytoplasmic protein coagulation. The mode of action of iodine and iodophors has, surprisingly, been little studied, but evidence to date suggests that they react with bacterial cytoplasmic protein. They will also combine with thiol groups in enzymes. Biocides already described, such as alkylating agents (Section 6.1) and cross-linking agents (Section 6.2), also combine with proteins.

The halogen iodine is bactericidal and sporicidal but is highly toxic and stains materials. The activity of low, but not of high, concentrations is reduced significantly by organic matter. Iodine is far more effective at acid than at alkaline pH, the active moiety being diatomic iodine (I_2) although hypoiodous acid (HI) makes some contribution. At alkaline pH, the formation of the hypoiodide (HI^-) ion, which possesses feeble activity, and of the inactive iodate (IO_3^-), iodide (I^-) and triiodide (I_3^-) ions explains the decreased efficacy of iodine as the pH rises. Iodophors (literally, iodine carriers) are compounds in which iodine is solubilized by means of an appropriate surface-active agent. They retain the germicidal action, but not the undesirable properties, of iodine, and are active over a wide pH range.

6.7 Nature and mechanisms of agents that interact with identifiable chemical groups

Diverse types of biocides react with identifiable chemical groups within the bacterial cell. Some of these biocides have already been described, e.g. alkylating agents (Section 6.1) and cross-linking agents (Section 6.2). Other types of biocides are included here.

6.7.1 *Oxidizing agents*

Hypochlorites are powerful antimicrobial agents, being bactericidal and sporicidal. Activity is decreased markedly by organic matter, and the hypochlorites are more active at acid than at alkaline pH because undissociated hypochlorous acid (HClO) is the active moiety. *N*-chloro (organic chlorine) compounds containing the =N—Cl group, e.g. chloramine-T, dichloramine-T, dichloroisocyanurates and trichloroisocyanurates, hydrolyse in water to produce an imino (=NH) group.

Oxidizing agents, such as halogens, may progressively oxidize thiol groups to disulphides (Fig. 3.21(a)), sulphoxides (Fig. 3.21(b)) or disulphoxides (Fig. 3.21(c)). The primary sites of cellular inactivation by chlorine-releasing agents are the thiol groups in the membrane and cytoplasmic regions of bacteria.

Whereas the first reaction may be reversible, the latter two are not. The halogens can also halogenate essential groups in proteins, such as amino groups, with the formation of halogenamines. Chlorine dioxide has been found to inhibit bacterial protein synthesis.

The most important peroxygens are hydrogen peroxide (H_2O_2) and peracetic acid (CH_3COOOH). Hydrogen peroxide (H_2O_2) is a powerful oxidizing agent, water-miscible and possessing bactericidal and sporicidal properties. Its activity results from the formation of free hydroxyl radicals ($^{\cdot}OH$) which oxidize thiol groups in enzymes and proteins. Effects elsewhere have also been noted, however, e.g. on the bacterial cell surface and on ribosomes (Section 6.5). Peracetic acid combines the active oxygen characteristics of a peroxide within an acetic acid molecule, existing with these in equilibrium. It decomposes ultimately to acetic acid and peroxide, which is further broken down to water and oxygen, and is claimed to be more powerful than hydrogen peroxide. Peracetic acid is believed to disrupt thiol groups in proteins and enzymes.

Ozone (O_3) possesses potent bactericidal and sporicidal properties, and could prove to be an important sterilizing agent. It reacts with amino acids, RNA and DNA, but its exact mechanism of action is unknown.

6.7.2 *Metal derivatives*

Derivatives of mercury, silver, copper and tin are used as antiseptics, disinfectants and preservatives. Inorganic mercurials such as mercuric chloride are now little used as biocides. However, organomercurials such as phenylmercuric nitrate (PMN), phenylmercuric acetate (PMA) and thiomersal (Fig. 3.27) are widely used as preservatives in the pharmaceutical and cosmetic fields. They are bactericidal but not sporicidal. As described earlier (Section 5.4.1.2, Fig. 3.20) they combine strongly with —SH groups in bacterial enzymes, an action that can be reversed by the addition of a thiol-containing compound.

The mode of action of silver salts resides in the Ag^+ ion, which reacts strongly with —SH groups in proteins (both functional and structural) in the bacterial cell to produce mercaptides (Fig. 3.28). Silver inhibits glucose, succinate and lactate

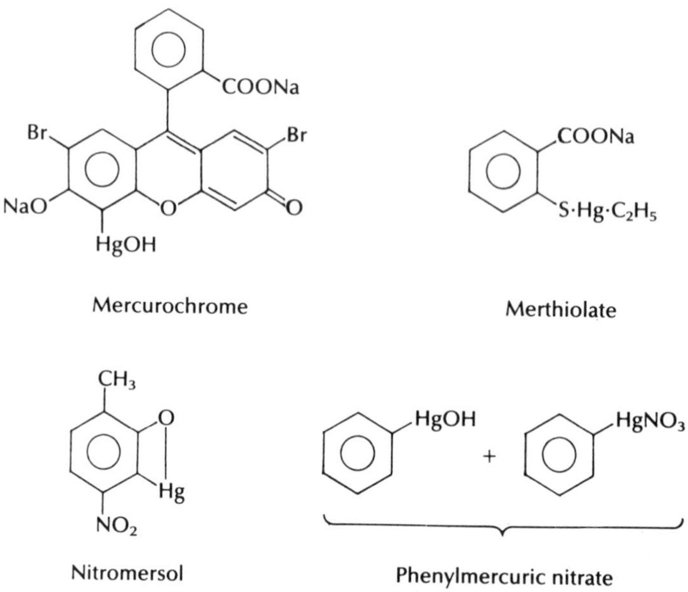

Figure 3.27 Organomercurials: mercurochrome, thiomersal (merthiolate), nitromersol and phenylmercuric nitrate.

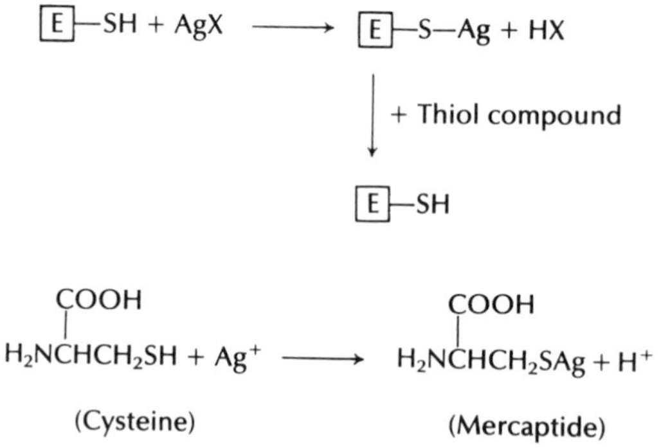

Figure 3.28 Interaction of Ag^+ with sulphydryl (thiol, $-SH$) groups to produce a mercaptide and its reversal by a thiol compound: E, enzyme; AgX, silver compound.

oxidation, this inhibitory effect being prevented by reduced glutathione. The thiol group derived from cysteine residues is essential for the activity of many enzymes. Silver salts also produce structural changes to the cell envelope of *Ps. aeruginosa*, and the Ag^+ ion reacts preferentially with the bases rather than the phosphate groups in DNA.

Sodium sulphadiazine (NaSD) is water soluble and is thus absorbed rapidly from wounds. Silver sulphadiazine (AgSD) and other compounds were produced in the 1960s in attempts to retard the absorption of sulphadiazine (SD). SD is a weak acid and reacts with silver nitrate to produce the water-insoluble AgSD. Unlike other silver salts, AgSD does not react rapidly with chloride or thiol groups or with protein, and unlike other sulphonamides its activity is not eliminated by *para*-(4-) aminobenzoic acid (PABA). AgSD promotes the rapid healing of wounds and is useful in the treatment of severe burns.

AgSD binds to cell components, especially DNA, as evidenced from studies with [110]Ag-labelled AgSD in which the label was found only in the DNA fraction. AgSD is not mutagenic and the fact that its activity is not reduced by PABA demonstrates that its mode of action differs from that of other sulphonamides. Unlike silver nitrate, AgSD produces surface protuberances (blebs) in sensitive bacteria.

Copper(II) salts combine with thiol groups in bacterial enzymes but are used mainly as fungicides and algicides.

6.8 Conclusions

It is difficult to ascribe a single target site to many of the biocides discussed in this section. The reasons for this are twofold: (i) several biocides are highly reactive and combine with several types of receptor molecules so that the mechanism of inactivation is often unclear; (ii) the paucity of information available for some of the biocides.

7
Combination of biocides

There are several recorded instances where a combination of biocides has been shown to have an enhanced antibacterial effect over each component used alone. For example, acid or alkali plus alcohol is sporicidal, whereas any one of these agents used alone does not kill spores.

In the medical context, it might be necessary to enhance disinfectant or antiseptic activity, whereas in the pharmaceutical or cosmetic context there is often a need to preserve complex formulations. A single preservative might be ineffectual and it is in such cases that a combination of preservatives might be beneficial.

7.1 Possible responses

By analogy with antibiotic combinations, the effect on bacteria of two biocidal agents acting together may be

(i) additive, in which the combined action is not greater than the activities of the individual compounds,

(ii) synergistic, in which the combined effect is greater than the sum of the individual effects of either agent acting alone, or

(iii) antagonistic, where the overall effect may be reduced

Fig. 3.29(a) shows the effects of two biocides, A and B, acting alone, whereas Fig. 3.29(b) depicts the three possible effects outlined above when A and B are acting in combination.

7.2 Measurement of synergy

There are several ways of measuring synergy.

(1) Minimum inhibitory concentrations (MICs) of all available combinations can be determined. The MIC of each agent (A, B) employed singly is determined, after which subMICs of A and B are used in combinations. From this, it is possible to obtain fractional inhibitory concentrations (FICs) of A and B:

$$\text{FIC of A} = \frac{\text{inhibitory concentration of A in mixture}}{\text{MIC of A alone}}$$

$$\text{FIC of B} = \frac{\text{inhibitory concentration of B in mixture}}{\text{MIC of B alone}}$$

From this $\Sigma\text{FIC} = \text{FIC(A)} + \text{FIC(B)}$. Then, if $\Sigma\text{FIC} = 1$, the effect is additive, if $\Sigma\text{FIC} = <1$, there is synergy, and if $\Sigma\text{FIC} = >1$, an antagonistic effect is obtained.

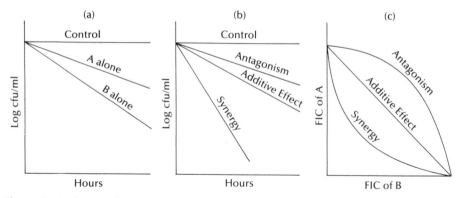

Figure 3.29 Bacterial responses towards two biocides (A, B) acting alone and in combination: (a), (b) bactericidal effects (in (a) the biocides are acting alone, in (b) in combination); (c) isobologram.

It is clear that a ΣFIC value can be obtained for each combination of A and B tested. It is also possible to plot an isobologram (Fig. 3.29(c)) of the results obtained, the shape of the curve expressing graphically the nature of the response. These procedures are identical to those which have been developed for assessing the *in vitro* efficacy of antibiotic combinations.

(2) Minimum bactericidal concentrations (MBCs) of all available combinations can be determined. By analogy with the first method, ΣFBC = FBC(A) + FBC(B), where FBC is the fractional bactericidal concentration.

(3) In the product preservation procedure the activities of two preservatives alone and in combination in, for example, a cosmetic or pharmaceutical formulation are compared. The method is, in essence, an extension of method (2), since synergy here involves a significant decrease in killing time for the combination compared with the individual preservative components. There is, however, the advantage of working with the products themselves.

7.3 Examples of combinations

Several examples are known in which synergy is produced from two biocides acting together. These include

(i) chlorocresol and phenylmercuric nitrate,
(ii) chlorhexidine and aromatic alcohols (Section 7.4)
(iii) the use of extremes of polymer length, e.g. $n = 4$ plus $n = 35$, of PHMB biocide formulations,
(iv) phenoxyethanol and a paraben, and
(v) lipophilic acids and fatty alcohols.

7.4 Mechanisms of synergy

Mechanisms of synergy are by no means well defined. It would be expected that biocides having the same mode of action would, in combination, produce an additive effect, e.g. methyl plus propyl parabens, whereas a mixture of two biocides with different mechanisms of action would provide a synergistic or antagonistic response. For example, phenol would disrupt the bacterial cytoplasmic membrane, thereby making phenylmercuric nitrate (example (i), Section 7.3) better able to reach its target site of −SH groups in cytoplasm-located enzymes and proteins.

Extensive studies have been undertaken with a mixture of chlorhexidine and aromatic alcohols (example (ii), Section 7.3). These have demonstrated that

(i) the uptake of ^{14}C-chlorhexidine, used alone, was maximal within 20 seconds although the rate of cell death was much slower,
(ii) neither benzyl alcohol (BZA) nor phenoxyethanol (POE) had any effect on chlorhexidine uptake,

(iii) unlabelled chlorhexidine had a marked effect on ^{14}C-benzyl alcohol uptake, but there was no direct link between uptake and cell death,

(iv) the lethal activity of moderate chlorhexidine concentrations was potentiated by BZA or PEA, and

 (v) there was an enhanced rate of leakage of ^{86}Rb from rubidium-loaded cells and K^+ and pentose (indicative of gross membrane damage) when chlorhexidine was used with an aromatic alcohol.

Taken as a whole, these findings imply that the bisbiguanide and BZA or PEA act synergistically at the level of the cytoplasmic membrane.

When permeabilizing agents (Section 4.2) are involved, the mechanism of synergy is a weakening of the outer membrane barrier in Gram-negative bacteria with greater uptake of a second agent.

8
Uptake of biocides by bacteria

Most biocides are bactericidal because of their effects on the cytoplasmic membrane and/or the innermost parts of the bacterial cell. This means that they must cross the cell wall of Gram-positive bacteria or the outer membrane of Gram-negative organisms. In contrast to antibiotics (see Chapter 2), there are no specific receptor molecules or permeases to assist biocide penetration. Most biocides enter Gram-positive bacteria readily, probably by passive diffusion and partitioning, as described for antibiotics (Fig. 2.39). Such organisms are frequently more sensitive to biocides than are Gram-negative cells.

The initial interaction of a biocide occurs at the bacterial cell surface. Such interaction has been studied predominantly by use of two procedures, adsorption and microelectrophoresis. The uptake of biocides can be measured by means of a radioactive chemical, e.g. ^{14}C-chlorhexidine gluconate, or by chemical analysis of the amount remaining in solution after mixing with a dense bacterial suspension. A plot of the amount taken up, e.g. as micrograms per milligram of dry weight against the equilibrium concentration, can be used to explain the nature of the interaction of the biocide and the cell surface. For example, Fig. 3.30 depicts various types of adsorption isotherms, which are considered further in Table 3.6. ^{14}C-chlorhexidine is rapidly bound to Gram-positive and -negative bacterial cells, being maximally bound within 30 seconds; in contrast, its bactericidal effect is slower, from which it has been concluded that damage to organisms is necessary before the compound reaches its target site(s) within the cell. In other words, the comparatively slow rate of kill could result from a slow passage across the outer membrane to inner membrane targets.

The surface of bacterial cells is negatively charged. Biocides that interact strongly with the cell surface can reduce the charge and even, in some cases,

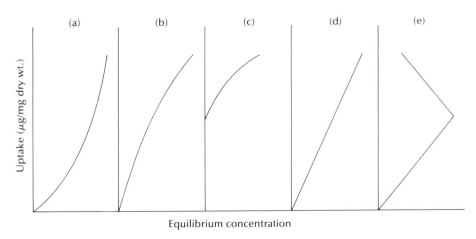

Figure 3.30 Adsorption isotherms (see text and Table 3.6).

reverse it (Fig. 3.31). This effect is pronounced with cationic biocides such as chlorhexidine.

Useful though adsorption isotherms and changes in electrophoretic mobility are, however, in assessing the effects of biocides on the cell surface, they have been of only marginal use in measuring the uptake of biocides into bacterial cells. A more comprehensive use of radioactive biocides with subsequent fractionation of treated cells might yield useful information. Alternatively, the energy-dispersive analysis of X-rays procedure may be used to attempt to ascertain the location of a biocide intracellularly.

As pointed out in Section 3.2, mycobacteria are less sensitive than cocci to biocidal action. It would be instructive to examine the uptake of biocides into mycobacteria and to compare this with other, less resistant, types of organisms.

Gram-negative bacteria are more complex than cocci because of the presence of an outer membrane (Chapter 1). The cell surface of smooth Gram-negative bacteria is hydrophilic in nature, a property that can be readily demonstrated by measuring the partitioning of cells into a water-immiscible hydrocarbon solvent. Deep rough (heptoseless) mutants, on the other hand, are much more hydrophobic. Thus, wild-type (smooth) strains are resistant to hydrophobic antibiotics and biocides whereas deep rough mutants are much more sensitive (Chapter 6). The entry of biocides into Gram-negative bacteria is not a well-researched topic. It is believed that cationic bactericides such as the QACs and chlorhexidine are able to promote their own entry by displacing divalent metal cations in the outer membrane. Nevertheless, QACs are considerably more effective against deep rough mutants than wild-type strains of *E. coli* whereas chlorhexidine shows almost equal activity against both. There is little evidence to date that OmpC and OmpF porins are utilized by biocides. Hydrophobic-type

Table 3.6 Types of adsorption isotherms

Adsorption isotherm pattern	Example(s)	Explanation
S	Monohydric phenols	Moderate intermolecular attraction, orientate vertically; solvent molecules compete strongly for substrate sites
L (Langmuir)	Resorcinol, QACs	As more sites on cell surface are filled, becomes increasingly difficult for biocide to find a vacant site; no tendency for multilayer formation
H (high affinity)	Iodine from iodophor	Biocide almost completely adsorbed
C (constant partition)	Phenols, chlorhexidine, alexidine	Biocide penetrates more readily into adsorbate than does the solvent
Z	Phenoxyethanol	Sharp break in isotherm, followed by an increasing uptake: biocide promotes breakdown in structure of adsorbate, thereby generating new adsorbing sites

biocides (phenolics and higher esters of *p*-hydroxybenzoic acid) utilize the hydrophobic lipid bilayer pathway but information about their mechanism of penetration across the outer membrane is sparse. Generally, it is likely that biocide uptake onto the cell wall/outer membrane is a passive process.

Many of the biocides described in this chapter affect the cytoplasmic membrane (Tables 3.4 and 3.5). Consequently, they are able to penetrate to the cytoplasm where further damage to nucleic acids and/or proteins may occur. Other biocides are not membrane-active but as they affect target sites deeper within the cell they must be able to cross the inner (cytoplasmic) membrane. The mechanism by which this is achieved is unknown.

9
Mechanisms of actions: general conclusions

Many of the biocides described in this chapter are potent antibacterial agents with an effect that often embraces more than one target site. This is exemplified in Fig. 3.32 and in Table 3.7, the latter summarizing the responses elicited at different biocide concentrations. The effect on different target sites contrasts with the

Table 3.7 Mechanisms of action of biocides[a]: a summary

Site of action[b]	1	2	3	4	5	6	7	8	9	10	11	12	13	14	15[c]	16	17	18
1. Cell wall/outer membrane																		
Lysis								?						?	?			
Cross-linking												L						
Increased permeability (Gram-negative)					L	L										L		
2. Cytoplasmic membrane																		
General membrane permeability (leakage)		L	L	L	L	?									I	L		L
Lysis (of protoplasts/spheroplasts)	L				I										L	I		
Membrane potentials										H							L	
Electron transport chain	L									L								L
ATPase					H					L								
Enzymes with thiol groups											L			L			L	
3. Cytoplasm																		
Alkylation				L			L	L	L	H			L	L	H			
Cross-linking								L	L									
Intercalation		L																
Coagulation					H				I	H		L	L		H	H	H	
Thiol groups				L			L		L			L	L	L				
Amino groups				L			L							L				
Ribosomes											L							

Key to headings:

1, acids (organic); 2, acridines; 3, alcohols; 4, β-propiolactone; 5, chlorhexidine; 6, EDTA; 7, ethylene oxide; 8, formaldehyde; 9, glutaraldehyde; 10, hexachlorophane; 11, hydrogen peroxide; 12, hypochlorites; 13, iodine and iodophors; 14, mercury compounds; 15, phenols; 16, QACs; 17, silver salts; 18, TCS.

[a] Activity is usually concentration dependent: L denotes activity elicited at low, H at high, concentrations; I, intermediate concentration; ?, unclear whether effect occurs.

[b] See also appropriate section of text.

[c] Some phenolics: see Section 5.1.1.

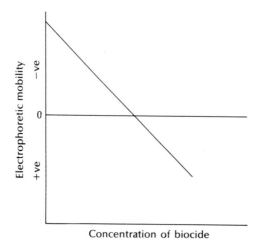

Figure 3.31 Electrophoretic mobility of bacterial cells and the reversal of surface charge at higher biocide concentrations.

situation for antibiotics which often have a specific molecular target and specific uptake systems for delivery to the target (Chapter 2). Furthermore, biocides are usually toxic to mammalian cells and lack the selectively toxic properties associated with antibiotics used as chemotherapeutic agents (Chapter 2). For this reason, these biocides are employed as antiseptics, disinfectants and preservatives and are not used systemically for the treatment of infections.

Further reading

General works on antisepsis, disinfection and preservation

Ascenzi, J. M. (1996). *Handbook of Disinfectants and Antiseptics*. Marcel Dekker, Inc., New York.

Block, S. S. (1991). *Disinfection, Sterilization and Preservation*. Fourth edition, Lea & Febiger, Philadelphia.

Branen, A. L. & Davison, J. M. (1983). *Antimicrobials in Foods*. Marcel Dekker, New York.

Gardner, J. F. & Peel, M. M. (1991). *Introduction to Sterilization, Disinfection and Infection Control*. Churchill Livingstone, Edinburgh.

Gould, G. W. (1989). *Mechanisms of Action of Food Preservation Procedures*. Elsevier Applied Science, London.

Hugo, W. B. (1971). *Inhibition and Destruction of the Microbial Cell*. Academic Press, London.

Kabara, J. J. (1984). *Cosmetic and Drug Preservation: Principles and Practice*. Marcel Dekker, New York.

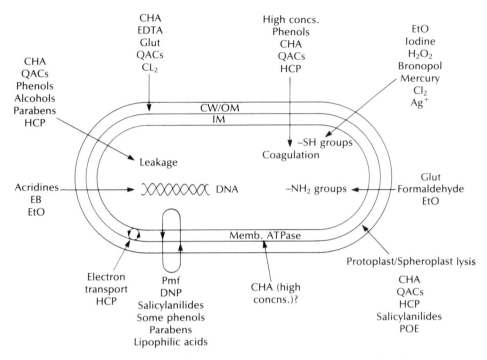

Figure 3.32 Target sites and effects of biocides. Note that many biocides have more than one target site. The figure should be read in conjunction with Table 3.7 which summarizes concentration-dependent effects. EDTA, ethylenediamine tetraacetic acid; Glut, glutaraldehyde; CHA, chlorhexidine diacetate (or gluconate); QACs, quaternary ammonium compounds; HCP, hexachlorophane; Cl_2, chlorine-releasing agents (e.g. hypochlorites); POE, phenoxyethanol; DNP, dinitrophenol; EB, ethidium bromide; EtO, ethylene oxide; CW, cell wall (Gram positive); OM, outer membrane (Gram negative); IM, inner (or cytoplasmic) membrane; PMF, proton-motive force.

Linton, A. H., Hugo, W. B. & Russell, A. D. (1987). *Disinfection in Veterinary and Farm Animal Practice*. Blackwell Scientific Publications, Oxford.

Lueck, E. (1980). *Antimicrobial Food Additives*. Springer-Verlag, New York.

Payne, K. R. (1988). *Industrial Biocides*. Critical Reports on Applied Chemistry, Volume 23. John Wiley & Sons, Chichester.

Russell, A. D., Hugo, W. B. and Ayliffe, G. A. J. (1992). *Principles and Practice of Disinfection, Preservation and Sterilization*. Second edition. Blackwell Scientific Publications, Oxford.

Russell, N. J. and Gould, G. W. (1991). *Food Preservatives*. Blackie, Glasgow and London.

General works on mechanisms of action

Albert, A. (1979). *Selective Toxicity*. Fifth edition. Methuen & Co., London.

Cherrington, C. A., Hinton, M., Mead, G. C. and Chopra, I. (1991). Organic acids: chemistry, antibacterial activity and practical applications. *Advances in Microbial Physiology* **32**: 87–108.

Gould, G. W. (1988). Interference with homeostatis-food. *FEMS Symposium*, No. 44, pp. 220–228. Bath University Press, Bath.

Hugo, W. B. (1992). Disinfection mechanisms. In *Principles and Practice of Disinfection, Preservation and Sterilization* (eds A. D. Russell, W. B. Hugo and G. A. J. Ayliffe). Second edition, pp. 187–210. Blackwell Scientific Publications, Oxford.

Russell, A. D. & Hugo, W. B. (1988). Perturbation of homeostatic mechanisms in bacteria by pharmaceuticals. *FEMS Symposium*, No. 44, pp. 206–219. Bath University Press, Bath.

Russell, A. D. & Hugo, W. B. (1994). Antimicrobial activity and action of silver. *Progress in Medicinal Chemistry* **31**: 351–371.

Russell, J. B. (1992). Another explanation for the toxicity of fermentation acids at low pH: anion accumulation versus uncoupling. *Journal of Applied Bacteriology* **73**: 363–370.

Salton, M. R. J. (1968). Lytic agents, cell permeability and monolayer penetrability. *Journal of General Physiology* **52**: 227S–252S.

Mechanisms of action: selected papers

Broxton, P., Woodcock, P. M., Heatley, F. & Gilbert, P. (1984). Interaction of some polyhexamethylene biguanides and membrane phospholipids in *Escherichia coli*. *Journal of Applied Bacteriology* **57**: 115–124.

Chawner, J. A. & Gilbert, P. (1989). A comparative study of the bactericidal and growth inhibitory activities of the bisbiguanides alexidine and chlorhexidine. *Journal of Applied Bacteriology* **66**: 243–252.

Chawner, J. A. & Gilbert P. (1989). Interaction of the bisbiguanides chlorhexidine and alexidine with phospholipid vesicles: evidence for separate modes of action. *Journal of Applied Bacteriology* **66**: 253–258.

Chopra, I., Johnson, S. C. & Bennett, P. M. (1987). Inhibition of *Providencia stuarti* cell envelope enzymes by chlorhexidine. *Journal of Antimicrobial Chemotherapy* **19**: 743–751.

Collier, P. J., Ramsey, A. J., Austin, P. & Gilbert, P. (1990). Growth inhibitory and biocidal activity of some isothiazolone biocides. *Journal of Applied Bacteriology* **69**: 569–577.

Eklund, P. (1985). The effect of sorbic acid and esters of *p*-hydroxybenzoic acid on the protonmotive force in *Escherichia coli* membrane vesicles. *Journal of General Microbiology* **313**: 73–76.

Lambert, P. A. & Hammond, S. M. (1973). Potassium fluxes. First indications of membrane damage in micro-organisms. *Biochemical and Biophysical Research Communications* **54**: 796–799.

Richards, R. M. E., Zing, J. Z., Gregory, D. W. & Marshall, D. (1993). Investigation of cell envelope damage to *Pseudomonas aeruginosa* and *Enterobacter cloacae* by dibromopropamidine isethionate. *Journal of Pharmaceutical Sciences* **82**: 975–977.

Salmond, C. V., Kroll, R. G. & Booth, I. R. (1984). The effect of food preservatives on pH homeostasis in *Escherichia coli. Journal of General Microbiology* **130**: 2845–2850.
Sofos, J. N., Pierson, M. D., Blocher, J. C. & Busta, F. F. (1986). Mode of action of sorbic acid on bacterial cells and spores. *International Journal of Food Microbiology* **3**: 1–17.

Mycobactericidal agents: selected publications

Best, M., Sattar, S. A., Springthorpe, V. S. & Kennedy, M. E. (1990). Effects of selected disinfectants against *Mycobacterium tuberculosis. Journal of Clinical Microbiology* **28**: 2234–2239.
Russell, A. D. (1992). Mycobactericidal agents. In *Principles and Practice of Disinfection, Preservation and Sterilization* (eds A. D. Russell, W. B. Hugo & G. A. J. Ayliffe). Second edition, pp. 246–253. Blackwell Scientific Publications, Oxford.

Enhancement of activity: selected publications

Ayres, H. M., Furr, J. R. & Russell, A. D. (1993). A rapid method of evaluating permeabilizing activity against *Pseudomonas aeruginosa. Letters in Applied Microbiology* **17**: 149–151.
Denyer, S. P., Hugo, W. B. & Harding, M. D. (1985). Synergy in preservative combinations. *International Journal of Pharmaceutics* **29**: 245–253.
Modha, J., Barrett-Bee, K. J. & Rowbury, R. J. (1989). Enhancement by cationic compounds of the growth inhibitory effect of novobiocin on *Escherichia coli. Letters in Applied Microbiology* **8**: 219–222.
Vaara, M. (1992). Agents that increase the permeability of the outer membrane. *Microbiological Reviews* **56**: 395–411.
Vaara, M. & Jaakkola, J. (1989). Sodium hexametaphosphate sensitizes *Pseudomonas aeruginosa*, several other species of *Pseudomonas* and *Escherichia coli* to hydrophobic drugs. *Antimicrobial Agents and Chemotherapy* **33**: 1741–1747.

CHAPTER FOUR

Sporistatic and sporicidal agents: their properties and mechanisms of action

1
Introduction

The bacterial spore is a complex entity consisting of one or two spore coats, a cortex and an inner spore core (protoplast), with an exosporium present in some types (see Chapter 1).

In this chapter, we shall consider how some chemicals, including antibiotics, destroy spores or inhibit their development. To encompass the topic adequately, it is necessary to describe the complex processes leading, first, to the development of a spore and then to the production of a vegetative cell.

2
Sporulation

Sporulation is a multiphase process leading to the production of a spore from a vegetative cell (summarized in Table 4.1 and Fig. 4.1). The process involves the formation of a refractile cell which is resistant to many treatments, both chemical and physical.

2.1 Stages in sporulation

There are seven stages (I–VII) in sporulation and stage 0 represents the end of logarithmic growth of the vegetative cell culture. There appears to be a link between the induction of sporulation and a specific stage in the DNA replication cycle. Furthermore the successful termination of existing rounds of DNA replication is essential for sporulation to occur.

In the pre-septation stage (stage I), the nuclear material in *Bacillus* spp. is present as an axial filament, although this is rarely observed in clostridia. Stage I terminates when a septum starts to form asymmetrically in the mother cell,

Table 4.1 Summary of stages in the sporulation process[a]

Stage	Characteristics
0	Vegetative cell.
I	Pre-septation: DNA in axial filament form. Extra-cellular products (including amylase, proteases and antibiotics) appear.
II	Septation: separation of chromosomes resulting in asymmetric cell formation.
III	Engulfment of forespore: membrane of developing spore becomes completely detached from that of mother cell to give the spore protoplast. Appearance of characteristic enzymes.
IV	Cortex formation begins to be laid down between the two membranes of the protoplast. Refractility begins to develop, commencement of peptidoglycan synthesis (see text in present chapter and in Chapter 7).
V	Synthesis of spore coats. DPA deposition, uptake of Ca^{2+}. Development of resistance to organic solvents (octanol, chloroform).
VI	Spore maturation: coat material becomes more dense, increase in refractility, development of heat resistance.
VII	Lysis of the mother cell, and liberation of the mature spore.

[a]This should be read in conjunction with Fig. 4.1. Additional information appears in the text.

resulting in the synthesis of the forespore membrane and the compartmentalization of DNA in stage II.

The forespore protoplast is engulfed in stage III, the result being the existence of the forespore as a discrete cell, bounded by two forespore membranes (see Chapter 7), the former later becoming the cytoplasmic membrane of the germinated spore.

Cortex synthesis takes place in stage IV. During this phase, peptidoglycan is laid down between the two membranes, possibly in two phases. The first phase involves the synthesis of vegetative-cell-type polymer and the second the formation of spore-specific peptidoglycan. In conditional cortexless mutants of *B. sphaericus*, the spore cortex cannot be detected unless the medium contains diaminopimelic acid (see Chapter 7).

Synthesis of the spore coats takes place in stage V, although deposition of at least part of these layers occurs during earlier stages. In addition, dipicolinic acid (DPA) accumulates and there is an uptake of calcium.

Stage VI is termed spore maturation. Here, the coat material becomes more dense in appearance, spore refractility increases and heat resistance develops. In addition, dehydration occurs and the spore shows resistance to ionizing and ultraviolet radiation. Liberation of the spore takes place in stage VII.

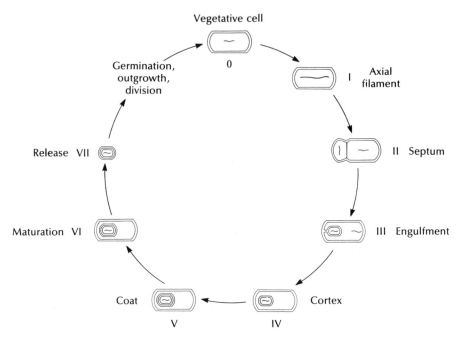

Figure 4.1 Stages in the sporulation process: 0, vegetative cell; I, axial filament formation (pre-septation); II, formation of septum; III, engulfment (encystment, envelopment) of forespore; IV, cortex formation; V, coat formation; VI, maturation (development of refractility and heat resistance); VII, release of forespore.

2.2 Initiation and commitment to sporulation

Commitment, a specific term, may be defined as 'the point of no return', i.e. the events associated with the developing system cannot be reversed. In contrast, initiation is a different term since it implies the commencement of the sporulation process, but not necessarily that the process is committed to forming a mature spore.

Early sporulation events can be overcome and growth resumed if the sporulating culture is diluted into fresh medium, whereas later the cells are committed to continue the sporulation process.

3
Germination

Activation is a treatment resulting in a spore which is poised for germination but which still retains most spore properties (e.g. heat resistance, lack of stainability,

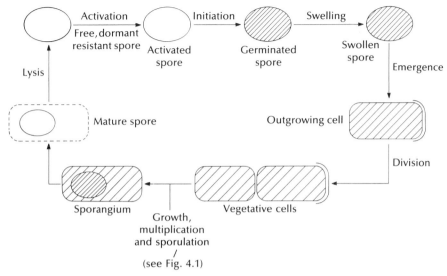

Figure 4.2 Diagrammatic representation of the cycle of bacterial endospore formation, germination and outgrowth. (Reprinted with permission from Gould (1984).)

refractility). Activation is thus responsible for the breaking of dormancy in spores but is reversible (Fig. 4.2). The most widely used procedure is heat activation in which spores are exposed to a sublethal heat treatment; it must, however, be pointed out that not all types of bacterial spores require heat activation for the breaking of dormancy, since many types undergo germination rapidly when placed in an appropriate germination medium.

Germination itself is an irreversible process and is defined as a change of activated spores from a dormant to a metabolically active state within a short period of time (Fig. 4.2). The first biochemical step in germination is termed a biological trigger reaction. This initiation process can be induced by metabolic or non-metabolic means, although it is now generally believed that the trigger reaction is allosteric in nature rather than metabolic, because the inducer does not need to be metabolized to induce germination. The most widely studied nutrient and non-nutrient germinants are L-alanine and calcium dipicolinate (CaDPA), respectively.

Initiation of germination is followed rapidly by various degradative changes in the spore, leading within a short period of time to outgrowth (Section 4). An early event is loss of heat resistance with a decrease in optical density a late marker. Intermediate events are changes in stainability, a decrease in refractility so that phase-bright spores take on the appearance of phase-dark forms (Fig. 4.3), a decrease in dry weight and the release of DPA.

(a)   (b)

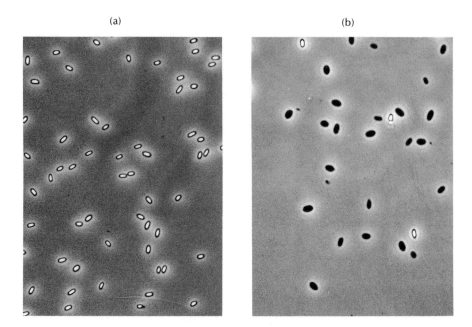

Figure 4.3   (a) Phase-bright spores, (b) phase-dark germinated spores.

Within the first 20–30 min of germination, all of the small acid-soluble proteins (SASPs; Chapter 1) are degraded to amino acids. This degradation is initiated by an endoprotease known as germination protease (GPR), an enzyme synthesized during sporulation just prior to SASP synthesis. There is also a complete reaction between 3-phosphoglycerate (3-PGA; Chapter 1) and phosphoglycerate mutase (PGM).

3.1 Germination (*ger*) mutants

It has been well demonstrated that *B. subtilis* spores will respond to at least two types of germinative stimuli:

(a) alanine (ALA) or certain analogues, e.g. valine;
(b) asparagine plus glucose, fructose and a potassium salt (AGFK).

By varying the germinant incorporated into an enrichment medium, different types of conditionally-defective mutants have been isolated. These have been classified (by phenotype and by map location) thereby defining a number of *ger* genes. Whereas *ger*A mutants germinate normally in AGFK but not in ALA, *ger*B mutants will not germinate in the former but will in the latter. As pointed out later (Section 5.3) antibiotics that inhibit specific biosynthetic processes, e.g. DNA, protein syntheses, are without effect on germination. Germination thus involves proteins already present in the mature spore. Most of the *ger* genes have been cloned and sequenced so that some of the proteins involved in the germination process have been defined.

It is not known whether or how these *ger* mutants could provide evidence about the mechanisms of inhibition of germination by antibacterial agents.

3.2 Control of germination

Inhibition and control of spore germination are important considerations in many fields, including food preservation, where control of clostridium species, and especially *Cl. botulinum*, is so important. Chemical antibacterial agents that act as germination inhibitors, as well as those possibly having an effect on the trigger mechanism, are considered in Section 5.3.

4
Outgrowth

Outgrowth is defined as the development of a vegetative cell from a germinated spore. It takes place in a synchronous and orderly manner when germination is carried out in a medium that supports vegetative growth. After germination, germinated spores become swollen and shed their coats to allow the young, vegetative cells to emerge, elongate and divide. There is a sequential alteration in cell structure, with an initial swelling followed by emergence from the spore coat, elongation of the emergent organism and, finally, cell division. During outgrowth, RNA synthesis occurs soon after the termination of the germination phase and is closely followed in *Bacillus* spp. by the onset of protein synthesis, and then DNA synthesis which occurs later. Dormant and newly germinated spores possess little or no functional mRNA. Spores do, however, contain a DNA-dependent RNA polymerase which is responsible for synthesizing the mRNAs necessary for transcription of early functions during outgrowth.

Cell wall synthesis commences after RNA and protein synthesis but before DNA synthesis and coincides with swelling of the germinated spore.

5
Mechanisms of action of sporistatic and sporicidal agents

Antibacterial agents that can be considered in this context include chemotherapeutic drugs and biocides (food and pharmaceutical preservatives, and antiseptics and disinfectants). Biocides can be classified into two groups depending

Table 4.2   Bactericidal, sporistatic and sporicidal properties of some antibacterial agents

Bactericidal agents that are sporistatic	Bactericidal agents that are sporicidal	Comment
Group A Phenols Organic acids and esters (parabens) QACs Biguanides Organomercurials Alcohols	None in group A	Even high concentrations for prolonged periods at ambient temperatures are not sporicidal; may be sporicidal at elevated temperatures.
Group B Glutaraldehyde Formaldehyde Iodine compounds Chlorine compounds Hydrogen peroxide Peroxyacids Ethylene oxide β-Propiolactone	All in group B	Low concentrations are sporistatic; usually much higher concentrations are needed for sporicidal effect.

on whether or not they are sporicidal (Table 4.2). Those in the first group are bactericidal but sporistatic, whereas those in the second group are bactericidal and sporicidal. The bacteriostatic and sporistatic concentrations of a given biocide are usually very similar, whereas sporicidal concentrations are normally much higher than bactericidal ones (Table 4.3). Like bactericidal activity, sporicidal efficacy may be enhanced at elevated temperatures.

5.1   Effects on sporulation

β-Lactam antibiotics inhibit the sporulation septation stage. There are, in fact, two periods of enhanced binding of these drugs during sporulation. The first increase in binding corresponds to the period of spore septum formation and the second to spore cortex formation. There are also two periods of peptidoglycan synthesis during the sporulation process with differences occurring in the structure of the peptidoglycan present in the cortex and the germ cell wall. The cortical peptidoglycan contains a muramic lactam, a unique spore constituent (Fig. 1.18). The two peaks of penicillin binding to sporulating cultures could be due either to the appearance of new penicillin-binding proteins (PBPs) that are specific to the spore itself or to changes in the amounts of PBPs that are also present in

Table 4.3 Activity of biocidal agents against spores and non-sporulating bacteria

Antibacterial agent	Bacteriostatic concentration (μg/ml)	Factor for sporistatic concentration[a]	Bactericidal concentration (μg/ml)	Factor for sporicidal concentration[b]
Benzalkonium chloride	2.5–5	0.3–1.25	20	>25
CPC	2.5–5	0.5–1	20	>25
Chlorhexidine salts	1	1	20	>25
Chlorocresol	200	1	1000	>4
Cresol	800	1.25	3000	>1.7
Phenol	2000	1	5000	>10
PMN	0.1–1	0.2–2	20	>10
Glutaraldehyde	—[c]	—[c]	500	40
Formaldehyde	20	1	<1000	>4–8
Hypochlorite	—[c]	—[c]	1–2	10–20

[a]Sporistatic concentration obtained by multiplying bacteriostatic concentration by factor listed.
[b]Sporicidal concentration obtained by multiplying bactericidal concentration by factor listed (in many cases, e.g. phenolics, not sporicidal at maximum solubility).
[c]Not applicable (interaction with both constituents produces meaningless figures).

vegetative cells of the organism. The latter is believed to be the correct interpretation.

Other antibiotics also inhibit septation (Fig. 4.4). These include D-cycloserine (a specific inhibitor of peptidoglycan synthesis in vegetative cells; see Chapter 2) and chloramphenicol, an inhibitor of protein synthesis (see Chapter 2). The latter also affects the morphology of spores during their formation, since the spores are rounder and smaller, and inhibits the incorporation of amino acids into the protein fraction of sporangia.

Rifampicin is an antibiotic that binds strongly to DNA-dependent RNA polymerase and acts as an inhibitor of RNA synthesis (Chapter 2). Rifampicin blocks spore development at stage III, the encystment (engulfment) stage (Fig. 4.4).

Effects of biocides on sporulation have not been widely studied. Although low levels of chlorhexidine inhibit the sporulation of *B. subtilis* cells, the mechanism involved is poorly understood.

5.2 Effects on mature spores

The antibiotics mentioned in Section 5.1 are not sporicidal, even at high concentrations, but this is hardly surprising since they are inhibitors of specific

	Stage		Antibiotic[a]
	I	Axial filament	
	II	Forespore septum	Pen, Cyclo
Enhance Pen-binding	III	Engulfment	Rif
capacity	IV	Cortex development	Pen, Cyclo
	V	Coat development	
	VI	Maturation	
	VII	Spore release	

Figure 4.4   Effect of antibiotics on the sporulation process. [a]Pen, benzylpenicillin; Cyclo, D-cycloserine; Rif, rifampicin. Antibiotics other than those listed also inhibit the septation stage (see text).

biosynthetic reactions and the spore is virtually metabolically inert. On the other hand, some bactericidal agents, e.g. certain aldehydes, alkylating agents, halogens and oxidizing agents, may be sporicidal. To define the basis by which these agents act, certain questions need to be addressed: whether (a) intact spores are lysed, (b) spore permeability is increased or decreased, (c) surface layers, cortex and core are affected, (d) mutant and coatless forms are more or equally sensitive than parent cells.

Answers to the above questions, together with knowledge about the mechanism of action of bactericides against non-sporing bacteria (Chapter 3), suggest the following mechanisms of sporicidal action (see also Tables 4.4 and 4.5).

5.2.1   Glutaraldehyde

This aldehyde is sporicidal at high concentrations. It is considerably more effective at alkaline than at acid pH, but stability is lost at higher pH fairly rapidly. Novel formulations have attempted to optimize both stability and sporicidal properties.

Interaction at acid and alkaline pH occurs to a considerable extent with the spore surface, but it is believed that at alkaline pH the aldehyde is better able to penetrate into the spore and has an enhanced interaction with amino groups.

The surface of bacterial spores is hydrophobic. Low concentrations of both acid and alkaline glutaraldehyde increase this surface hydrophobicity, presumably as a result of the extensive interaction of glutaraldehyde with the outer spore layers. It is likely that the acid form resides at the cell surface whereas the alkalinating agent, e.g. sodium bicarbonate, assists the increased penetration of the alkaline form into the spore. The major initial effect of bicarbonate is believed to be on the spore exterior, although it is not sporicidal.

Glutaraldehyde is thus likely to seal outer spore layers, with penetration of alkaline dialdehyde into the spore. It also interacts strongly with the cortex and spore protoplast. Penetration and reaction of glutaraldehyde with the cortex may be assisted by the action of divalent metals.

Table 4.4 Sporicidal activity of some aldehydes

Aldehyde	Chemical name	Chemical structure	Sporicidal activity
Formaldehyde	Methanal	H·CHO	Moderate
Glyoxal	Ethanedial	CHO·CHO	Only at 10%
Malonaldehyde	Propanedial	CHO·CH$_2$·CHO	Slight
Succinaldehyde[a]	Butanedial	CHO·(CH$_2$)$_2$·CHO	Slight
Glutaraldehyde	Pentanedial	CHO·(CH$_2$)$_3$·CHO	High[b]
Adipaldehyde	Hexanedial	CHO·(CH$_2$)$_4$·CHO	Slight

[a]One formulation contains both succinaldehyde and formaldehyde and is more active than formaldehyde alone.
[b]Long periods of contact may be necessary.

Table 4.5 Mechanisms of sporicidal action

Sporicidal agent	Site or mechanism of action	Comment
Alkali	Inner spore coat	Outer coat unaffected
Chlorine compounds	Cortex and core	Effect on coats also
Iodine compounds	Presumably, core protein	Further studies needed
Ethylene oxide	Alkylation of core protein and DNA	Both contribute to spore inactivation
β-Propiolactone	Alkylation of core protein and DNA	
Glutaraldehyde	Cortex and core	Effect on coats also
Hydrogen peroxide	Spore core (DNA?)	Effect on coats also
Lysozyme[a]	Cortex	β,1–4 links in peptidoglycan[b]
Nitrous acid[a]	Cortex	At muramic acid residues[b]

[a]Only effective vs coatless spores.
[b]See Fig. 1.18.

5.2.2 Formaldehyde (methanal)

This monoaldehyde probably penetrates into the spore where it combines with RNA, DNA and amino groups in protein. It is much less effective as a sporicidal agent than glutaraldehyde and this is probably related to its weaker interaction with target molecules. In fact, although formaldehyde has long been considered as a sporicidal agent, some doubt has been cast on this belief. It has been possible by appropriate thermal treatments to revive formaldehyde-treated spores, i.e. to resuscitate them from what would have been inactivation.

5.2.3 Other aldehydes

Of the other aldehydes that have been studied (Table 4.4), glyoxal is sporicidal only at high concentrations (10%), whereas malonaldehyde, succinaldehyde and adipaldehyde have only slight activity. Apart from formaldehyde, which is a monoaldehyde, all the compounds listed in Table 4.4 are dialdehydes. It has been proposed that the distance between the two aldehyde groups in glutaraldehyde is optimal for interaction of these groups with target amino and other groups in proteins, enzymes and nucleic acids and hence for sporicidal activity.

A newly introduced aldehyde, orthophthalaldehyde, is claimed to be bactericidal and sporicidal but no information about its mechanism of sporicidal action has been presented to date.

5.2.4 Alkylating agents

The epoxide ethylene oxide is a gaseous sporicide. Its action is slow but can be accelerated by a rise in temperature. The most important factor governing its activity is relative humidity, although this is a complex relationship depending both on the water content of the organism and on the atmosphere surrounding spores (the 'microenvironment') rather than the overall humidity.

β-Propiolactone (BPL) in both liquid and vapour phases is sporicidal under suitable conditions. Relative humidity is the most important factor influencing the activity of BPL vapour, although again the moisture content and location of water in the spore are of paramount importance.

Ethylene oxide and β-propiolactone probably kill spores by combining with specific groups in proteins and by alkylation of guanine in DNA (Figs 3.24 and 3.25).

5.2.5 Chlorine-releasing agents

There are various types of chlorine-releasing agents (CRAs), e.g. sodium and calcium hypochlorites, sodium dichloroisocyanurate (NaDCC) and chloramine-T. Recent studies have improved our knowledge of the effects of CRAs on spores and of the manner in which they are believed to achieve their sporicidal action.

There are three possible target sites, i.e. the spore coat(s), cortex and core. CRAs release coat protein and increase spore sensitivity to the enzyme lysozyme, the target site of which is cortex peptidoglycan (see Chapter 1, Fig. 1.18). The extent of coat protein extraction appears to correlate with sporicidal activity, with sodium hypochlorite being more effective on both counts than sodium dichloroisocyanurate (NaDCC). Chloramine-T releases some coat protein but is sporicidal only at very high concentrations. The presence of sodium hydroxide enhances CRA-induced coat extraction. However, coatless spores retain their viability and thus an effect of CRAs on the coats *per se* is unlikely to explain their mechanism of action.

Hypochlorites induce DPA leakage, suggesting an increase in spore permeability and a site of action on the cortex. The cortex controls the water content of the core and hence the heat resistance of spores; pretreatment of spores with sublethal concentrations of chlorine increases their sensitivity to moist heat, a finding that supports the contention of an action of hypochlorites on the cortex. Furthermore, sodium hypochlorite produces a substantial release of cortex hexosamine, the extent increasing with increasing concentration of available chlorine. NaDCC releases less hexosamine, but in the presence of sodium hydroxide it induces a release equivalent to that from hypochlorite-treated spores. Chloramine-T, even in the presence of alkali, has little effect on hexosamine release.

Thus, the relative sensitivity of spores to antibacterial agents that exert an oxidizing action is related to the ability of these compounds to produce coat and cortex degradation. The result of such degradation would allow chlorine to reach the spore core and cause death by oxidation of essential proteins.

The sporicidal activity of CRAs is generally attributed to undissociated hypochlorous acid (HOCl) and not the hypochlorite ions (OCl$^-$) with which it is in equilibrium. NaDCC dissociates in water to yield two HOCl molecules with a pH-dependent equilibrium being set up between HOCl and OCl$^-$ as with Na OCl solutions. In solutions buffered to the same pH, the degree of dissociation of HOCl and thus sporicidal activity should be the same in both cases. In fact, as pointed out above, NaOCl is a more powerful bactericidal and sporicidal agent. It has been suggested that such differences may be attributable to differences in chemical structure, dissociation equilibria and activity as *N*-chlorinating agents, thereby affecting ability (as pointed out above) to produce coat and cortex degradation and hence an effect on the spore core.

5.2.6 *Iodine-releasing agents*

The mechanism of the sporicidal action of iodine is not completely understood. However, iodine can bind to bacterial proteins and oxidize them.

Iodine, in aqueous or alcoholic solution, and iodophors are effective sporicides. The concentration of free iodine (I$_2$) in iodine solutions and in iodophors determines sporicidal activity. Antiseptic strength iodine solutions are not regarded as sporicidal.

Apparently contradictory results have been obtained with Lugol's iodine solution and an iodophor, polyvinylpyrrolidine–iodine (PVP-I), because, above a certain concentration, bactericidal and sporicidal activity is reduced markedly.

Their relative sporicidal activity can, in fact, be explained by considering the chemistry of aqueous solutions. There are at least eight separate equilibrium reactions in such solutions; however, since it is deemed that non-complexed iodine

(I_2) is responsible for the antibacterial activity, only two equilibria need be considered, i.e.

$$I_2 \rightleftharpoons I + I^-$$ (1)

$$I_2 + I^- \rightleftharpoons I_3^-$$ (2)

According to Oswald's dilution law, as the dilution of an aqueous I_2–KI solution (Lugol's) increases, the concentration of I_2 decreases as dissolution of the I_3^- species increases in order that k remains constant. Thus as the concentration of available iodine decreases, so the concentration of non-complexed iodine also decreases thereby reducing the rate of sporicidal activity.

The equilibrium situation is more complex in the presence of PVP. PVP chains form complexes with iodine, in addition to which the PVP-I coils formed by the non-ionic surfactant associate reversibly, non-complexed iodine being retained in the spaces between the units. As the mixture is further diluted, these complexes dissociate into smaller subunits. The number of spaces available for non-complexed iodine decreases and so the concentration of non-complexed iodine increases. The amount of non-complexed iodine initially increases with increasing total available iodine up to a maximum value (about 0.1% by weight PVP-I), and then increases upon further dilution. Sporicidal activity of PVP-I shows a similar pattern with an increased effect as PVP-I concentration rises up to a maximum value of 0.05% by weight PVP-I (about 45 ppm available iodine). At PVP-I concentrations above 0.1% by weight (about 90 ppm available iodine) there is a decreasing rate of kill comparable with very low PVP-I levels. This again suggests a decrease in non-complexed iodine concentration or, conversely, an increase in iodine complexation. A summary is provided in Fig. 4.5.

5.2.7 Hydrogen peroxide

Its target site remains a matter for conjecture, with some evidence suggesting the outer spore layers and other evidence the spore core. Copper (Cu^{2+}) ions potentiate the sporicidal action of peroxide and are bound to the core, providing a tentative conclusion that the core may be the major site of peroxide action.

Hydrogen peroxide removes coat protein from *Cl. bifermentans* but prior coat removal markedly increases its effectiveness against these spores, although *B. cereus* spores are affected to a smaller extent. Activation of peroxide to hydroxyl radicals (˙OH) is necessary for sporicidal action and this might explain the synergistic effect observed with the combined use of peroxide and ultraviolet radiation.

Dithiothreitol (DTT) is a disulphide-bond-reducing agent that substantially removes the outer coat. DTT-treated spores of *Cl. perfringens* are much more susceptible to peroxide-induced lysis in the presence of Cu^{2+} ions than are untreated spores and this lysis is reduced in the presence of ˙OH scavengers. Peroxide and Cu^{2+} alone do not produce lysis of cortical fragments but do so in

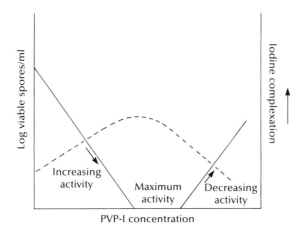

Figure 4.5 Sporicidal activity of the iodophor, polyvinyl-pyrrolidone-iodine (PVP-I). Solid line, sporicidal activity; broken line, content of non-complexed iodine.

combination. It has been suggested that peroxide may react with Cu^{2+} bound to cortex peptidoglycan, thereby generating ˙OH radicals. These would be formed at the region near the germ cell wall and be responsible for causing protoplast lysis.

Thus, peroxide affects spore coats in some organisms but this is insufficient to explain its sporicidal action. Its major effects are undoubtedly on the cortex and core, with the latter tentatively being pinpointed as its major target site. The sporicidal activity of hydrogen peroxide probably results from generation of hydroxyl radicals which cleave the DNA backbone within the core. This mechanism of action is also consistent with the observation that spores $(\alpha^- \beta^-)$ deficient in α/β-type small acid-soluble proteins (SASPs: Section 3, see also Chapter 1) are much more sensitive to peroxide than are mature spores.

5.2.8 Peracetic acid

Peracetic acid has sporicidal activity. Furthermore, it has the advantage of eventually breaking down to innocuous decomposition products, oxygen and acetic acid. Its effects against obligate anaerobes are, in fact, potentiated by one of these (oxygen). Although its mechanism of sporicidal action is unknown, peracetic acid might disrupt sulphydryl ($-SH$) and disulphide ($S-S$) bonds.

5.2.9 Ozone

Ozone is sporicidal, and because it is converted ultimately to oxygen there are no toxic residues. Ozone probably kills by interacting with amino acids, RNA and DNA, but the exact mechanism is unknown.

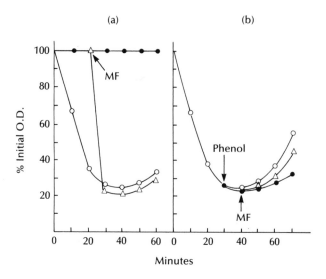

Figure 4.6 Reversibility by membrane filtration (MF) of the germination-inhibitory effect of 0.15%w/v phenol on *B. subtilis* spores: (a) phenol added at zero time; (b) phenol added at 30 min; O——O, control (phenol absent): ●——●, phenol treatment without filtration; △——△, phenol treatment followed by filtration, 10 or 20 min later. The initial decrease in optical density represents germination, the subsequent increase denotes outgrowth, which is followed (not shown here) by vegetative cell multiplication.

Clearly, much remains to be learned about the mechanism of action of sporicidal agents, and whether these mechanisms differ substantially from their effects on non-sporulating bacteria.

　　A summary of current information on the mechanisms of action of sporicidal agents is presented in Table 4.5.

5.3　Effects on germination

Several inhibitors prevent spore germination. They include phenols and cresols, parabens, alcohols, glutaraldehyde and formaldehyde (Tables 4.2, 4.3). An example of the effect of phenol is presented in Fig. 4.6(a). It is noticeable that amongst these agents (Fig. 4.7) only glutaraldehyde and formaldehyde are sporicidal. The effects of inhibitors of spore germination may be reversible, as demonstrated for phenol in Fig. 4.6(a,b). Thus, there appears to be a loose binding to sites on the spore surface, since washing is sufficient to dislodge this antibacterial agent (also cresols, parabens, alcohols and formaldehyde at low concentrations). As might be expected from a powerful cross-linking agent, however, the effects of glutaraldehyde on spore germination are not readily reversible. Low concentra-

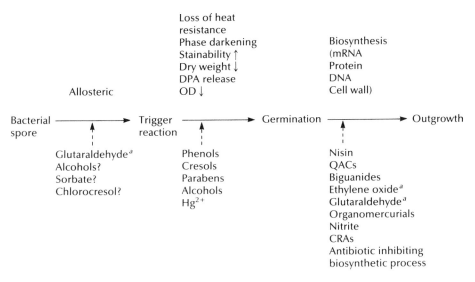

Figure 4.7 Sites of action of antibacterial agents during germination and outgrowth. Note that some agents, e.g. glutaraldehyde, can act at more than one stage. [a], sporicidal agent when used at high concentrations. ↑, increase; ↓, decrease; OD, optical density; CRAs, chlorine-releasing agents.

tions of both acid and alkaline forms of the dialdehyde exert an early effect on germination.

As pointed out in Section 3, initiation of germination is followed by rapid degradative changes. Thus, antibiotics that inhibit specific biosynthetic processes are without effect on germination. The reasons for the lack of effect of QACs and chlorhexidine on the germination process are unknown.

5.3.1 *Inhibition of the trigger reaction*

Some antibacterial agents inhibit the L-alanine-induced trigger reaction. There are four possible mechanisms of inhibition (Fig. 4.8): (a) inhibition of uptake of L-alanine by competition for binding sites on the spore, (b) prevention of passive diffusion of L-alanine into the spore, (c) sealing of the spore surface, and (d) a later, unexplained, inhibition of the L-alanine-stimulated trigger effect. Glutaral-dehyde at high concentrations causes (c), whereas (a) appears to be unaffected. Mechanism (b) might occur as a consequence of (c). Sorbic acid probably inhibits the trigger reaction, although the mechanism is unknown; it affects a number of sites on germinating and developing spores of *Cl. botulinum* rather than acting on a single site. Sorbic acid is a competitive inhibitor of L-alanine- or L-cysteine-induced germination, this effect being reversible.

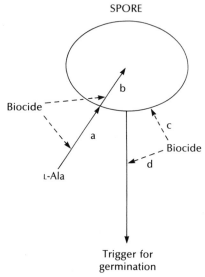

Figure 4.8 Possible mechanisms of inhibition of the trigger reaction. See text for comments.

5.4 Effects on outgrowth

As previously stated (Section 4), outgrowth is the development of a vegetative cell from a germinated spore. During outgrowth, several biosynthetic processes are stimulated and it is, therefore, not surprising that various antibiotics are inhibitory during these stages. Thus, β-lactams inhibit a late stage involving synthesis of vegetative cell-type peptidoglycan, whereas the earliest stages of mRNA, protein and DNA syntheses are inhibited by, respectively, actinomycin D, chloramphenicol or tetracycline, and mitomycin C (Fig. 4.9).

Some disinfectant-type compounds are also effective during outgrowth. These include the following (Fig. 4.7).

(a) QACs and chlorhexidine are sporistatic and not sporicidal. They are bound strongly to spores but do not inhibit germination.
(b) Parabens inhibit outgrowth only at concentrations higher than those active at the germination stage.
(c) Chlorine prevents outgrowth at moderate, but germination only at high, concentrations.
(d) Sublethal concentrations of ethylene oxide inhibit outgrowth, but not germination.
(e) Organomercury preservatives, such as phenylmercuric nitrate, are sporistatic agents.

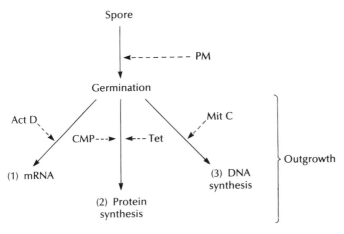

Figure 4.9 Effect of antibiotics on germination and outgrowth: Act D, actinomycin D; CMP, chloramphenicol; Mit C, mitomycin C; PM, polymyxin; Tet, tetracycline.

(f) Nisin, tylosin and subtilin have been considered for use as food preservatives. Nisin is produced by *Streptococcus lactis*; it is not firmly adsorbed by spores and is not sporicidal although it is inhibitory, probably by virtue of its effect on outgrowth. Subtilin has a similar action, and tylosin also is inhibitory and not sporicidal. Their possible usefulness as preservatives thus resides in their ability to inhibit rather than to destroy spores. Tylosin inhibits protein synthesis in non-sporulating bacteria and might have a similar effect during outgrowth. The antibacterial action of nisin is restricted to its action on outgrowing spores, because the growth of vegetative cells of many *Bacillus* spp. is unaffected by much higher nisin concentrations.

(g) Glutaraldehyde inhibits outgrowth at concentrations well below those needed for sporicidal activity. It is thus an inhibitor of both germination and outgrowth.

(h) Sodium nitrite has an unusual, not fully explained, effect on bacterial spores. When heated in laboratory media at temperatures in excess of 90 °C, nitrite is more inhibitory to clostridial spores than unheated or filter-sterilized nitrite. This effect, known as the Perigo effect, is also observed in some, but not all, cooked meats to which the salt has been added. Outgrowth is inhibited by nitrite. Because the effect of nitrite is pH dependent, it has been proposed that undissociated nitrous acid is the active form of the preservative. Current opinion, however, is that nitric oxide (NO) is the active form: this reacts with iron found in a variety of functional proteins, e.g. the haem iron of cytochrome oxidase in aerobic bacteria. In clostridia, a non-haem iron (probably pyruvate: ferredoxin oxidoreductase, PFR) is a target. Nitrite also inhibits other enzymes, particularly those containing −SH groups, but this inhibition occurs only at high concentrations.

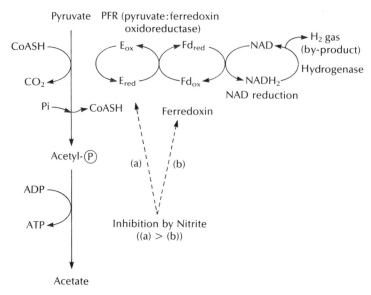

Figure 4.10 The phosphoroclastic system and inhibition by sodium nitrite: $\textcircled{P}$, high-energy phosphate; CoASH, coenzyme A; E_{ox}, oxidized pyruvate:ferredoxin oxidoreductase; E_{red}, reduced oxidoreductase.

These conclusions are based, in part, on the enhancement of the bacteriostatic activity of nitrite by the reducing agent ascorbic acid and the involvement of ferric complexes in the reaction of nitrite with foods. Ferredoxins, iron-containing bacterial proteins, are essential for electron transport, metabolic activity and energy production in *Cl. botulinum*. Inhibition of the phosphoroclastic system, one metabolic pathway requiring ferredoxins and other iron proteins, reduces the ability of the cell to germinate and outgrow. Nitrite inhibits ferredoxin and, especially, PFR (Fig. 4.10). Nitrite has a much greater effect on hydrogen production (hydrogenase is particularly sensitive: Fig. 4.10) from *Cl. botulinum* if autoclaved with ferrous sulphate and cysteine prior to the addition of the organism. It is believed that a nitrosyl–cysteyl ferrate complex is formed which is similar to, or identical with, a nitrite reaction in certain types of canned meats; the anticlostridial effect of this complex might explain the nature of the Perigo effect alluded to above.

5.5 Biocide-induced sublethal spore injury

Spore injury can be expressed during germination or outgrowth or during growth following outgrowth. Germination and outgrowth are distinct developmental events and a number of types of injury have been reported. For instance, hypochlorite injures spores of *Cl. bifermentans* so that they become susceptible to lysozyme-induced germination. Sublethal spore damage may be manifested as an increased susceptibility to 'stressing agents' (such as alkali, non-ionic, anionic and cationic agents) that are not sporicidal.

Little is known about the manner in which biocides produce sublethal spore damage and at which stage such injury is expressed. Spores can be considered as being irreversibly damaged, i.e. killed, when a key lethal target site (sites) is (are) inactivated beyond any possibility of repair. Less critical sites will also be damaged, so that survivors of a sublethal biocide treatment will be deficient in some of these secondary sites. This will be expressed as an increased degree of injury to a subsequent stressing procedure.

Possible mechanisms involved in the repair of biocide-induced sublethal injury are considered in Chapter 7.

6
Conclusions

Comparatively few antibacterial compounds show sporicidal activity although all are sporistatic, inhibiting germination and/or outgrowth. Studies on mechanisms of action demonstrate that the cortex, spore membranes and spore protoplast are major target sites. Nevertheless, much less information is available about the manner of inactivation of spores than of non-sporulating bacteria. There is considerable scope for further investigations leading to improved knowledge of modes of sporicidal action, since this is one approach to the ultimate development of better sporicides.

It is clear that disinfectants and preservatives are generally inhibitors of either germination or outgrowth. Where an agent inhibits both processes, it is often the case that wide concentration differences are necessary for the duality of action. What has yet to be properly examined, however, is the reason for the different effects. Why, for example, should some inhibitors but not others prevent the degradative changes that are a feature of germination? Is their effect linked to the type and degree of binding to the spore? Are some, but not other, disinfectants capable of preventing the binding of L-alanine associated with the trigger reaction of germination? Answers to such questions would be illuminating.

Further reading

General works on sporicidal and sporistatic agents

Bloomfield, S. F. & Arthur, M. (1994). Mechanisms of inactivation and resistance of spores to chemical biocides. *Journal of Applied Bacteriology (Symposium Supplement)* **76**: 91S–104S.

Cook, F. K. & Pierson, M. D. (1983). Inhibition of bacterial spores by antimicrobials. *Food Technology* **37**(11): 114–126.

Gould, G. W. (1984). Injury and repair mechanisms in bacterial spores. In *The Revival of Injured Microbes* (eds M. H. E. Andrew & A. D. Russell). Society for Applied Bacteriology Symposium Series No. 12, pp. 199–220. Academic Press, London.

Gould, G. W., Russell, A. D. & Stewart-Tull, D. E. S. (eds) (1994). *Fundamental and Applied Aspects of Bacterial Spores. Journal of Applied Bacteriology (Symposium Supplement)*.

Hurst, A. & Gould, G. W. (1983). *The Bacterial Spore*, Volume 2. Academic Press, London.

Russell, A. D. (1982). *The Destruction of Bacterial Spores*. Academic Press, London.

Russell, A. D. (1990). Bacterial spores and chemical sporicidal agents. *Clinical Microbiology Reviews* **3**: 99–119.

Sporicidal and sporistatic agents: selected papers

Gorman, S. P., Hutchinson, E. P., Scott, E. M. & McDermott, L. M. (1983). Death, injury and revival of chemically treated *Bacillus subtilis* spores. *Journal of Applied Bacteriology* **54**: 91–99.

Power, E. G. M. & Russell, A. D. (1989). Uptake of L-(^{14}C)-alanine to glutaraldehyde-treated and untreated spores of *Bacillus subtilis*. *FEMS Microbiology Letters* **66**: 271–276.

Power, E. G. M., Dancer, B. N. & Russell, A. D. (1989). Possible mechanisms for the revival of glutaraldehyde-treated spores of *Bacillus subtilis* NCTC 8236. *Journal of Applied Bacteriology* **67**: 91–98.

Russell, A. D., Jones, B. D. & Milburn, P. (1985). Reversal of the inhibition of bacterial spore germination and outgrowth by antibacterial agents. *International Journal of Pharmaceutics* **25**: 105–112.

Sofos, J. N., Pierson, M. D., Blocher, J. C. & Busta, F. F. (1986). Mode of action of sorbic acid on bacterial cells and spores. *International Journal of Food Microbiology* **3**: 1–17.

Stewart, G. S. A. B., Johnstone, K., Hagelberg, E. & Ellar, D. J. (1981). Commitment of bacterial spores to germinate. A measure of the trigger reaction. *Biochemical Journal* **198**: 101–106.

Williams, N. D. & Russell, A. D. (1991). The effects of some halogen-containing compounds on *Bacillus subtilis* endospores. *Journal of Applied Bacteriology* **70**: 427–436.

General works on spores, genetics and germination

Berkeley, R. C. W. & Ali, N. (1994). Classification and identification of endospore-forming bacteria. *Journal of Applied Bacteriology (Symposium Supplement)* **76**: 1S–8S.

Foster, S. J. & Johnstone, K. (1990). Pulling the trigger, the mechanism of bacterial spore germination. *Molecular Microbiology* **4**: 137–141.

Johnstone, K. (1994). The trigger mechanism of spore germination: current concepts. *Journal of Applied Bacteriology (Symposium Supplement)* **76**: 17S–24S.

Moir, A., Kemp, E. H., Robinson, C. & Corfe, B. M. (1994). The genetic analysis of bacterial spore germination. *Journal of Applied Bacteriology (Symposium Supplement)* **76**: 9S–16S.

Moir, A. & Smith, D. G. (1990). The genetics of bacterial spore germination. *Annual Review of Microbiology* **44**: 531–553.

CHAPTER FIVE

Genetic and biochemical basis of acquired resistance to chemotherapeutic antibiotics

1
Introduction

1.1 The distinction between intrinsic and acquired resistance

Antibiotics have been available for the treatment of bacterial infections for some 50 years. However, even during the initial period surrounding the commercial development of benzyl penicillin, it was realized that certain bacteria were not killed by the antibiotic, i.e. that antibiotic-resistant bacteria existed. Today, two broad categories of antibiotic resistance are recognized: intrinsic (or intrinsic insusceptibility) and acquired. These categories also apply to biocides (see Chapters 6 and 7). The term 'intrinsic' is used to imply that inherent features of the cell are responsible for preventing antibiotic action and to distinguish this situation from acquired resistance, which occurs when resistant strains emerge from previously sensitive bacterial populations, usually after exposure to the agent concerned. Intrinsic resistance is usually expressed by chromosomal genes, whereas acquired resistance may result from mutations in chromosomal genes or by acquisition of plasmids and transposons. In the clinical setting, acquired antibiotic resistance results essentially from the selective pressure exerted on bacteria during the administration of antibiotics for chemotherapy.

Intrinsic resistance mechanisms can complicate chemotherapy, for example by restricting the choice of agents available for treatment of certain infections. In particular this applies to infections caused by *Ps. aeruginosa* and mycobacteria, where features of the cell envelope in these organisms result in low permeability of the cell to many agents effective against other bacteria. Nevertheless, acquired antibiotic resistance poses the greatest threat to successful chemotherapy because of its variable and largely unpredictable nature. Consequently, this chapter considers mainly the genetic and biochemical basis of acquired resistance to antibiotics. Readers wishing to gain information on intrinsic antibiotic resistance mechanisms should consult the chapter by Godfrey & Bryan (1984) cited at the end of this chapter under 'Further Reading, Review Articles'.

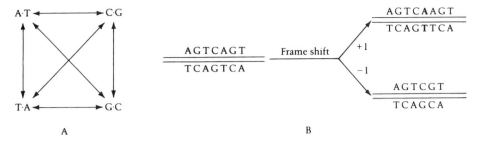

Figure 5.1 Classes of microlesion mutations. A, base pair mutations. Horizontal and vertical lines indicate transversions; diagonal lines indicate transitions. B, frameshift mutations illustrated by possible changes in a length of double-stranded DNA. (Reproduced, with permission, from Ingraham *et al.* (1983) (for reference see 'Further Reading', Chapter 1).)

1.2 Genetic determinants of acquired antibiotic resistance

Antibiotic resistance can be determined by genes that reside in the host cell chromosome, on plasmids or on transposons. The genetic basis of these mechanisms is outlined below. More comprehensive treatments of the topics can be found by consulting 'Further Reading' at the end of this chapter.

1.2.1 *Resistance determined by chromosomal genes*

It is well established that resistance to certain antibiotics can be acquired by chromosomal mutations, i.e. changes in the base sequence of DNA. These mutations can be divided into two broad categories: microlesions, in which a single base pair has been altered, and macrolesions, in which more extensive changes have occurred. Both categories of mutations can be further subdivided.

Microlesions comprise transition, transversion or frameshift mutations (Fig. 5.1). Transition mutations involve base pair changes in which one purine is substituted for another purine, and consequently one pyrimidine for another pyrimidine. Transversions involve substitution of a purine for a pyrimidine and vice versa, whereas addition or loss of one or two base pairs constitutes a frameshift mutation. Macrolesions involve deletions, duplications, inversions and translocations (insertions) (Table 5.1). In many cases, the precise molecular basis of the mutational events leading to antibiotic resistance are known (see later sections in this chapter).

1.2.2 *Resistance determined by plasmids*

Plasmids, i.e. extrachromosomal genetic elements that replicate independently of the chromosome, frequently carry genes that confer antibiotic resistance. The evolution and existence of plasmid-determined resistance mechanisms can be

Table 5.1   Macrolesions of DNA

Type	Molecular change[a]	
Deletion	abcdefghi	abc–ghi[b]
Duplication	abcdefghi	abcdef–defghi
Inversions	abcdefghi	abc–fed–ghi
Translocations (insertions)	abcdefghi	uvw–def–xyz

[a]Letters are meant to indicate genes on double-stranded DNA.
[b]The dash (–) indicates improper junction as in abc–ghi.
Reproduced, with permission, from Ingraham *et al.* (1983) (for reference see 'Further Reading', Chapter 1).

attributed to a number of factors. (a) In the absence of selection pressure by an antibiotic, the majority of cells in a particular population need not maintain plasmids, thereby reducing the biochemical stress on the cell that would otherwise be required for replication and expression of plasmid DNA. Therefore, it is not necessarily essential for every member of a particular species to maintain a particular resistance plasmid. Provided that certain organisms maintain such plasmids, selective pressure following exposure to an antibiotic will ensure that the plasmid-carrying (resistant) progeny will survive and replicate. (b) Genes encoded by plasmids are mobile because plasmids can be transferred both within and between certain species. Thus plasmids can be acquired from other bacteria in addition to inheritance from mother cells. In naturally occurring systems, plasmid transfer occurs by either conjugation or transduction. Conjugation is a process requiring cell-to-cell contact whereby DNA is transferred from a donor bacterium to a recipient. Many Gram-negative bacteria and some Gram-positive bacteria are able to conjugate. The ability to conjugate is normally encoded by conjugative plasmids, many of which also carry antibiotic resistance genes. Although some resistance plasmids are non-conjugative, they may often be transferred (mobilized) to a recipient if they co-inhabit a cell with a conjugative plasmid. Transduction involves the transfer of genes by bacterial viruses (bacteriophages) and plays an important role in the natural transmission of antibiotic resistance plasmids amongst strains of *S. aureus* and of *Strep. pyogenes*. Since the process depends on donors and recipients possessing common, surface-located, bacteriophage receptors, transduction is generally limited to related species and is not effective as a means of plasmid transfer across species boundaries. (c) Plasmids are frequent vectors of transposons (see Section 1.2.3).

1.2.3   *Resistance determined by transposons*

Transposons are mobile DNA sequences capable of transferring (transposing) themselves from one DNA molecule (the donor) to another (the recipient).

Table 5.2 Properties of some antibiotic resistance transposons

Transposon	Size (kilobase pairs)	Resistance encoded
Found in Gram-negative bacteria		
Tn1	5.0	Ampicillin
Tn2	5.0	Ampicillin
Tn3	5.0	Ampicillin
Tn5	5.1	Kanamycin
Tn7	14.0	Streptomycin, trimethoprim
Tn9	2.7	Chloramphenicol
Tn10	9.3	Tetracycline
Tn21	19.0	Streptomycin, sulphonamides (mercury)[a]
Tn1721	11.2	Tetracycline
Found in staphylococci		
Tn551	5.3	MLS group[b]
Tn552	6.1	Penicillin
Tn554[c]	6.7	MLS group, spectinomycin
Tn4001	4.7	Gentamicin, trimethoprim, kanamycin
Tn4002	6.7	Penicillin
Tn4003	3.6	Trimethoprim
Tn4201	6.6	Penicillin
Found in streptococci		
Tn916	16.4	Tetracycline
Found in enterococci		
Tn1546	10.8	Glycopeptides

[a]Resistance to mercury is described in Chapter 6.
[b]MLS group: macrolides, lincosamides and streptogramins.
[c]Tn554 is unusual among transposons in that it does not possess inverted or direct repeat sequences at its termini.

Unlike plasmids, transposons are not able to replicate independently and must be maintained within a functional replicon (e.g. plasmid or chromosome). Transposons contain at their ends short regions that in any particular transposon are almost identical. These regions, or repeats, as they are termed, can lie in the same direction with respect to each other (direct repeats) or, more commonly, in the opposite direction (inverted repeats). The terminal repeats are believed to serve as recognition sequences for transposition enzymes (transposases) in their role of fusing the ends of the transposon with the recipient DNA. The central, or core, regions of transposons lying between the repeated ends frequently carry antibiotic resistance genes (Table 5.2), in addition to genes necessary for the process of transposition itself.

Transposition does not involve the normal host mechanism for recombining

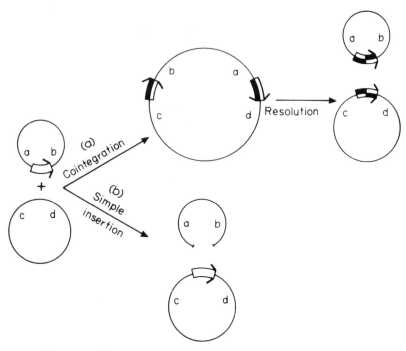

Figure 5.2 Replicative and conservative transposition. The transposable element is indicated by the box. The donor replicon is lettered ab and the target replicon cd. Replicative transposition is shown to involve fusion of the replicons to give a cointegrate. This can be resolved by site-specific recombination between the duplicated copies of the transposable element. The outcome of conservative transposition is simple insertion of the element into the target replicon: the donor replicon may be destroyed or undergo other fates. (Reproduced, with permission, from Wilkins (1988).)

homologous DNA molecules, i.e. the process is *recA* independent. For some elements (such as Tn3) the process of transposition is replicative and involves co-integration or fusion of donor and recipient replicons, which are coupled by two similarly oriented copies of the transposon. The co-integrate is subsequently resolved by transposition encoded resolvase protein (Fig. 5.2). Although certain so-called composite (or class 1) transposons, i.e. Tn5 and Tn10, transpose by a replicative process to give stable co-integrates (Fig. 5.2, path a), movement of these elements more usually involves a conservative, non-replicative mechanism that can result in destruction of the donor replicon following movement of the transposon (Fig. 5.2, path b).

The existence of transposons that confer antibiotic resistance is one factor accounting for the emergence of multiply resistant (multiresistant) bacteria. Since transposons do not require extensive DNA homology to insert into the recipient

Table 5.3 Mechanisms of acquired antibiotic resistance

Mechanism	Examples
(1) Alteration (antibiotic inactivation).	Resistance to aminoglycosides, β-lactams, fosfomycin and chloramphenicol.
(2) Target site in the cell is insensitive to the inhibitor but still able to perform its normal physiological function.	Resistance to aminoglycosides, β-lactams, glycopeptides, macrolides, quinolones, rifampicin, trimethoprim, tetracycline and mupirocin.
(3) Decreased antibiotic accumulation: (a) Impaired uptake (b) Enhanced efflux.	Resistance to many antibiotics. Resistance to tetracycline, macrolides, chloramphenicol and quinolones.
(4) Bypass of antibiotic-sensitive step by duplication of the target site, the second version being insusceptible to drug action.	Resistance to methicillin, sulphonamides, trimethoprim and mupirocin.
(5) Overproduction of target so that higher antibiotic concentrations are needed to inhibit bacterial growth.	Resistance to trimethoprim.
(6) Absence of an enzyme–metabolic pathway.	Resistance to isoniazid in mycobacteria.

molecule, it is possible for bacteria to acquire several different resistance genes by a series of transposon insertions in resident plasmids.

1.3 Biochemical mechanisms of antibiotic resistance

A variety of biochemical mechanisms for antibiotic resistance have been described, the most important of which are summarized in Table 5.3. However, it should be noted at the outset that resistance to a particular antibiotic can result from the combined expression of several of the listed mechanisms. For instance, the efficacy of a β-lactam antibiotic against a Gram-negative organism will be determined by the diffusion rate of the antibiotic across the outer membrane, its susceptibility to any periplasmic β-lactamase that may be present, and finally its affinity for target penicillin-binding proteins (PBPs) located in the cytoplasmic membrane. Consequently, β-lactam resistance may evolve by affecting one or more of these parameters.

The sections that follow discuss the basis of acquired bacterial resistance to the antibiotics described in Chapter 2. As before, the antibiotics are grouped into four classes, i.e. as inhibitors of nucleic acid, protein and peptidoglycan synthesis and of membrane integrity. Acquired resistance of mycobacteria to specific anti-mycobacterial agents is considered separately in Section 6.

2
Resistance to inhibitors of nucleic acid synthesis

2.1 Compounds that interrupt nucleotide metabolism

2.1.1 Sulphonamides

Both chromosomal and plasmid-mediated resistance to sulphonamides have been described.

Chromosomal resistance can result from two mechanisms. The first involves hyperproduction of *p*-aminobenzoic acid (PABA) that overcomes the metabolic block imposed by the inhibition of dihydropteroate synthetase (DHPS). Resistance of this type was observed in certain organisms (e.g. *S. aureus*) soon after the introduction of sulphonamides for therapeutic purposes. Although resistance probably results from chromosomal mutation, the nature of the change respon-sible for PABA hyperproduction has not been examined. A second type of chromosomal resistance involves mutation of DHPS (e.g. in *Strep. pneumoniae*) to produce an altered enzyme for which sulphonamides have a lower affinity than the wild-type enzyme.

Plasmid-mediated resistance to sulphonamides involves a bypass of the drug-sensitive step by duplication of the corresponding target enzyme, the second (plasmid-encoded) version conferring resistance. Two different types (I and II) of plasmid-encoded sulphonamide-resistant DHPS enzymes have been found in Gram-negative bacteria. These enzymes bind sulphonamides about 10 000-fold less efficiently than the chromosomally encoded (sensitive) enzyme, but resistance is achieved without sacrificing the efficiency with which natural substrate is bound.

2.1.2 2,4-Diaminopyrimidines

Chromosomal-, plasmid- and transposon-encoded resistances to the 2,4-diamino-pyrimidine antibiotic trimethoprim have been reported in various bacterial species. Chromosomal mutations have been reported in *E. coli* that cause overproduction of dihydrofolate reductase (DHFR). This leads to trimethoprim resistance because a higher inhibitor concentration is needed inside the cell to decrease the residual enzyme activity to a level below that required to sustain tetrahydrofolic acid synthesis. Furthermore, mutation to enzyme overproduction can act in concert with other mutations rendering the DHFR less susceptible to inhibition by trimethoprim. A clinical *E. coli* isolate of this type, resistant to more than 1000 μg trimethoprim/ml, has been examined in detail. Various mutations were defined in the chromosomal DHFR gene (three transitions, four transversions and one nucleotide addition) that collectively lead to more efficient transcription and translation of the enzymes. A further transversion occurred within the coding region of the gene that resulted in substitution of glycine for tryptophan at amino acid position 30 in the enzyme. This change causes about a threefold increase in resistance of the enzyme to inhibition by trimethoprim.

Plasmid- and transposon-mediated resistance to trimethoprim have been found in a variety of Gram-positive and Gram-negative bacteria. Resistance involves a bypass of the antibiotic-sensitive step by duplication of the chromosomally encoded target DHFR enzyme, the plasmid- or transposon-encoded version conferring resistance. Ten different trimethoprim-resistant bacterial DHFR enzymes have been identified. These enzymes contain altered active sites which render them resistant to trimethoprim.

2.2 Resistance to compounds that inhibit enzymic processes in nucleic acid synthesis

2.2.1 Inhibitors of RNA polymerase

As discussed in Chapter 2, rifampicin inhibits RNA synthesis in bacteria by binding to the β subunit of DNA-dependent RNA polymerase. In *E. coli* acquired resistance to rifampicin results from amino acid substitutions, or small insertions and deletions, within three short highly conserved regions of the β subunit of RNA polymerase. The majority of mutations occur within region II between amino acid residues 507 and 534 (Fig. 5.3). Similar alterations within the corresponding region of the RNA polymerase from strains of *M. tuberculosis* and *M. leprae* are associated with acquired resistance to rifampicin in these organisms (Fig. 5.3).

2.2.2 Inhibitors of DNA gyrase

As discussed in Chapter 2 the quinolone antibiotics inhibit bacterial DNA gyrase activity. Acquired resistance to the quinolones in several organisms (e.g. *E. coli*, *S. aureus*, *Campylobacter jejuni*, *M. tuberculosis*, and *M. smegmatis*) results from point mutations located within a part of *gyr*A (encoding the A subunit of DNA gyrase) termed the quinolone-resistance-determining region (QRDR) (Fig. 5.4). These mutations have been detected alone and in combination, and the level of resistance to quinolones is related to the number and type of mutations accumulated in the QRDR. Exactly how the mutations confer resistance is unknown, but they probably result in conformational changes in DNA gyrase following association of the A and B subunits to form the functional enzyme.

Two other types of chromosomal mutations that confer quinolone resistance have been reported in *E. coli*. *nor*B mutants show low level resistance to some quinolones and other unrelated antibiotics as a consequence of decreased OmpF

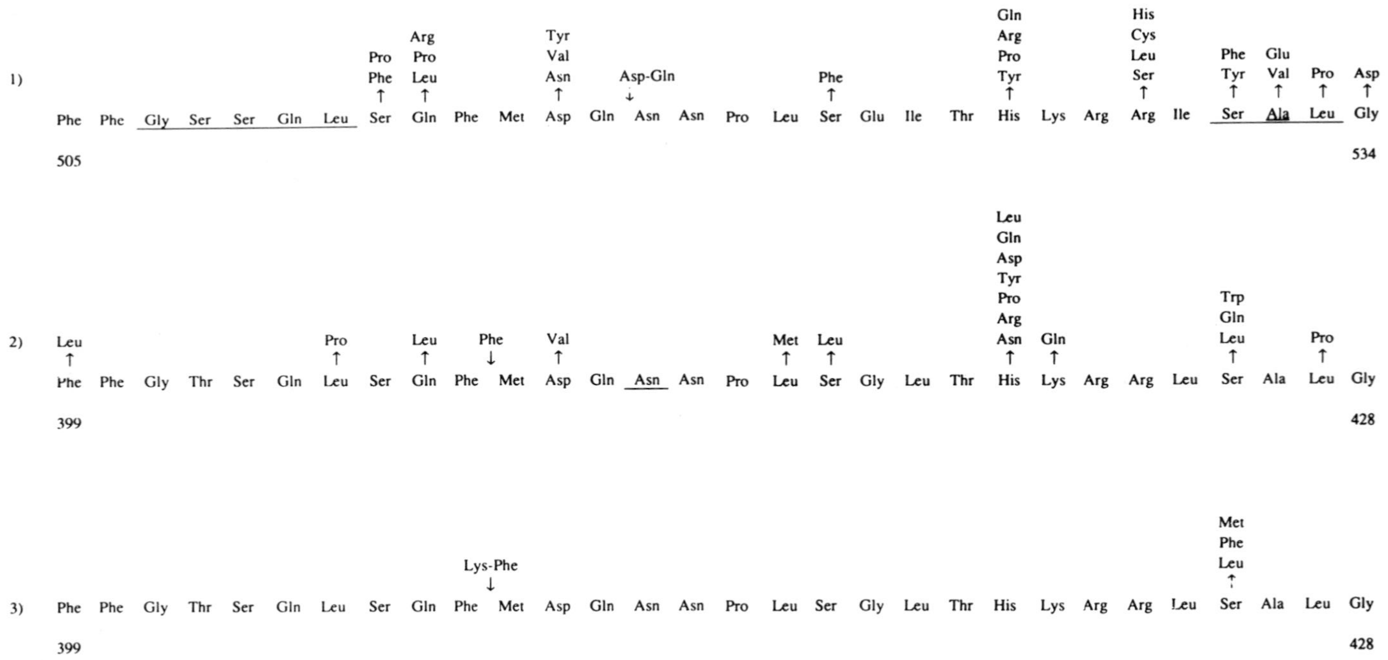

1)

Phe Phe Gly Ser Ser Gln Leu Ser Gln Phe Met Asp Gln Asn Asn Pro Leu Ser Glu Ile Thr His Lys Arg Arg Ile Ser Ser Ala Leu Gly

       Phe↑   Leu↑   Asn↑   Asp-Gln→   Phe↑   Tyr↑   Leu↑   Tyr↑ Val↑ Pro↑

       Pro   Arg   Tyr   Gln   His   Phe Glu

505

534

2)

Phe Phe Gly Thr Ser Gln Leu Ser Gln Phe Met Asp Gln Asn Asn Pro Leu Ser Gly Leu Thr His Lys Arg Arg Leu Ser Ala Leu Gly

399

428

3)

Phe Phe Gly Thr Ser Gln Leu Ser Gln Phe Met Asp Gln Asn Asn Pro Leu Ser Gly Leu Thr His Lys Arg Arg Leu Ser Ala Leu Gly

399

428

Figure 5.3 Amino acid substitutions associated with acquired resistance to rifampicin in the *β* subunit of RNA polymerase from *E. coli* (1), *M. tuberculosis* (2) and *M. leprae* (3). Upward arrows indicate amino acid substitutions, downward arrows insertions and underlined residues deletions.

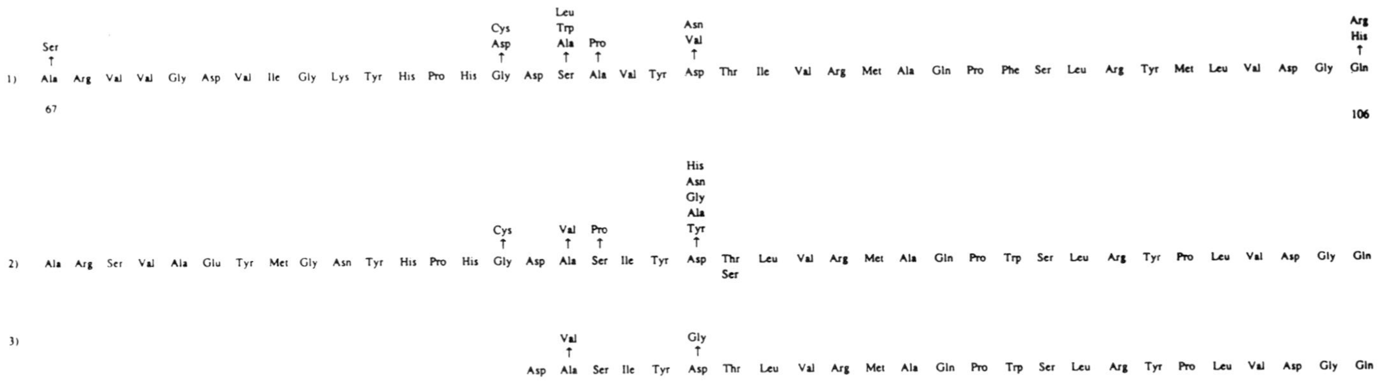

Figure 5.4 Amino acid substitutions associated with acquired resistance to fluoroquinolones in the A subunit of gyrase from *E. coli* (1), *M. tuberculosis* (2) and *M. smegmatis* (3). Upward arrows indicate amino acid substitutions. Codon 88 in *M. tuberculosis* gyrA may display a serine or a threonine in fluoroquinolone-susceptible strains. The GyrA numbering system for *E. coli* has been adopted, amino acid residues 67–106 constituting the quinolone resistance determining region (QRDR).

porin content and *nor*C mutants are less susceptible to certain quinolones (e.g. norfloxacin and ciprofloxacin), but hypersusceptible to others. *nor*C mutants are altered in both OmpF porin content and lipopolysaccharide structure. However, *nor*C mutations do not map in the *omp*F structural gene, but appear to affect a locus that regulates OmpF production. Mutations that produce similar phenotypes to *nor*B and *nor*C have also been identified in other members of the Enterobacteriaceae, e.g. *Klebsiella*, *Enterobacter* and *Serratia*.

Efflux-based resistance to quinolones has recently been described in clinical isolates of *S. aureus* and *Proteus vulgaris*. The gene mediating resistance in *S. aureus*, *nor*A, encodes a membrane protein that displays homology with other transport proteins coupled to the electrochemical proton gradient. A possible pathway for the selection of organisms expressing efflux-based resistance to quinolones has been suggested by recent studies. Several organisms express endogenous chromosomally encoded efflux systems that are to some extent able to remove quinolones from the cell. Selection pressure, exerted by the clinical use of quinolones, may have resulted in the emergence of resistant strains carrying acquired mutations within the endogenous transport system that improve affinity of the efflux system for quinolones.

3
Resistance to inhibitors of protein synthesis

3.1 Mupirocin

As discussed in Chapter 2 mupirocin inhibits isoleucyl tRNA synthetase, thereby leading to depletion of charged isoleucyl tRNA and cessation of protein synthesis. Because it is metabolized *in vivo*, mupirocin is restricted to topical use and it is within isolates of the skin pathogen *S. aureus* that acquired resistance to the antibiotic has been reported.

Resistant staphylococcal strains fall into two categories: those expressing high level resistance (i.e. up to 1000-fold more resistant than sensitive strains) and those expressing moderate level resistance (i.e. up to 60-fold more resistant than sensitive strains). High level resistance is associated with possession of two isoleucyl tRNA synthetases, the normal resident chromosomal enzyme (mupirocin sensitive) and a second mupirocin-resistant enzyme which is usually plasmid encoded. The sequence of the gene encoding the resistant enzyme differs substantially from the native resident gene indicating acquisition from an external, but as yet unidentified, source. Staphylococcal strains exhibiting moderate level resistance do not contain the gene encoding high level resistance and possess only a single resistant isoleucyl tRNA synthetase which has presumably arisen by one or more point mutations in the resident chromosomal gene.

3.2 Aminoglycoside–aminocyclitol group

Acquired resistance to these antibiotics can arise by mechanisms 1 (altered anti-biotic), 2 (altered target site) and 3a (impaired uptake) described in Table 5.3.

The most widespread mechanism of resistance involves modification of the antibiotics by bacterial enzymes that are either plasmid or transposon encoded (Table 5.2). There are three classes of enzymes that modify amino-glycoside–aminocyclitol (AGAC) antibiotics: acetyltransferases (AACs), adenylyl-transferases (AADs) and phosphotransferases (APHs) (Fig. 5.5 and Table 5.4). AACs use acetylCoA as a cofactor, whereas in the phosphorylation and nucleotidylation reactions ATP is the cofactor. The enzymes have been further divided into subtypes (Table 5.4) on the basis of the sites they modify in the antibiotics. For example AAC(6′) enzymes acetylate the 6′-amino group on aminohexose I of susceptible antibiotics (Fig. 5.5).

Unlike other drug resistance mechanisms involving enzymatic inactivation (see, for example, β-lactamases: Section 4.5.3), only small amounts of AGAC antibiotics are modified. This has led to the hypothesis that resistance is achieved by modification of the antibiotic during the process of transport into the cell so that resistance to a particular AGAC antibiotic is dictated by competition between the rates of drug uptake and drug modification. If accumulation occurs at a greater rate than modification, active drug will reach the ribosomes and protein synthesis will cease. However, if the rate of drug modification exceeds that of transport, modified drug is accumulated but does not inhibit protein synthesis, and the organism is resistant. The ability to modify a particular AGAC molecule will depend on the amount of modifying enzyme per cell, and its catalytic ef-ficiency.

AGAC resistance can also be expressed by mechanism 2 (Table 5.3). For instance, mutations in the *rps*L gene of *E. coli* K-12 lead to high level resistance to streptomycin by altering the nature of ribosomal protein S12 thereby preventing the antibiotic from binding to its target. Similar types of chromosomal mutation occur in other bacterial species, e.g. clinical isolates of *S. aureus*.

Acquired resistance to streptomycin in *M. tuberculosis* also arises by mechanism 2 and is associated with mutations in 16S ribosomal RNA, ribosomal protein S12, or a combination of both. Expression of antibiotic resistance arising from point mutations in ribosomal RNA genes is recessive in the majority of bacteria because multiple (7–10) rRNA operons exist. However, slow-growing mycobacteria, such as *M. tuberculosis*, are an exception, possessing only one rRNA operon. Accordingly, direct expression of rRNA mutations occurs in slow-growing mycobacteria of which resistance to streptomycin and macrolides (see Section 3.5.2.1) are examples. Resistance to streptomycin in *M. tuberculosis* can result from single-base substitutions in nucleotides 491, 512, 903 or 904 of 16S ribosomal RNA (for the corresponding *E. coli* numbering add 10). By analogy with *E. coli*, mutations in region 903–904 probably prevent the binding of streptomycin to the

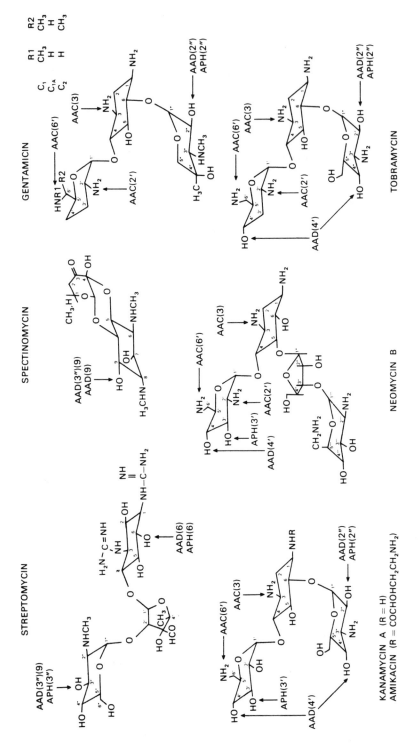

Figure 5.5 Enzymic modifications of aminoglycoside–aminocyclitol antibiotics. The sites of acetylation (AAC), phosphorylation (APH) and adenylylation (AAD) are indicated by arrows.

Table 5.4 Aminoglycoside-modifying enzymes

Enzyme	Modification of									Organisms where found
	Strepto-mycin	Spectino-mycin	Neo-mycin B and C	Kana-mycin A	Amikacin	Tobra-mycin	Genta-micin C sissomicin	Netil-micin	Apra-mycin	
APH(3")	+	−	0	0	0	0	0	0	0	Gram-negative and Gram-positive organisms
APH(6)	+	0	0	0	0	0	0	0	0	Pseudomonas
APH(3')	0	0	+	+	Variable	0	0	0	0	Gram-negative and Gram-positive organisms
APH(2")	0	0	0	+	±	+	+	±	0	Gram-positive organisms
AAD(3")(9)	+	+	0	0	0	0	0	0	0	Gram-negative organisms
AAD(6)	+	0	0	0	0	0	0	0	0	Staphylococci
AAD(9)	−	+	0	0	0	0	0	0	0	Staphylococci
AAD(4')(4")	0	0	+	+	+	+	0	0	0	Staphylococci
AAD(2")	0	0	0	+	Variable	+	+	±	0	Gram-negative organisms
AAC(3)I	0	0	−	−	−	+	+	±	−	Gram-negative organisms
AAC(3)II	0	0	−	±	−	±	+	+	−	Gram-negative organisms
AAC(3)III	0	0	+	+	−	+	+	±	−	Gram-negative organisms
AAC(3)IV	0	0	+	+	0	+	+	+	+	Gram-negative organisms
AAC(2')	0	0	+	0	0	+	+	+	0	Providencia
AAC(6')I	0	0	+	+	+	+	Variable[a]	+	0	Gram-negative organisms
AAC(6')II	0	0	+	+	+	+	Variable[a]	+	0	Moraxella
AAC(6')III	0	0	+	+	±	+	Variable[a]	+	0	Pseudomonas
AAC(6')IV	0	0	±	+	+	+	Variable[a]	+	0	Gram-positive organisms

Symbols: +, modified; −, not modified; ±, poorly modified; 0, substituent necessary for modification absent.

[a] Gentamicin C_1, 0; gentamicins C_{1A} and C_2 and sissomicin, +.

Reproduced, with permission, from Phillips & Shannon (1984).

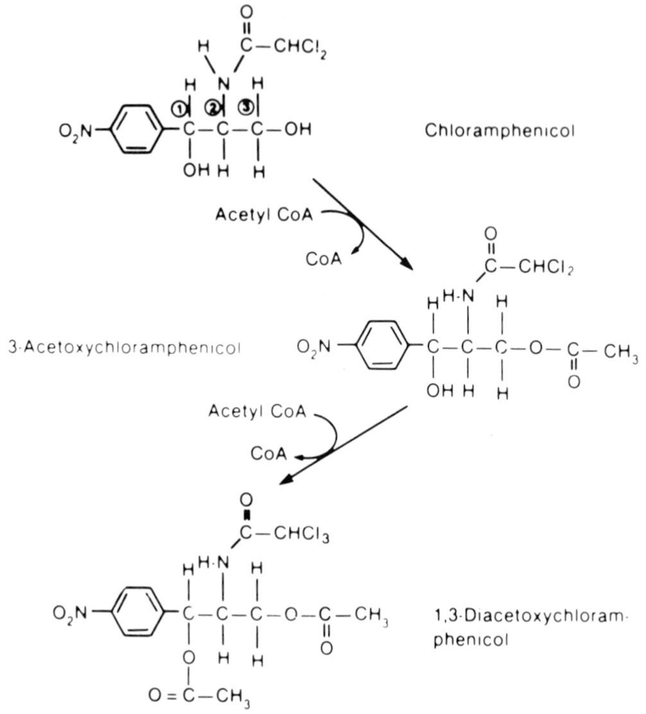

O
‖
H   C–CHCl₂
\ /
H   N   H
①   ②   ③
O₂N–⟨⟩–C–C–C–OH   Chloramphenicol
OH H   H

Acetyl CoA

CoA

3-Acetoxychloramphenicol

O
‖
C–CHCl₂
H H·N   H
O₂N–⟨⟩–C–C–C–O–C–CH₃
OH H   H   O

Acetyl CoA

CoA

O
‖
C–CHCl₃
H H·N   H
O₂N–⟨⟩–C–C–C–O–C–CH₃   1,3-Diacetoxychloram-
O   H   H   O   phenicol
|
O=C–CH₃

Figure 5.6 Modification of chloramphenicol by acetyltransferase.

ribosome, whereas the mutations at positions 491 and 512 may interfere with the conformational perturbations caused by the binding of streptomycin to the ribosome (see Chapter 2, Section 3.4.2.2).

In organisms other than the mycobacteria, acquired resistance due to mechanism 3a (i.e. impaired uptake) has been reported with mutations affecting the coupling of energy to membrane transport processes.

3.3 Chloramphenicol

Acquired resistance to chloramphenicol is frequently due to inactivation of the drug. Inactivation is mediated by plasmid- or transposon-encoded chloramphenicol acetyltransferases (CATs) that convert the drug to 3-acetoxychloramphenicol followed by conversion to 1,3-diacetoxychloramphenicol, the final inactivation product (Fig. 5.6). The acetoxy derivatives are antibiotically inactive because they fail to bind to the ribosomal target. Several types of plasmid-encoded CATs are found that have been characterized with respect to catalytic properties, electrophoretic mobility and reactivity to antisera. The enzymes are tetramers of identical subunits, the monomeric polypeptides having molecular weights in the range 23–25 kDa. The type I enzyme has been most studied and the complete amino acid sequence of its subunits is known. A histidine residue at position 193 (Fig. 5.7) plays a critical role in the catalytic modification of chloramphenicol and is likely to be located at the active site of the enzyme. The type III enzyme also contains a region sharing homology with the segment running between amino acids 190 and 200 in the type I enzyme, the catalytic histidine residue being located at residue 188 in the case of the type III molecule (Fig. 5.7). Other CATs (Fig. 5.7) also contain histidine at their active sites.

Although the majority of plasmids conferring chloramphenicol resistance in *E. coli* encode CATs, at least one example of a plasmid-encoded non-enzymic resistance mechanism has been described. This type of resistance, encoded by the gene *cml*A (contained in transposon Tn1696) involves active efflux of chloramphenicol mediated by the membrane-located CmlA protein.

In Gram-negative bacteria low-level resistance to chloramphenicol can arise by mutational loss of outer membrane porins through which the drug normally diffuses to reach the periplasm.

Finally, strains resistant to chloramphenicol by virtue of general mechanism 2 (Table 5.3) i.e. possession of drug-resistant ribosomes, have also been described.

3.4 Fusidic acid

As noted in Chapter 2, fusidic acid is a steroid antibiotic that prevents bacterial protein synthesis by inhibiting functions associated with translocation factor protein (G factor or EFG).

Gram-negative bacteria are intrinsically resistant to fusidic acid by virtue of poor antibiotic penetration across the outer membrane. However, acquired resistance to fusidic acid does occur in these organisms (e.g. the Enterobacteriaceae; see below), further elevating the level of resistance. Acquired resistance also occurs in Gram-positive bacteria that do not express intrinsic resistance to the antibiotic.

Acquired resistance results from either chromosomal mutations or possession of plasmids. Chromosomal mutants invariably have a modified G factor which has decreased affinity for the drug. In *S. aureus*, plasmid-mediated resistance to fusidic acid may involve decreased uptake of antibiotic across the cytoplasmic membrane (i.e. mechanism 3a, Table 5.3), but the molecular basis of resistance is unknown. The mechanism of plasmid-determined resistance to fusidic acid in the Enterobacteriaceae is also not fully understood and indeed is somewhat puzzling. Many plasmids confer resistance to fusidic acid, but the determinant in plasmid R100 has been studied in most detail. Surprisingly, the gene encoding resistance to fusidic acid also encodes a type I CAT (Section 3.3). Firm evidence has been obtained that the CAT itself confers fusidic acid resistance and that a separate *fus*

Primary structures of polypeptides

Enzyme type	1	5	10	15	20	190	195	200 → C-terminus
I (Tn9)	Met Glu Lys Lys Ile	Thr	Gly Tyr Thr Thr Val Asp Ile	Asp Ile Ser Gln Trp His Arg Lys Glu ---	Gln Val His	His Ala Val Cys Asp Gly Phe His ---		
II		Met	Asn Phe Thr Arg Ile	Asp Len Asn Thr Trp Asn	not determined	Gln Val His His Ala Val Cys Asp Gly Gly Phe His ---		
III		Met	Asn Tyr Thr Lys Phe	Asp Val Lys Asn Trp Val Arg Arg Glu ---	Gln Val His His Ala Val Cys Asp Gly Tyr His ---			
C (pC221)		[Met]	Thr Phe Asn Ile Ile	Lys Leu Glu Asn Trp Asp Arg Lys Glu ---	Gln Val His His Ala Val Cys Asp Gly Tyr His ---			
(pC194)		Met	Asn Phe Asn Lys Ile	Asp Leu Asp Asn Trp Lys Arg Lys Glu ---	Gln Val His His Ser Val Cys Asp Gly Tyr His ---			
B. pumilus		Met	Thr Phe Asn Ile Ile	Lys Leu Glu Asn Trp Asp Arg Lys Glu ---	Gln Val His His Ala Val Cys Asp Glu Tyr His ---			

Figure 5.7 Amino acid sequences surrounding the active site histidine residues (marked with an arrow) in various bacterial chloramphenicol acetyltransferases. The type C enzyme determined by plasmid pC221 is synthesized with an N-terminal methionine residue, but this is removed from the protein after translation. (Reproduced, with permission, from Shaw (1984).)

product is not translated from an initiation codon internal to the *cat* message. However, fusidic acid is not inactivated or modified by the enzyme, which appears to have a binding domain that sequesters a variety of aromatic compounds that are not necessarily closely related structurally.

3.5   Macrolides, lincosamides and streptogramins (MLS group)

3.5.1   *Common mechanism of resistance*

As noted in Chapter 2, MLS antibiotics arrest protein synthesis by binding to the 50S ribosomal subunit. Resistance mechanisms specific to individual members of the MLS antibiotics occur (see below) but, in addition, resistance to all these antibiotics can be conferred by a single mechanism involving mono- or di-methylation of an adenine residue in 23S rRNA. Determination of the site of methylation indicates that an analogous residue, corresponding to position 2058 of the *E. coli* rRNA, is modified by different rRNA methylases in both Gram-positive and Gram-negative bacteria. For example, three distinct RNA methylase genes (*ermA*, *ermB*, *ermC*) have been reported in staphylococci, all of which confer complete cross-resistance to MLS antibiotics. Methylation prevents the drugs from binding to the 50S ribosomal subunit probably as a consequence of a conformational change in the 23S rRNA. Genes specifying MLS resistance by rRNA methylation are carried by plasmids and transposons.

Recently a new resistance phenotype (MS) was observed in clinical isolates of *S. aureus*, in which cells are resistant to macrolides (M) and streptogramins (S) but remain sensitive to lincosamides. The gene responsible, *msr*A, is unrelated to the *erm*A, B, and C methylase genes. *msr*A encodes a 55 kDa protein containing two ATP binding sites which resemble the multidrug resistant P-glycoprotein (Mdr) of tumour cells which mediates resistance to antibiotics by drug efflux. *msr*A therefore probably confers resistance to MS antibiotics by a mechanism of drug efflux.

3.5.2   *Mechanisms of resistance to individual MLS antibiotics*

3.5.2.1   *Macrolides*

Three different chromosomal mutations in *E. coli* that affect ribosomal proteins can confer resistance to the macrolides. Mutants designated *ery*A show an alteration in protein L4 which leads to loss of macrolide binding by ribosomes. The *ery*A locus is therefore probably the structural gene for protein L4. The second type of mutant, designated *ery*B, confers a change in protein L22, but the *ery*B locus does not correspond to the structural gene for L22. The third class of mutation, *ery*C, has been reported to affect maturation of ribosomal RNA and a 30S ribosomal subunit protein. Therefore the mechanisms of macrolide resistance conferred by *ery*B and C mutations are presently unclear.

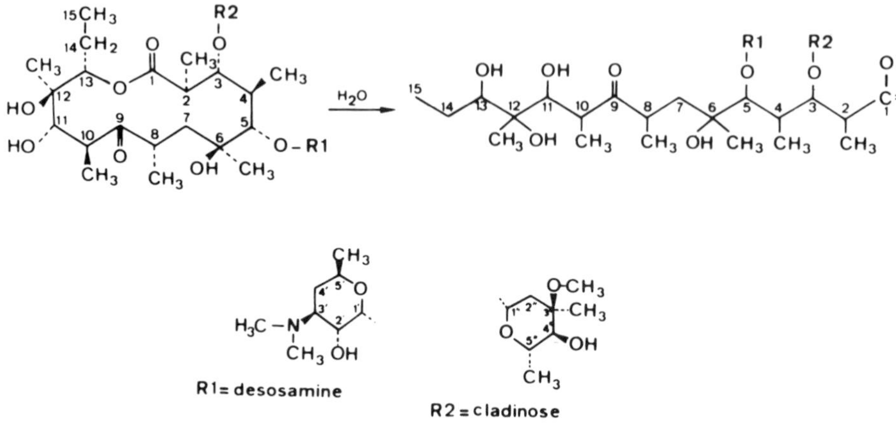

Figure 5.8 Enzymatic hydrolysis of erythromycin.

Two of the newer macrolides, clarithromycin and azithromycin, have been effectively used in the therapy of infections caused by *Mycobacterium avium* and *M. intracellulare*. However, prolonged monotherapy leads to the emergence of resistant strains with a 30- to 60-fold decrease in susceptibility to the antibiotics. Acquired resistance in clinical isolates is associated with single point mutations at nucleotides 2058 and 2059 in 23S ribosomal RNA. Since macrolides are known to bind directly to the 2058–2062 region in *E. coli* 23S rRNA (see Chapter 2, Section 3.4.6), the point mutations in the mycobacteria described above are likely to be responsible for resistance in these organisms. As for streptomycin resistance in *M. tuberculosis* (see Section 3.2), expression of macrolide resistance in *M. avium* and *M. intracellulare* depends on a low number of rRNA genes.

Plasmid-mediated mechanisms of resistance to 14-membered macrolides (e.g. erythromycin and oleandomycin) that correspond to general mechanism 1 (Table 5.3) have also been described. Inactivation (mechanism 1) of erythromycin and oleandomycin is widespread in enterobacteria highly resistant to these antibiotics and results from hydrolysis of the lactone ring in the antibiotics by plasmid-encoded esterases (Fig. 5.8). Inactivation is restricted specifically to 14-membered macro-lides. The nucleotide sequences of two plasmid genes, *ere*A and *ere*B, encoding esterases types I and II have recently been determined. Although both genes occur in clinical isolates of *E. coli*, the corresponding proteins are different. The type I esterase contains 349 amino acid residues and type II 419 amino acids. Furthermore, comparison of the amino acid sequences indicates that the proteins are unrelated.

Plasmid-mediated inactivation of erythromycin has also recently been detected in streptococci and staphylococci. However, the genes mediating resistance in these Gram-positive organisms are not homologous with either *ere*A or *ere*B.

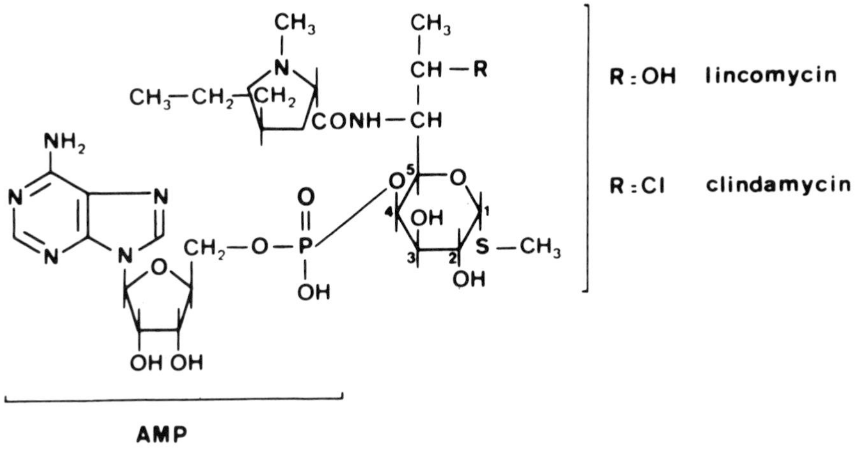

Figure 5.9 Structures of lincosamides inactivated by enzymic nucleotidylation at position 4 of the molecules.

3.5.2.2 *Lincosamides*

Plasmid-mediated inactivation of lincosamides occurs in a variety of resistant staphylococcal species. Inactivation results from enzymic nucleotidylation at position 4 of the antibiotics (Fig. 5.9). Two closely related enzymes are responsible for nucleotidylation, each containing 161 amino acid residues and showing 91% homology with each other.

3.5.2.3 *Streptogramins*

Resistance to streptogramin antibiotics in *S. aureus* can result from inactivation by plasmid-encoded enzymes. Streptogramin A is inactivated by an *O*-acetyltransferase and streptogramin B by a hydrolase.

3.6 Resistance to tetracyclines

3.6.1 *Resistance from expression of plasmid- or transposon-encoded efflux systems*

Eight genetic determinants (*tet*A through *tet*F, *tet*K and *tet*L) have been described in bacteria that encode tetracycline efflux proteins. Total nucleotide sequences are available for the *tet*A–*tet*D, *tet*K and *tet*L genes which encode a set of hydrophobic proteins ranging in size from 459 amino acids (TetK) to 394 amino acids (TetD).

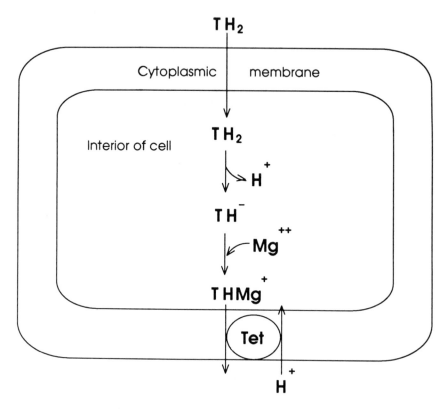

Figure 5.10   Proposed mechanism for tetracycline uptake (see also Chapter 2) and efflux across the bacterial cytoplasmic membrane. Mg^{++}, divalent magnesium cation; TH_2 and TH^-, protonated and deprotonated tetracycline, respectively; TH Mg^+, magnesium–tetracycline chelate complex. Tet proteins confer resistance to tetracycline by mediating expulsion of TH Mg^+ from the cell in exchange for a proton (H^+).

Each efflux protein has an even number of membrane-spanning α-helices with the *N*-terminus of the protein located at the inner face of the cytoplasmic membrane.

   Efflux is dependent on the proton-motive force (PMF: see Chapters 1 and 3) and involves an electrically neutral proton–tetracycline antiport system with exchange of a monocationic magnesium–tetracycline chelate complex for a proton (Fig. 5.10). Functional domains within tetracycline efflux proteins have not yet been established. However, it is assumed that a substrate (tetracycline) binding site fluctuating between high and low affinity states and a proton transfer site whose protonation–deprotonation affects the affinity of the binding site are present in the efflux proteins.

3.6.2 *Resistance from expression of plasmid- or transposon-encoded ribosomal protection factors*

Recently, two types of ribosomal protection factors have been described, TetM and TetO, both of which are plasmid or transposon encoded. The *tet*M resistance system occurs naturally in certain streptococci, gonococci and *Ureaplasma urealyticum*, whereas *tet*O has been described in *Campylobacter jejuni*. The TetM and TetO proteins probably act in a catalytic manner to modify the tetracycline binding site on the 30S ribosomal subunit. This might involve methylation of either ribosomal RNA or ribosomal protein, thereby rendering ribosomes insensitive to tetracycline.

3.6.3 *Other acquired mechanisms of tetracycline resistance*

Chromosomal mutations in *E. coli* leading to loss of the outer membrane porin OmpF, through which the antibiotic normally diffuses, confer low level resistance to tetracycline (and other unrelated compounds).

4
Resistance to antibiotics that inhibit peptidoglycan synthesis

4.1 D-cycloserine

As noted in Chapter 2, D-cycloserine is transported across the bacterial cytoplasmic membrane by the D-alanine transport system. In *E. coli* this transport system is encoded by the chromosomal gene *cyc*A which is involved in accumulation of D-alanine, D-glycine and D-serine as well as D-cycloserine. Mutations in *cyc*A confer resistance to cycloserine as well as defects in the transport of the other molecules.

In streptococci, transport mutants analogous to those in *E. coli* have been isolated as well as resistant mutants which produce more of the target enzymes inhibited by D-cycloserine. Mutants with up to five times more synthetase or eight times more racemase than normal can occur. The enzymes in these mutants are identical to those of the parent strain except in quantity. Acquired resistance to cycloserine in *M. tuberculosis* has been attributed to point mutations in the synthetase, but the mutants have not been characterized in detail.

4.2 Fosfomycin

As described in Chapter 2, fosfomycin acts at the level of phosphoenol-pyruvate:UDP-*N*-acetylglucosamine enoylpyruvil transferase, an enzyme involved in the biosynthesis of peptidoglycan.

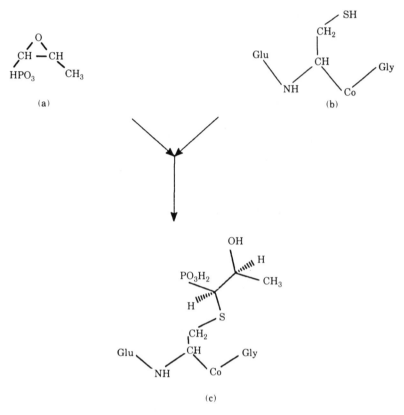

Figure 5.11 Conversion of (a) fosfomycin to (c) an inactive compound following combination with (b) glutathione.

Resistance to the antibiotic has been reported in several types of Gram-negative bacteria and occurs principally by general mechanisms 1 (drug alteration) and 3a (impaired uptake) (Table 5.3). Mechanisms of type 3a (impaired uptake) involve chromosomal mutations in the hexose-6-phosphate or L-glycerophosphate uptake systems by which fosfomycin is transported into susceptible bacteria.

Resistance mediated by mechanism 1 and encoded by the gene *for-r* confers about a 2000-fold increase in resistance. The *for-r* genetic determinant is common to a variety of plasmids and, at least in one case, this determinant is also known to be located in a transposon termed Tn2921. Fosfomycin is modified intracellularly by combination with glutathione to produce a derivative lacking antibiotic activity (Fig. 5.11). The modifying enzyme is located in the cytoplasm with subunits of molecular weight 16 kDa, active only as a dimer.

4.3 Bacitracin

As noted in Chapter 2, bacitracin forms a complex with the membrane-bound pyrophosphate form of the lipid carrier molecule involved in transferring disaccharide–pentapeptide units to the nascent peptidoglycan chain.

Gram-negative bacteria are intrinsically resistant to bacitracin so that discussion of acquired resistance to this antibiotic is only relevant for Gram-positive organisms. Bacitracin-resistant mutants of *S. aureus* have been isolated in the laboratory, but the mutations appear to revert at high frequency because resistance is readily lost on removal of the selective pressure. Clinical isolates of Gram-positive bacteria resistant to bacitracin have not been reported which may reflect the unstable nature of resistance mentioned above.

4.4 Glycopeptide antibiotics

As noted in Chapter 2, glycopeptide antibiotics interfere with glycan unit insertion by combining directly with peptidoglycan, in particular to the acyl-D-alanyl-D-alanine terminus of peptidoglycan precursors.

Acquired resistance to glycopeptides occurs in the enterococci, the genes conferring resistance residing within transposon Tn1546. Conjugal transfer of various plasmids that have acquired Tn1546 contributes to the spread of glycopeptide resistance genes in enterococci. Tn1546 encodes two key proteins (VanA and VanH) that are responsible for changing the pathway of peptidoglycan synthesis to produce a modified peptidoglycan structure no longer able to bind glycopeptides. VanH is an NADPH-dependent dehydrogenase that catalyses synthesis of the D-hydroxy acid, D-lactate, that forms a depsipeptide D-Ala-D-Lac replacing D-Ala-D-Ala in peptidoglycan (Fig. 5.12). VanA is a ligase of broad substrate specificity that catalyses the synthesis of D-Ala-D-Lac (Fig. 5.12). Cell wall assembly with the modified depsipeptide precursor relies on the resident chromosomal enzymes but results in a substitution that prevents binding of glycopeptides to cell wall components thereby allowing peptidoglycan polymerization in the presence of the antibiotics. The origin of the glycopeptide resistance genes in Tn1546 is unknown, but they may be derived from *Lactobacillus* or *Leuconostoc* spp. since these organisms are resistant to glycopeptides and contain D-specific α-keto acid reductases with properties similar to VanH.

4.5 β-Lactam antibiotics

4.5.1 Introduction

Acquired resistance to β-lactam antibiotics can arise by three different mechanisms: (1) in Gram-negative organisms through reduction in permeability

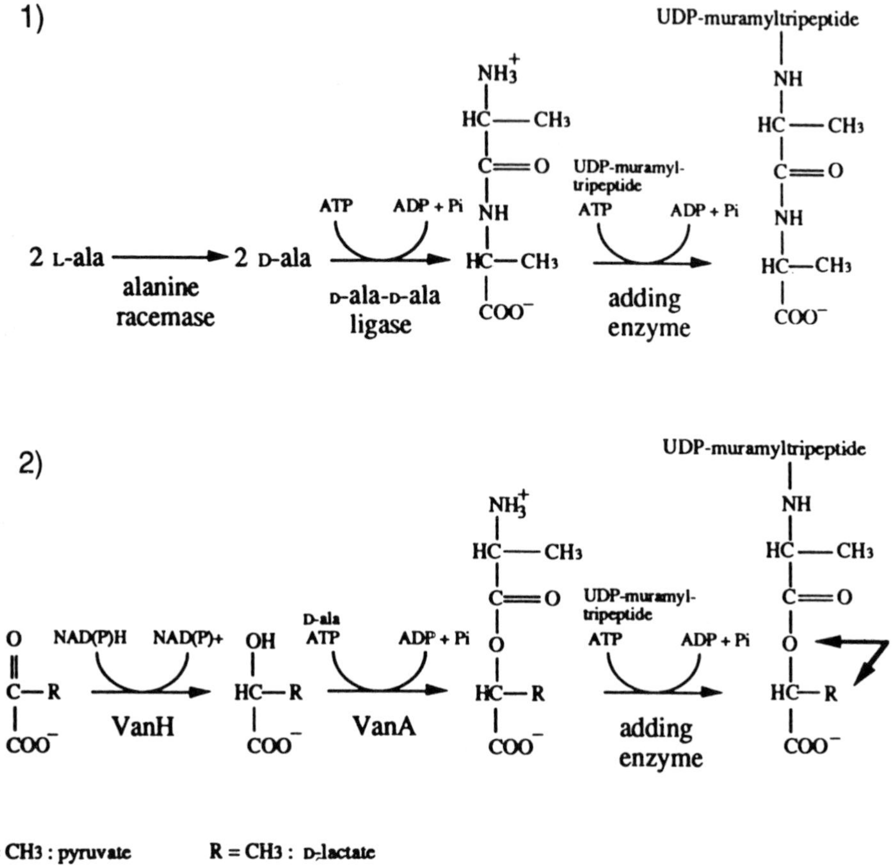

1)

2)

R = CH3 : pyruvate   R = CH3 : D-lactate

Figure 5.12 Pathways for the synthesis of cytoplasmic peptidoglycan precursors in the enterococci. (1) Synthesis of UDP-muramyl pentapeptide in enterococci susceptible to glycopeptides. (2) Alternative pathway involving incorporation of D-lactate at the *C*-terminal position of peptidoglycan precursors of enterococci resistant to glycopeptides. Boldface arrows indicate chemical groups that prevent binding of glycopeptides to peptidoglycan precursor analogues.

of the outer membrane to the antibiotic, (2) by synthesis of beta-lactamases, and (3) by modification of one or more PBPs. These mechanisms, either separately or jointly, account for acquired resistance to β-lactams.

4.5.2 Decreased β-lactam accumulation by virtue of outer membrane changes

It has been known for many years that changes in the Gram-negative outer membrane may affect the influx rate of β-lactams and thereby affect the resistance level. In particular, mutational loss of porins (e.g. OmpF and OmpC), through

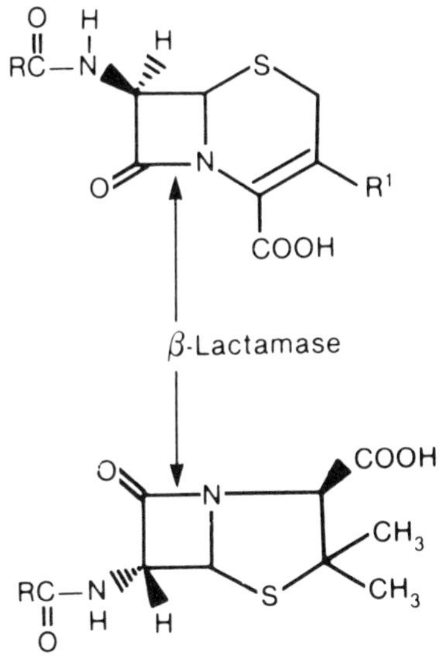

Cephalosporin

β-Lactamase

Penicillin

Figure 5.13   Interaction of cephalosporins and penicillins with β-lactamases. In cephalosporins, opening of the β-lactam ring and expulsion of R^1 is followed by general disintegration of the molecule. In penicillins, opening of the β-lactam ring occurs.

which many β-lactams normally diffuse, provides low levels of β-lactam resistance.

4.5.3   β-Lactamase synthesis

β-Lactamases hydrolyse the cyclic amide bond in β-lactam molecules (e.g. see Fig. 5.13), thereby rendering the drugs unable to bind to bacterial PBPs. In the case of Gram-negative bacteria the enzymes are synthesized within the cell and are then secreted into the periplasmic region. Resistance results from the strategic location of β-lactamases between the antibiotic penetration barrier (the outer membrane) and the antibiotic targets (PBPs) located in the cytoplasmic membrane whereby the β-lactamases can sequentially destroy antibiotic molecules as they enter the periplasm. Therefore, in Gram-negative bacteria resistance due to β-lactamase production is predominantly a single-cell phenomenon. In contrast, β-lactamases produced by Gram-positive bacteria are mainly excreted from the cell so that resistance is a population phenomenon, i.e. the excreted enzyme spreads into the external environment and can reduce the level of β-lactam to a concentration that permits growth of both enzyme-producing and non-enzyme-producing bacteria.

Bacterial β-lactamases are extremely heterogeneous with respect to both structure and substrate profiles. Over the years, many classification schemes have

Table 5.5 General classification scheme for bacterial β-lactamases

Group	Subtitle	Preferred substrates[a]	Inhibited by		Representative enzyme(s)
			CA[b]	EDTA	
1	CEP-N	Cephalosporins (B)	No	No	Chromosomal enzymes from Gram-negative bacteria
2a	PEN-Y	Penicillins (A)	Yes	No	Gram-positive penicillinases
2b	BDS-Y	Cephalosporins (B), penicillins (A)	Yes	No	TEM-1, TEM-2
2b'	EBS-Y	Cephalosporins (B), penicillins (A), cefotaxime (B)	Yes	No	TEM-3, TEM-5
2c	CAR-Y	Penicillins (A), carbenicillin (A)	Yes	No	PSE-1, PSE-3, PSE-4
2d	CLX-Y	Penicillins (A), cloxacillin (A)	Yes[c]	No	OXA-1, PSE-2
2e	CEP-Y	Cephalosporins (B)	Yes	No	*Proteus vulgaris*
3	MET-N	Variable	No	Yes	*Bacillus cereus* II, *Pseudomonas maltophilia* L1
4	PEN-N	Penicillins (A)	No	?[d]	*Pseudomonas cepacia*

[a]In relation to the β-lactam classification scheme illustrated in Fig. 2.27 the preferred substrates are classified as penams (A) and cephems (B).
[b]10 μM clavulanic acid.
[c]Inhibition by clavulanic acid may occur at higher concentrations for some members of the group.
[d]Variable.
Reproduced, with permission, from Bush (1989).

been proposed for these enzymes. However, the general classification scheme of Bush (Table 5.5), published in 1989, is the most suitable at present.

Apart from the group 3 enzymes, all other β-lactamases contain serine at their active sites. β-Lactamases containing serine inactivate β-lactams by forming an acyl enzyme intermediate with the serine residue in the active centre of the enzyme. Eventually, a hydrolysed (penicilloic acid type) β-lactam is released, the reaction scheme conforming to that shown in Fig. 2.32.

Many bacterial β-lactamases are plasmid or transposon encoded, but the group 1 β-lactamases are predominantly chromosomal. However, recent reports indicate the mobilization of group 1 encoding genes into transferable plasmids. In some species (e.g. *E. coli*), enzyme is produced at a low level and is not inducible, whereas in others, e.g. *Citrobacter freundii*, *Enterobacter cloacae* and *Ps. aeruginosa*, enzyme production is normally low, but can be induced to levels several hundred times higher after exposure of bacteria to a β-lactam. Furthermore, mutations can occur in the regulatory genes controlling expression of these normally inducible β-lactamases to produce resistant organisms synthesizing high levels of β-lactamase constitutively. Such mutations, which lead to enhanced expression of the β-lactamases, are of considerable clinical importance since they have been responsible for the rapid development of bacterial resistance during therapy to a number of the newer β-lactams, until recently regarded as β-lactamase-stable antibiotics.

Class 3 enzymes exhibit zinc-dependent activity and have been loosely described as 'carbapenemases' since they have the ability to hydrolyse all β-lactam antibiotics including carbapenems. Currently these enzymes, usually encoded by chromosomal genes, are found in less common pathogenic organisms. However, plasmid-mediated carbapenemase activity has recently been reported in *Ps. aeruginosa* and the possible spread of this enzyme could have serious consequences for the usage of all β-lactam antibiotics, including the carbapenems.

4.5.4 Alterations in the nature of PBPs that lead to resistance

4.5.4.1 Changes in target PBPs rendering them insensitive to β-lactams, but still able to perform peptidoglycan synthesis

Since β-lactam antibiotics are analogues of the cell wall substrate, mutations in PBPs affecting binding of the inhibitor (and thus potentially conferring resistance) might be expected to be lethal as binding of the natural peptidoglycan substrate would also be affected. Indeed, laboratory studies suggest that large changes in the ability of a PBP to discriminate between the binding of an inhibitor and the structurally analogous substrate cannot be achieved by single amino acid substitutions. Therefore, when it has occurred, the development of PBP-based resistance has arisen by recombination, involving the introduction of multiple amino acid substitutions, rather than individual point mutations.

Acquired resistance to penicillin in *Streptococcus pneumoniae* provides a clear example of this type of mechanism. Organisms resistant to penicillin have several PBPs of altered size and decreased affinity for penicillins. Molecular analysis of PBP2 genes from penicillin-susceptible and -resistant organisms revealed that the gene from susceptible strains was uniform in sequence, whereas those from resistant isolates had a mosaic structure, containing regions identical to those in susceptible strains and regions up to 23% divergent in sequence. The modified PBP2 genes thus appear to have arisen by block replacement of parts of the pneumococcal PBP2 gene with homologous regions from some other species, probably by DNA transformation.

4.5.4.2 Bypass of β-lactam-susceptible PBPs by duplication of target enzyme, the second version being insusceptible to antibiotic

The most important example of this type of resistance mechanism (mechanism 4, Table 5.3) concerns β-lactam resistance in clinical *S. aureus* isolates mediated by the *mec* determinant. Resistance results from the synthesis of a unique PBP (molecular weight 74 000) designated PBP2' or PBP2a that has a low affinity for β-lactam antibiotics. PBP2 is the only functional PBP at concentrations of β-lactams sufficient to inhibit the normal complement of PBPs in sensitive cells. The *mec* determinant confers resistance to all β-lactam antibiotics, including β-lactamase resistant compounds such as methicillin. The origin of the *mec* determinant is unknown, but may have been transferred to a single strain of *S. aureus* and then disseminated worldwide by clonal descent.

5
Resistance to antibiotics that inhibit membrane integrity—polymyxin

Plasmid-determined resistance to polymyxin has not been described, but chromosomal mutants of *Ps. aeruginosa* resistant to polymyxin (and the divalent ion chelator EDTA: see Chapter 6) have been isolated. Resistance is associated with an increase in the content of an outer membrane protein (H1) which apparently decreases the requirement for divalent cations in the outer membrane. Since the initial binding of polymyxin to sensitive cells depends on displacement of divalent cations from the outer membrane, it is suggested that protein H1 replaces cations at sites in the outer membrane which would otherwise be susceptible to the antibiotic.

Chromosomal mutations conferring resistance to polymyxin also occur in Gram-negative enteric bacteria such as *S. typhimurium* and *E. coli*. In these organisms the molecular basis of resistance differs from that of *Ps. aeruginosa*. In *E.coli* and *S. typhimurium* resistance to polymyxin is accompanied by a decrease in the net ionic charge of outer membrane lipopolysaccharide following substitution of phosphate groups in the molecule by aminoethanol and aminocarabinose.

These charges are responsible for decreased binding of polymyxin to the outer membrane, resulting in decreased susceptibility to polymyxin.

6
Resistance to antimycobacterial drugs

6.1 Introduction

This section deals with mechanisms of acquired resistance to specific antimycobacterial agents. Mechanisms of mycobacterial resistance to broad-spectrum agents (e.g. quinolones, rifampicin, macrolides) that also have a role in the chemotherapy of mycobacterial infections have been considered earlier in this chapter.

6.2 Capreomycin

As noted in Chapter 2 the capreomycin complex inhibits protein synthesis in *M. tuberculosis* by an unknown mechanism. Spontaneous mutation frequencies of 10^{-3} have been reported for capreomycin suggesting that single point mutations may confer resistance. Capreomycin-resistant *M. tuberculosis* isolates display cross-resistance to the aminoglycoside antibiotic kanamycin which appears to bind directly to 16S ribosomal RNA. It is therefore tempting to assume that resistance to capreomycin in *M. tuberculosis* may arise from nucleotide changes in the target ribosomal RNA. However, this hypothesis is currently unproven.

6.3 Clofazimine

Acquired resistance to clofazimine, used in the chemotherapy of leprosy, has been reported. However, the molecular basis of resistance in *M. leprae* is unknown.

6.4 Ethambutol

In *M. tuberculosis* acquired resistance to ethambutol arises with spontaneous mutation frequencies of about 10^{-6}. Although the mechanism of resistance has not been explored, a possible explanation is mutation of a target enzyme involved in arabinogalactan synthesis.

6.5 Ethionamide

Resistance to ethionamide arises spontaneously in mycobacteria with a mutational frequency of about 10^{-7}. Resistance has been correlated with a single amino acid substitution in the protein InhA, resulting in replacement of serine with alanine at position 94 of the protein. The InhA protein therefore appears to be a target for ethionamide and the point mutation conferring resistance may reduce affinity of the protein for the drug. This hypothesis is consistent with the likely role of InhA which appears to be involved in mycolic acid biosynthesis at the level of fatty acid metabolism. The mutation in *inhA* conferring resistance to ethionamide also confers cross-resistance to isoniazid, another antimycobacterial agent that targets mycolic acid biosynthesis.

6.6 Isoniazid

As noted in Chapter 2 (Section 6.6) the *kat*G gene of *M. tuberculosis* is probably involved in the conversion of isoniazid to one or more inhibitory molecules that target the protein InhA. Indeed, evidence supporting this theory on the mechanism of action of isoniazid derives in part from genetic studies on *kat*G. For example, deletions of *kat*G are associated with isoniazid resistance in both laboratory and clinical *M. tuberculosis* isolates and transformation of *kat*G into isoniazid-resistant mutants of *M. smegmatis* or *M. tuberculosis* restores sensitivity to isoniazid. Mutations in *kat*G do not confer cross-resistance to either pyrazinamide or ethionamide which are structural analogues of isoniazid.

In addition to mutations that affect the level of production of *kat*G and therefore expression of resistance to isoniazid, resistance to isoniazid (and ethionamide) also arises by point mutation in the gene *inh*A (see this chapter, Section 6.5). Although *kat*G and *inh*A mutations confer isoniazid resistance, some clinical isolates of *M. tuberculosis* display high-level resistance to isoniazid that is not associated with mutation in either *kat*G or *inh*A. The nature of the mutation(s) conferring resistance in these strains is unknown.

6.7 Pyrazinamide

As noted in Chapter 2 (Section 6.7) pyrazinamide is converted to pyrazinoic acid by an intracellular nicotinamidase. Reduced levels of nicotinamidase activity have been reported in some pyrazinamide-resistant isolates of *M. tuberculosis*, but the molecular mechanism has not been investigated.

6.8 Thiacetazone

Acquired resistance to thiacetazone has been reported in *M. tuberculosis*, but the mechanism is unknown.

7
Conclusions

It is now well recognized that acquisition of resistance determinants on plasmids and transposons is particularly important in the evolution of antibiotic-resistant bacteria. In evolutionary terms, acquisition of plasmid- or transposon-located resistance genes offers one major advantage over resistance based on chromosomal mutation: acquisition of a resistance determinant by a recipient cell provides it with pre-evolved genes refined to express resistance at high level. Furthermore, resistance determinants contained in transposons can become established in diverse bacterial species in which the original plasmid vectors themselves may be unable to replicate. Inducibility is another phenomenon frequently exhibited by pre-evolved resistance determinants, i.e. enzyme or other gene product levels increase following exposure of bacteria to antibiotics specifically inactivated by the determinant. Although we have not considered induction of resistance in detail in this book, the ability to 'switch on' resistance only when the need arises (i.e. when the cell is threatened by an antibiotic) is clearly another example of the refined nature of many pre-evolved resistance determinants. Readers wishing to learn more about the nature of induction as applied to resistance systems should consult the review articles cited at the end of this chapter.

Despite the undoubted importance of plasmid- and transposon-mediated antibiotic resistance, acquired resistance resulting from changes in chromosomal genes, either by point mutation or homologous recombination events, has major clinical significance. Resistance to the quinolones mediated by mutations in *gyr*A, to rifampicin mediated by mutations in *rpo*B, and to penicillin in *Strep. pneumoniae* mediated by recombination events in PBP2 constitute important examples of acquired resistance mediated by chromosomal genes.

Interestingly, acquired resistance to antibiotics in the mycobacteria appears to result exclusively from chromosomal mutations with no convincing evidence for plasmid-mediated mechanisms. In the case of those antibiotics that bind to ribosomal RNA, it is evident that expression of mutations in mycobacterial rRNA genes confers resistant phenotypes, in contrast to the majority of bacteria where such mutations are recessive. Therefore it may be unnecessary for mycobacteria to import genes that confer resistance by other mechanisms to antibiotics acting at the ribosomal level. More broadly it has been suggested that the absence of resistance plasmids from species of mycobacteria that are well adapted to a parasitic role (particularly *M. tuberculosis*, *M. africanum*, *M. bovis* and *M. leprae*) relates to their existence within closed lesions in human or animal hosts, thereby preventing contact with other bacteria that might transmit resistance determinants to them.

The diversity of mechanisms used by bacteria to evade the action of antibiotics and the rapidity with which bacteria acquire resistance are depressing from the viewpoint of achieving successful therapy. Nevertheless, studies on the genetic and biochemical basis of antibiotic resistance have themselves suggested ways to circumvent it. This topic is considered further in Chapter 8.

Further reading

Review articles

Arthur, M. & Courvalin, P. (1993). Genetics and mechanisms of glycopeptide resistance in enterococci. *Antimicrobial Agents and Chemotherapy* **37**: 1563–1571.

Bugg, T. D. H. & Walsh, C. T. (1992). Intracellular steps of bacterial cell wall peptidoglycan biosynthesis: enzymology, antibiotics and antibiotic resistance. *Natural Product Reports* **9**: 199–215.

Bush, K. (1989). Characterization of beta-lactamases. *Antimicrobial Agents and Chemotherapy* **33**: 259–263.

Cambau, E. & Gutman, L. (1993). Mechanisms of resistance to quinolones. *Drugs* **45** (Supplement 3): 15–23.

Chopra, I. (1992). Efflux-based antibiotic resistance mechanisms: the evidence for increasing prevalence. *Journal of Antimicrobial Chemotherapy* **30**: 737–739.

Chopra, I., Hawkey, P. M. & Hinton, M. (1992). Tetracyclines, molecular and clinical aspects. *Journal of Antimicrobial Chemotherapy* **29**: 245–277.

Clewell, D. B., Senghas, E., Jones, J. M., Flannagan, S. E., Yamamoto, M. & Gawron-Burke, C. (1988). Transposition in *Streptococcus*: structural and genetic properties of the conjugative transposon Tn916. In *Transposition*, 43rd Symposium of the Society for General Microbiology (eds A. J. Kingman, K. F. Chater & S. M. Kingsman) pp. 43–58. Cambridge University Press.

Courvalin, P. (1990). Resistance of enterococci to glycopeptides. *Antimicrobial Agents and Chemotherapy* **34**: 2291–2296.

Eady, E. A., Ross, J. I. & Cove, J. H. (1990). Multiple mechanisms of erythromycin resistance. *Journal of Antimicrobial Chemotherapy* **26**: 461–465.

Foster, T. J. (1983). Plasmid-determined resistance to antimicrobial drugs and toxic metal ions in bacteria. *Microbiological Reviews* **47**: 361–409.

Georgopapadakou, N. H. (1993). Penicillin-binding proteins and bacterial resistance to β-lactams. *Antimicrobial Agents and Chemotherapy* **37**: 2045–2053.

Godfrey, A. J. & Bryan, L. E. (1984). Intrinsic resistance and whole cell factors contributing to antibiotic resistance. In *Antimicrobial Drug Resistance* (ed. L. E. Bryan) pp. 113–145. Academic Press, New York.

Hackbarth, C. J. & Chambers, H. F. (1989). Methicillin-resistant staphylococci: genetics and mechanisms of resistance. *Antimicrobial Agents and Chemotherapy* **33**: 991–994.

Huovinen, P., Sundstram, L., Swedeberg, G. & Skold, O. (1995). Trimethoprim and sulfonamide resistance. *Antimicrobial Agents and Chemotherapy* **39**: 279–289.

Jacobs, R. F. (1994). Multiple-drug-resistant tuberculosis. *Clinical Infectious Diseases* **19**: 1–10.

Leclercq, R. & Courvalin, P. (1991). Bacterial resistance to macrolide, lincosamide, and streptogramin antibiotics by target modification. *Antimicrobial Agents and Chemotherapy* **35**: 1267–1272.

Levy, S. B. (1992). Active efflux mechanisms for antimicrobial resistance. *Antimicrobial Agents and Chemotherapy* **36**: 695–703.

Livermore, D. M. (1992). Carbapenemases. *Journal of Antimicrobial Chemotherapy* **29**: 609–613.

Lyon, B. R. & Skurray, R. (1987). Antimicrobial resistance of *Staphylococcus aureus*. *Microbiological Reviews* **51**: 88–134.

Mitchison, D. A. (1984). Drug resistance in mycobacteria. *British Medical Bulletin* **40**: 84–90.

Murphy, E. (1988). Transposable elements in *Staphylococcus*. In *Transposition*, 43rd Symposium of the Society for General Microbiology (eds A. J. Kingsman, K. F. Chater & S. M. Kingsman) pp. 59–89. Cambridge University Press.

Payne, D. J. & Amyes, S. G. B. (1991). Transferable resistance to extended-spectrum β-lactams: a major threat or minor inconvenience? *Journal of Antimicrobial Chemotherapy* **27**: 255–261.

Phillips, I. & Shannon, K. (1984). Aminoglycoside resistance. *British Medical Bulletin* **40**: 28–35.

Shaw, W. V. (1984). Bacterial resistance to chloramphenicol. *British Medical Bulletin* **40**: 36–41.

Smith, J. T. & Amyes, S. G. B. (1984). Bacterial resistance to antifolate chemotherapeutic agents mediated by plasmids. *British Medical Bulletin* **40**: 42–46.

Spratt, B. G. (1994). Resistance to antibiotics mediated by target alterations. *Science* **264**: 388–393.

Suarez, J. E. & Mendoza, M. C. (1991). Plasmid-encoded fosfomycin resistance. *Antimicrobial Agents and Chemotherapy* **35**: 791–795.

Weisblum, B. (1995). Erythromycin resistance by ribosome modification. *Antimicrobial Agents and Chemotherapy* **39**: 577–585.

Wilkins, B. M. (1988). Organization and plasticity of enterobacterial genomes. *Journal of Applied Bacteriology (Symposium Supplement)* **65**: 51S–69S.

Zhang, Y. & Young, D. B. (1994). Molecular genetics of drug resistance in *Mycobacterium tuberculosis*. *Journal of Antimicrobial Chemotherapy* **34**: 313–319.

Research papers

Banerjee, A., Dubnau, E., Quermard, A., Balasubramanian, V., Um, K. S., Wilson, T., Collins, D., de Lisle, G. & Jacobs, W. R. (1994). inhA, a gene encoding a target for isoniazid and ethionamide in *Mycobacterium tuberculosis*. *Science* **263**: 227–230.

Gilbart, J., Perry, C. R. & Slocombe, B. (1993). High-level mupirocin resistance in *Staphylococcus aureus*: evidence for two distinct isoleucyl-tRNA synthetases. *Antimicrobial Agents and Chemotherapy* **37**: 32–38.

Hodgson, J. E., Curnock, S. P., Dyke, K. G. H., Morris, R., Sylvester, D. R. & Gross, M. S. (1994). Molecular characterisation of the gene encoding high-level mupirocin resistance in *Staphylococcus aureus* J2870. *Antimicrobial Agents and Chemotherapy* **38**: 1205–1208.

Honore, N. & Cole, S. T. (1994). Streptomycin resistance in mycobacteria. *Antimicrobial Agents and Chemotherapy* **38**: 238–242.

Meier, A., Kirschner, P., Springer, B., Steingrube, V. A., Brown, B. A., Wallace, R. J.

& Bottger, E. C. (1994). Identification of mutations in 23S rRNA gene of clarithromycin-resistant *Mycobacterium intracellulare*. *Antimicrobial Agents and Chemotherapy* **38**: 381–384.

Nummila, K., Kilpelainen, I., Zahringer, U., Vaara, M. & Helander, I. M. (1995). Lipopolysaccarides of polymyxin B-resistant mutants of *Escherichia coli* are extensively substituted by 2-aminoethanol pyrophosphate and contain aminoarabinose in lipid A. *Molecular Microbiology* **16**: 271–278.

Takiff, H. E., Salazar, L., Guerrero, C., Phillipp, W., Huang, W. M., Kreiswirth, B., Cole, S. T., Jacobs, W. R. & Telenti, A. (1994). Cloning and nucleotide sequence of *Mycobacterium tuberculosis* gyrA and gyrB genes and detection of quinolone resistance mutations. *Antimicrobial Agents and Chemotherapy* **38**: 773–780.

Williams, D. L., Waguespack, C., Eisenach, K., Crawford, J. T., Portaels, F., Salfinger, M., Nolan, C. M., Abe, C., Sticht-Groh, V. & Gillis, T. P. (1994). Characterization of rifampin resistance in pathogenic mycobacteria. *Antimicrobial Agents and Chemotherapy* **38**: 2380–2386.

CHAPTER SIX

Genetic and biochemical basis of resistance to antiseptics, disinfectants and preservatives

1
Introduction

Antimicrobial activity and mechanisms of action of various types of antiseptics, disinfectants and preservatives were considered in Chapter 3. This chapter discusses ways in which non-sporing bacteria survive exposure to chemicals employed as biocides.

The term 'resistance' is a well-defined concept when applied to antibiotic resistance (Chapter 5). When applied to antiseptics, disinfectants and preservatives, however, the term is less clearly defined, and is often used to describe a bacterial strain that is not susceptible to a concentration of antibacterial agent used in practice. It is also used to denote a strain that is not killed or inhibited by a concentration of biocide that kills or inhibits the majority of strains of that organism.

Some authors restrict the terms 'resistance' and 'resistant' to instances where the genetic and biochemical basis for resistance is known, and recommend the alternative terms 'tolerance' and 'tolerate' where the basis of insusceptibility has not been established. Although there is some merit in these proposals, we believe that two sets of terminology are confusing. Consequently, as with antibiotics, 'resistance' and 'resistant' have been used throughout this chapter and Chapter 7 to denote insusceptibility of bacteria and spores to biocides. Two major mechanisms of resistance will be considered; intrinsic and acquired. Biofilms have an important role in conferring intrinsic resistance to biocides, and their description forms an important aspect of this chapter (Section 2.5). The effects of biocides on plasmid transfer and other possible means of counteracting bacterial resistance are presented in Chapter 8.

1.1 Distinction between intrinsic and acquired resistance

In general, the mechanisms of bacterial resistance to antiseptics, disinfectants and preservatives are poorly understood when compared with knowledge of antibiotic resistance mechanisms (Chapter 5). However, as for antibiotics, resistance mechanisms can be considered as either natural (innate, intrinsic) or acquired. Specific examples within each group will be discussed where relevant. As with antibiotics, intrinsic resistance is usually expressed by chromosomal genes, whereas acquired resistance results from genetic changes in a cell and arises either by mutations in chromosomal genes or by the acquisition of genetic material from another cell.

Apart from a few specific instances, such as acquired resistance to some metals (Section 3.1.1) and cationic agents (Section 3.1.2), the intrinsic mechanisms of biocide resistance have been more widely studied. Usually, the latter results from exclusion of a biocide, although enzymatic inactivation of a biocide is another possible intrinsic resistance mechanism. Examples of intrinsic resistance by an exclusion mechanism (sometimes termed cell impermeability) are provided by Gram-negative bacteria (Sections 2.2 and 2.6), mycobacteria (Section 2.7) and bacterial spores (Chapter 7). Physiological (phenotypic) adaptations of an organism in response to changes in growth environment can modulate sensitivity to biocides.

Acquired resistance to biocides arises either as a consequence of chromosomal gene mutation (a biocide then acting as a means of selecting the mutant) or by the acquisition of plasmids and transposons. The possibility exists, but has yet to be shown conclusively, that acquired biocide resistance arises from selective pressures exerted by the widespread usage, particularly in hospitals, of antiseptics and disinfectants. If this is so, then an analogous situation to the chemotherapeutic use of antibiotics (see Chapter 8) has arisen.

2
Intrinsic biocide resistance

2.1 Introduction

Intrinsic resistance to biocides is often found with Gram-negative bacteria and is associated with the composition and structure of the outer layers of these cells (Section 2.2). An initial stage in the action of biocides involves their binding to the surface layers of bacteria (Chapter 3). This is followed by passage across the cell wall or outer membrane to the cytoplasmic membrane or deeper into the cell, wherever the target site resides. In Gram-positive bacteria, no specific receptor molecules or permeases exist to assist biocide penetration and the *Bacillus megaterium* cell wall is for example permeable to molecules with molecular weights up to 30 000 Da. Thus, most biocides appear to enter Gram-positive bacteria readily and such organisms are generally more sensitive to these agents than are Gram-negative cells (Table 6.1). Gram-positive bacteria, e.g. staphylococci, can

Table 6.1 Comparative responses of Gram-positive and Gram-negative bacteria to some antiseptics, disinfectants and preservatives

Antibacterial agent	MIC[a] (μg/ml) against			
	S. aureus	E. coli	Ps. aeruginosa	P. vulgaris
Chlorhexidine diacetate	0.5	1	5–60	12.5–25
Propamidine isethionate	1	64	256	256
Dibromopropamidine isethionate	1	4	32	128
Cetrimide	0.4	12.5	64–128	
Hexachlorophane	0.05	100	>100	>100

[a]MIC, minimum inhibitory concentration.

express resistance to some biocides when grown in broth containing glycerol (Section 2.3). The consequent increase in wall lipid acting as a barrier to biocide penetration is analogous to the intrinsic resistance presented by the outer membrane of Gram-negative bacteria (see below). The outer membrane of Gram-negative bacteria limits the intracellular entry of many biocides thereby conferring intrinsic resistance. In addition some organisms survive biocide treatment by producing a glycocalyx. Both of these aspects will be considered in this chapter, as will the intrinsic resistance of mycobacteria.

2.2 Role of the outer membrane of Gram-negative bacteria

The outer membrane of Gram-negative bacteria plays an important role in conferring resistance to many biocides (and antibiotics: see Chapter 5). The structure of the outer membrane was considered in Chapter 1. Basically, the cell surface of smooth Gram-negative bacteria is hydrophilic in nature, a property that can be readily demonstrated by measuring the partitioning of cells into a water-miscible hydrocarbon solvent. Deep rough (heptoseless) mutants, on the other hand, tend to be much more hydrophobic. Thus, wild-type (smooth) strains are resistant to hydrophobic biocides (and antibiotics) whereas deep rough mutants are sensitive. The basis of this difference is explained below, from which it will become clear that outer membrane mutants, which are genetically hypersensitve to a biocide, are of considerable value in evaluating the nature of intrinsic resistance in wild-type strains.

A distinction must be drawn between low molecular weight (less than about 600) hydrophilic molecules which can readily enter via the aqueous porins and

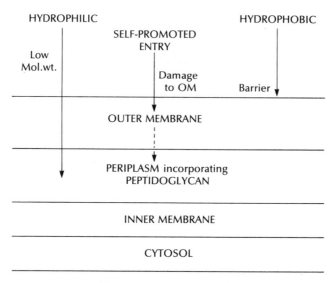

Figure 6.1 Interaction of biocides with the Gram-negative cell envelope: diagrammatic representation of uptake pathways and exclusion barrier. Demonstrated are a hydrophilic biocide of low molecular weight, a hydrophobic biocide and a biocide that promotes its own entry. OM, outer membrane. For additional information, see Fig. 6.2.

hydrophobic molecules which diffuse across the outer membrane bilayer (Fig. 6.1; see also Chapter 2). The porin system is present in both smooth and rough strains and uptake of hydrophilic biocides is thus not impeded by the presence of complete lipopolysaccharide (LPS) molecules. In wild-type bacteria, however, the intact LPS molecules prevent ready access of hydrophobic molecules to the cell interior. In smooth cells, the intact LPS shields phospholipids which are not present in the outer leaflet of the outer membrane. In deep rough strains, which lack the O-specific side chain and most of the core polysaccharide (Figs 6.2 and 6.3), and in EDTA-treated cells, patches of phospholipid appear in the outer leaflet (Fig. 6.4) thereby permitting diffusion of hydrophobic molecules across what is essentially a phospholipid bilayer.

The role of the outer membrane in intrinsic resistance of enteric bacteria to biocides is illustrated by the quaternary ammonium compounds (QACs) and amidines. These compounds are considerably less active against wild-type than deep rough strains of *E. coli* and *Salm. typhimurium* (Table 6.2). However, in the case of chlorhexidine salts the outer membrane of wild-type *Salm. typhimurium*, but not *E. coli*, confers intrinsic resistance to the antiseptic (Table 6.2).

P
GlcNAc
Glc
Glc
Glc
Hep
Hep
$(KDO)_3$
Lipid A
Gal
Hep
Hep
Rha
Etn
Strain
Heptoseless
CE1021 and D21f1
D21e7
Wild-type and CE1002

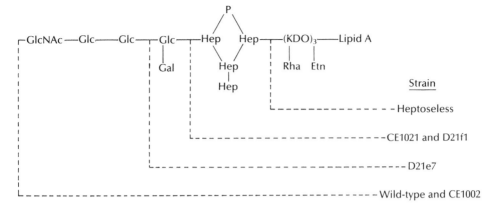

Figure 6.2 Lipopolysaccharide (LPS) of wild-type and envelope mutant strains of *E. coli*. GlcNAc, *N*-acetylglucosamine; Hep, L-glycero-D-manno-heptose; KDO, 2-ketodeoxyoctonate; Rha, rhamnose; Etn, ethanolamine; P, phosphate.

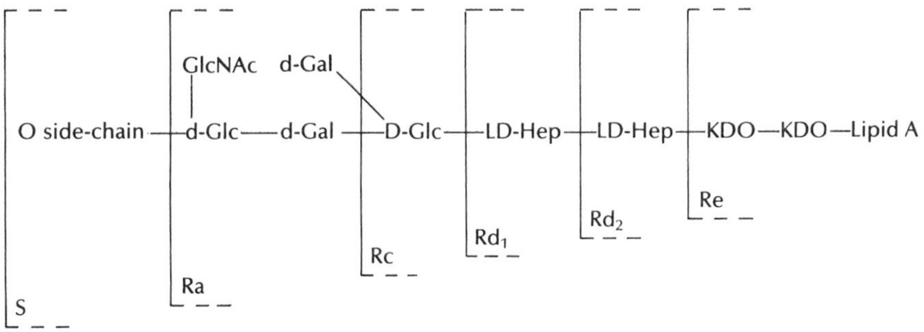

GlcNAc
d-Gal
O side-chain
d-Glc
d-Gal
D-Glc
LD-Hep
LD-Hep
KDO
KDO
Lipid A
Re
Rd_2
Rd_1
Rc
Ra
S

Figure 6.3 LPS of wild-type and envelope mutant strains of *Salm. typhimurium*. Abbreviations as for *E. coli* LPS (Fig. 6.5). Additionally, d-Gal is D-galactose.

2.2.1 Outer membrane barrier and intrinsic resistance to membrane-active biocides

Biocides with a target site in the cytoplasmic (inner) membrane are usually, if rather loosely, termed 'membrane-active' agents (Chapter 3). To reach their target these compounds must traverse the outer membrane. Limitation of their access by the outer membrane may result in intrinsic resistance.

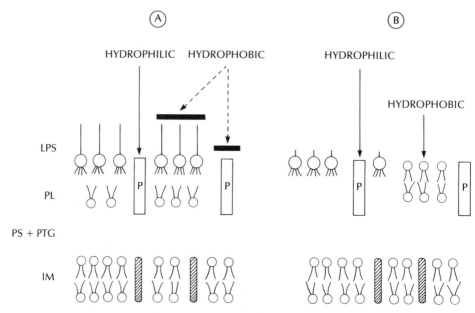

Figure 6.4 Comparison of intracellular penetration of hydrophilic and hydrophobic molecules into (a) smooth and (b) deep rough Gram-negative bacteria: P, porin; LPS, lipopolysaccharide; PL, phospholipid; PS, periplasmic space (periplasm): PTG, peptidoglycan; IM, inner membrane; bar, inner membrane protein.

Table 6.2 Susceptibility of wild-type and envelope mutant strains of Gram-negative bacteria to some cationic agents

Type of biocide	E. coli	Salm. typhimurium
QACs Amidines	Deep rough mutants much more sensitive	
Chlorhexidine	Deep rough mutants and wild-type strain show same order of sensitivity	Deep rough mutants rather more sensitive than wild type
Polyhexamethylene biguanides (PHMBs)	Cell envelope provides significant exclusion barrier, but does not confer complete resistance	Not studied

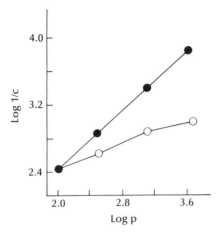

Figure 6.5 Structure–activity relationships for hydroxybenzoates acting against some *Escherichia coli* strains. log $1/C$ is the logarithm to base 10 of the reciprocal of the MIC molar value and log P is the logarithm to base 10 of the partition coefficient. ○, PC0479 (wild type); ●, D21f2 (deep rough).

2.2.1.1 Parabens

The parabens (Chapter 3) are widely used as preservatives in the food, pharmaceutical and cosmetic industries. They inhibit Gram-positive and Gram-negative bacteria but are only slowly bactericidal. Activity increases as the homologous series of methyl (Me), ethyl (Et), propyl (Pr) and butyl (Bu) esters of *para-* (4-) hydroxybenzoic acid is ascended, but this is accompanied by a corresponding decrease in solubility. Wild-type strains of *E. coli* and *Salm. typhimurium* are intrinsically more resistant to the four esters than are deep rough mutants, with the Me ester the least, and the Bu ester the most, active against any individual strain. This is clearly shown in Fig. 6.5, which depicts the response of a wild-type *E. coli* strain and its deep rough mutant to the four esters. The logarithm to base 10 of the reciprocal of the MIC (shown as log $1/C$) is plotted against the logarithm to base 10 of the partition coefficient (log P) in octanol:H_2O. A similar response is apparent when a series of well-characterized mutants of *Salm. typhimurium* is examined (Fig. 6.6).

 Uptake probably proceeds by a general dissolution of an ester into the cell with no specific sites existing for binding at the cell surface. The deficiency of LPS in deep rough mutants resulting in decreased intrinsic resistance, i.e. increased sensitivity, to the parabens is due to phospholipid patches appearing in the outer leaflet of the outer membrane. These aid the penetration of an ester, and especially the most hydrophobic one (the Bu ester), across the outer membrane to the target site at the inner membrane.

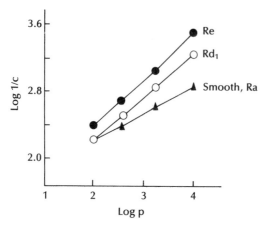

Figure 6.6   Plot of the logarithm to base 10 of the reciprocal of molar inhibitory concentrations (log $1/C$ values) vs partition coefficients (log P) for methyl, ethyl, propyl and butyl parabens vs strains of *Salmonella typhimurium*.

2.2.1.2 *Phenols and cresols*

Bacterial resistance to phenolics decreases in the order phenol > cresol > chlorocresol. Intrinsic resistance in Gram-negative bacteria is probably related to the ease with which these compounds cross the outer membrane, since deep rough mutants are more sensitive to an individual phenolic, and especially the most hydrophobic (chlorocresol) of the three cited, than are wild-type strains.

2.2.1.3 *Chlorhexidine*

Chlorhexidine is a widely used antiseptic, disinfectant and preservative effective against Gram-negative and Gram-positive bacteria, except mycobacteria (Section 2.7) and bacterial spores (Chapter 7). Activities against most staphylococci and some Gram-negative organisms such as *E. coli* are comparable. This suggests that the biguanide readily penetrates the *E. coli* outer membrane, i.e. that this structure does not confer substantial intrinsic resistance to chlorhexidine (see also Section 2.3). This contrasts markedly with the situation for other cationic agents such as the QACs (Section 2.2.1.4) and amidines (Section 2.2.2.1). However, certain Gram-negative bacteria, e.g. *Proteus* spp. and *Providencia stuartii*, exhibit high levels of intrinsic resistance to chlorhexidine. Here, intrinsic resistance is probably related to the nature of the outer membrane, but the basis of resistance is unknown. As noted later (Section 2.6.1.3) the gross chemical compositions of cell envelopes from chlorhexidine-resistant and -sensitive strains of *Prov. stuartii* are very similar. Nevertheless, spheroplasts of chlorhexidine-resistant *Prov. stuartii* are lysed by the biguanide, suggesting that the outer membrane in these organisms is indeed responsible for intrinsic resistance.

2.2.1.4 *Quaternary ammonium compounds*

The LPS in the outer membrane acts as a barrier to the entry of QACs into Gram-negative bacteria. This has been demonstrated by comparing the sensitivities to QACs of wild-type and envelope mutants with deletions in LPS. The barrier mechanism of intrinsic QAC resistance could result from shielding of phospholipid molecules beneath the LPS in wild-type strains or could arise by an interaction of the cationic biocides with anionic groups on LPS thereby reducing the amount of 'free' QAC available for penetration into the cell.

QACs such as cetrimide are also believed to promote their own entry into Gram-negative bacteria by virtue of their effect on the outer membrane. Nevertheless, the outer membrane undoubtedly acts as a penetration barrier to these agents.

2.2.2 **Outer membrane barrier and intrinsic resistance to other biocides**

2.2.2.1 *Amidines*

Gram-negative bacteria are intrinsically resistant to amidines such as propamidine isethionate (PI) or dibromopropamidine isethionate (DBPI). The outer membrane is a permeability barrier to PI and DBPI, a conclusion reached in part from studies with wild-type and LPS mutants of both *E. coli* and *Salm. typhimurium*. The exact mechanism for this intrinsic resistance is unknown. DBPI will itself damage the outer membrane of Gram-negative bacteria but as with the QACs (Section 2.2.1.4) this may be insufficient to prevent the membrane from acting as a barrier.

2.2.2.2 *Triphenylmethane dyes*

Gram-negative bacteria are intrinsically more resistant to dyes such as crystal violet than are Gram-positive organisms. Crystal violet is a hydrophobic agent and is therefore excluded by the Gram-negative outer membrane (Fig. 6.1). Wild-type cells of *Salm. typhimurium* are considerably more resistant than deep rough mutants and these and other findings demonstrate that intrinsic resistance is associated with the outer membrane.

2.2.2.3 *Acridines*

Some strains of *P. mirabilis* are more resistant to acriflavine than others. The basis of this resistance (apparently intrinsic) has not been investigated.

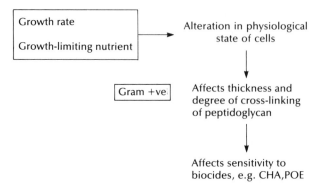

Figure 6.7   Cell surface changes and intrinsic resistance to biocides in *B. megaterium*: CHA, chlorhexidine diacetate; POE, phenoxyethanol.

2.3   Cell wall–cell envelope changes and modulation of intrinsic resistance to biocides

The cell wall of Gram-positive bacteria consists of a highly cross-linked peptidoglycan network into which are incorporated teichoic and teichuronic acids. The peptidoglycan acts as a molecular sieve, this property depending on the thickness and the degree of cross-linking within the macromolecule. These can vary depending on the physiological status of the cells, which in turn is influenced by the growth rate and by any growth-limiting nutrient. For example, the sensitivity of *B. megaterium* cells to chlorhexidine and phenoxyethanol alters when changes in growth rate and nutrient limitation are made. Since lysozyme-induced protoplasts remain sensitive to these membrane-active agents (Chapter 3, Section 5.2.1), it is clear that the cell wall is responsible for the modified response in whole cells (Fig. 6.7).

When staphylococci are repeatedly subcultured in media containing glycerol, the 'fattened' cells become less susceptible to the action of certain biocides. Enhanced levels of cellular lipid protect cells from pentylphenol and *n*-hexylphenyl, but not from lower phenols in this series or tetrachlorosalicylanilide or hexachlorophane.

Modulation of Gram-negative cell envelope composition can also be achieved by changes in growth rate and nutritional conditions. Changes in both the outer membrane and the inner membrane can occur, e.g. in phospholipid, porins, LPS and cations. Not unexpectedly, changes in susceptibility to biocides are observed:

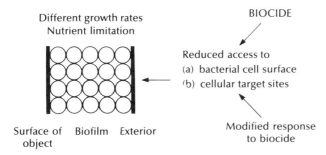

Figure 6.8   Biofilm production and bacterial susceptibility to biocides.

thus, carbon-limited cultures are most sensitive to chlorhexidine, but most resistant to QACs.

The overall hydrophobicity and fluidity of the cell envelope are affected by changes in its composition and consequently the ability of compounds to traverse the envelope changes. It is unlikely that a single component is involved (as originally believed). A complex interaction between all the components in the envelope and the biocide probably occurs. These interactions will then modify the penetration of the biocide through the envelope.

The composition and plasticity of the cell wall or cell envelope are thus altered by phenotypic (physiological) adaptation whereby intrinsic resistance to a biocide is enhanced or, in some instances, decreased.

2.4   Role of slime in intrinsic resistance to biocides

In nature, *S. aureus* may exist as mucoid strains, with a slime layer around the cells. Non-mucoid strains are killed more rapidly than mucoid strains by chloroxylenol, cetrimide and chlorhexidine, but there is little difference in response with phenols or chlorinated phenols. Removal of slime by washing cells phenotypically renders them as sensitive to the biocides. Slime therefore has a protective role and confers resistance to pathogenic staphylococci. This could act either (a) as a physical barrier to biocide penetration or (b) as a loose layer interacting with, or absorbing, the biocide.

2.5   Role of the glycocalyx and biofilm production in intrinsic resistance to biocides

The association of bacteria (or other microorganisms) with solid surfaces leads to the generation of a biofilm, which is defined as a consortium of bacteria organized within an extensive exopolysaccharide exopolymer (glycocalyx). Biofilms may consist of (i) monocultures, (ii) several diverse species, or (iii) mixed phenotypes

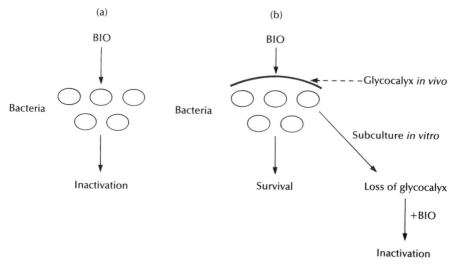

Figure 6.9 Comparison of (a) absence and (b) presence of glycocalyx in bacterial response to a biocide (BIO).

of a given species. The third example suggests that bacteria in different parts of a biofilm experience different nutrient environments thereby affecting their physiology. Within the depths of the biofilm, growth rates are likely to be reduced as a consequence of nutrient limitation. The phenotypes of sessile organisms found in biofilms may thus differ considerably from those of the 'free-floating' (planktonic) cells found, for example, in liquid cultures. This point is particularly relevant when it is realized (Fig. 6.8) that nutrient limitation may alter the bacterial cell surface with changes in growth rate occurring and consequent modified sensitivity to antibacterial agents. Slow-growing organisms are particularly recalcitrant to many biocides.

Interaction of bacteria with surfaces is initially reversible and eventually irreversible. Irreversible adhesion is initiated by the binding of bacteria to the surface through expolysaccharide glycocalyx polymers. Sister cells then arise by cell division and are bound within the glycocalyx matrix. The development of adherent microcolonies is thereby initiated, leading eventually to the production of a continuous biofilm on the colonized surface. As emphasized above, bacteria within such a biofilm reside in specific microenvironments that differ from cells grown under normal laboratory conditions.

Bacteria within a biofilm may be much less sensitive to biocides (and antibiotics) than planktonic cells in a laboratory culture (Fig. 6.9). There are several possible reasons (Table 6.3).

(a) Access of a biocide to the underlying cells is prevented by the glycocalyx; the glycocalyx prevents access to the bacterial surface, which depends on the nature

Table 6.3 Biofilms and bacterial responses to antiseptics and disinfectants

Mechanism of resistance associated with biofilms	Comment
(1) Exclusion or reduced access of biocide to underlying bacterial cell	Depends on (i) nature of biocide (ii) binding capacity of glycocalyx towards biocide (iii) rate of growth of microcolony relative to biocide diffusion rate
(2) Modulation of microenvironment	Associated with (i) nutrient limitation (ii) growth rate
(3) Increased production of degradative enzymes by attached cells	Mechanism unclear at present

of the biocide, its binding capacity to the glycocalyx and the rate of growth of the biofilm microcolony in relation to the diffusion rate of the biocide across the biofilm.

(b) Highly reactive biocides, such as iodine, iodine-releasing agents and isothiazolones, react chemically with the glycocalyx so that the antibacterial concentration is effectively reduced. In contrast, however, glutaraldehyde appears to have a dual role, in that it not only penetrates a biofilm but also kills cells protected by that biofilm. Furthermore, it appears that the dialdehyde accelerates the natural detachment rate of organisms from the biofilm (referred to as an 'enhanced erosion rate mechanism').

(c) Modulation of the microenvironment may produce changes in the chemical composition of the cell envelope and/or affect growth rate. Both can influence susceptibility to antibiotics and biocides. For example, the activity of bisbiguanides, QACs and substituted phenols decreases with reduced growth rate, and this is clearly more significant with sessile organisms than for bacteria growing planktonically in batch-type (laboratory) cultures.

(d) Attached cells can increase production of enzymes that degrade antibacterial agents.

The importance of biofilm production and the glycocalyx in conferring intrinsic resistance to biocides is illustrated by several examples.

(1) Bacteria can produce biofouling and corrosion of pipes in the industrial environment.

(2) Gram-negative pathogens grow as biofilms in the catheterized bladder and are able to survive concentrations of chlorhexidine that are effective against organisms in non-catheterized individuals (Fig. 6.10). The permeabilizer

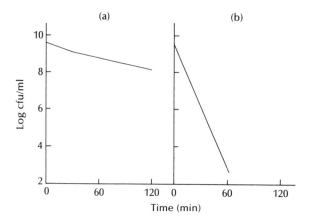

Figure 6.10   Effect of chlorhexidine (200 μg/ml) on *E. coli* (a) as a biofilm on a silicone surface and (b) in suspension. (Based on Stickler, D. J. & Hewett, P. (1991) *European Journal of Clinical Microbiology and Infectious Diseases* **10**: 416–421).

EDTA (Chapter 3) has only a temporary potentiating effect in the catheterized bladder, bacterial regrowth subsequently occurring.

(3) A glycocalyx associated with *Ps. aeruginosa* shields the cells from the effects of iodophors.

(4) Resistance to chlorine in staphylococci isolated from poultry processing plants has been ascribed to biofilm production since bacteria cultured in the laboratory remain fully sensitive to the disinfectant.

(5) *Ps. cepacia* freshly isolated from the hospital environment is often considerably more resistant than when grown in artificial culture media and a glycocalyx may be associated with intrinsic resistance of this organism to chlorhexidine.

(6) *Legionella pneumophila* is often found in hospital water distribution systems and cooling towers. Chlorination in combination with continuous heating (60 °C) of incoming water is usually the most effective disinfectant measure. However, because of biofilm production, contaminating organisms may be less susceptible to this treatment.

Subculture *in vitro* (under planktonic conditions) of bacteria growing as a biofilm leads to loss of the glycocalyx and often to an increased sensitivity to a biocide (Fig. 6.9).

2.6 Intrinsic resistance of Gram-negative bacteria

Having discussed the general role of the outer membrane as a means of excluding biocide entry (Section 2.2), the extent to which this resistance mechanism contributes towards intrinsic resistance in specific types of Gram-negative bacteria is now considered.

2.6.1 *Enterobacteriaceae*

The family Enterobacteriaceae encompasses a range of important pathogens and spoilage organisms. It includes members of the genera *Escherichia*, *Salmonella*, *Proteus*, *Providencia*, *Serratia*, *Klebsiella*, *Shigella* and *Yersinia*. Generally, they are less sensitive to biocides than Gram-positive bacteria such as *Staphylococcus aureus* but more sensitive than certain non-Enterobacteriaceae such as *Pseudomonas aeruginosa* (Table 6.1). Members of the genera *Proteus* and *Providencia* frequently show high resistance to cationic biocides such as chlorhexidine.

2.6.1.1 Escherichia coli

E. coli is more resistant to QACs, triphenyl methane dyes and diamidines than *S. aureus* and markedly more resistant to salicylanilides, carbanilides and hexachlorophane (hexachlorophene). Studies with deep rough *E. coli* mutants demonstrate that this resistance is intrinsic in nature. However, *E. coli* is only slightly less sensitive than *S. aureus* to chlorhexidine.

2.6.1.2 Proteus *spp.*

Members of the genus *Proteus* are unusually intrinsically resistant to high concentrations of chlorhexidine and other cationic bactericides, and are more resistant to EDTA than most other types of Gram-negative bacteria. Intrinsic resistance to (a) the cationic biocides may be caused by a less acidic type of LPS, so that biocide binding is reduced, and (b) EDTA may be due to the reduced divalent cation content of the *Proteus* outer membrane or inaccessibility of these cations to the chelator.

2.6.1.3 Providencia *spp.*

Prov. stuartii displays high-level intrinsic resistance to cationic bactericides, especially chlorhexidine. The mechanism of intrinsic chlorhexidine resistance is unknown but may relate to the nature of the outer membrane in this organism which effectively excludes the antiseptic. The cell envelopes of chlorhexidine-resistant strains and of chlorhexidine-sensitive mutants derived from them have very similar gross chemical compositions. It thus seems likely that subtle changes in their structural arrangement could account for differences in susceptibility to chlorhexidine.

2.6.1.4 Salmonella *spp.*

Mutants of *Salm. typhimurium* have provided useful information concerning the role of the outer membrane in conferring intrinsic resistance to biocides (Fig. 6.3, Table 6.2). Deep rough strains, with Re-type LPS, are considerably more sensitive than smooth strains to QACs, diamidines and parabens (especially the butyl ester) and even more sensitive to chlorhexidine, suggesting that LPS has an important role in intrinsic resistance of wild-type cells to these biocides. However, supersensitive mutants of *Salm. typhimurium* have been isolated that have the same LPS composition as the parent strain and similar amounts of LPS are released by EDTA or polycations. This implies that components other than LPS also contribute towards intrinsic resistance to these compounds in *Salm. typhimurium.*

2.6.1.5 Serratia *spp.*

Hospital isolates of *Ser. marcescens* may be highly resistant to chlorhexidine, hexachlorophane liquid soaps and detergent creams. The outer membrane probably determines resistance to the biocides, although it has been suggested that the inner membrane also has a role with respect to chlorhexidine resistance.

2.6.2 *Pseudomonads*

Considerable differences exist in the responses of pseudomonads to biocides. This is particularly true between *Ps. aeruginosa* and *Ps. cepacia* on the one hand and *Ps. stutzeri* on the other.

2.6.2.1 Ps. aeruginosa

Ps. aeruginosa displays higher levels of resistance to many biocides, especially QACs, than other Gram-negative bacteria. The organism is capable of surviving high concentrations of QACs and has occasionally been found as a contaminant in solutions of cetrimide and benzalkonium chloride.

   As with other Gram-negative organisms, the outer membrane is undoubtedly responsible for conferring intrinsic resistance. However, a factor of considerable importance is the cation content of this membrane, the Mg^{2+} content being greatest in *Ps. aeruginosa*. This confers strong LPS–LPS links which may relate to the exceptional biocide-resistant properties displayed by this organism. In support of this is the fact that spheroplasts of *Ps. aeruginosa* are lysed by cetrimide and chlorhexidine.

2.6.2.2 Ps. cepacia

Ps. cepacia is intrinsically resistant to a number of biocides, notably benzalkonium chloride and chlorhexidine. By acting as a permeability barrier, the outer membrane probably confers intrinsic resistance to these agents.

2.6.2.3 Ps. stutzeri

Ps. stutzeri is mentioned here not because of intrinsic resistance but because strains are often, but not invariably, intrinsically sensitive to a range of biocides (including chlorhexidine and QACs). *Ps. stutzeri* contains less wall muramic acid than other strains of pseudomonads and appears to be unique in this respect. Additional comparative studies with *Ps. stutzeri* and other pseudomonads could yield useful information about mechanism(s) of intrinsic resistance in the latter organisms.

2.7 Intrinsic resistance of mycobacteria to biocides

2.7.1 *Important types of mycobacteria*

Mycobacteria (acid fast bacilli) are responsible for various types of infections, such as tuberculosis (aetiological agent, *Mycobacterium tuberculosis*) and leprosy (*M. leprae*). They are highly hydrophobic, because of their waxy cell walls (Section 2.7.2). Environmental ('atypical') mycobacteria are usually saprophytes of soil and water but may be opportunistic pathogens. The most important opportunistic pathogens of man are the avian tubercle bacillus, *M. avium*, and the closely related *M. intracellulare*, which are usually grouped together, as the MAI complex. They cause lymphadenopathy, especially in AIDS patients. Two of the rapidly growing species, *M. chelonei* and *M. fortuitum*, are also well-known pathogens of man.

2.7.2 *Cell wall composition*

Mycobacteria are generally more resistant than other non-sporing bacteria to bactericides. This intrinsic resistance is undoubtedly linked to their cell wall composition; they possess a high wall lipid content and their high resistance has been claimed to be related to the amount of waxy material present. Mycobacterial walls contain several components:

(a) a covalent skeleton comprising two covalently linked polymers, peptidoglycan and an arabinogalactan mycolate (Fig. 6.11; Table 6.4);
(b) free lipids, which can be removed by neutral solvents;
(c) peptides which can be removed by proteolytic enzymes.

Table 6.4   Cell wall composition of mycobacterial strains

Cell wall component	Chemical composition	Comment
Covalent skeleton	Peptidoglycan	Contains *N*-glycolmuramic acid
		Two types of interpeptide linkage
	Arabinogalactan mycolate	D-arabinose, D-galactose and mycolic acid
Lipids	Free lipids	
	Wax D	
	Cord factors	
Peptides	Non-peptidoglycan amino acids	Removed by treatment with proteolytic enzymes
	Poly-α-L-glutamic acid	
Glucan		Present in some strains

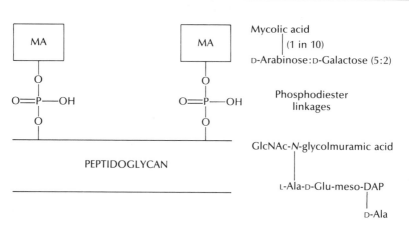

Figure 6.11   Cell wall skeleton of mycobacteria. MA, mycolate of arabinolactan. See also Figs 1.9 and 1.10, which show lipid and porin involvement and mycolic acids.

In some strains, a glucan may be present. The related genera, *Nocardia* and *Corynebacterium*, possess a covalent skeleton with the same general structure.

Mycobacterial peptidoglycan consists of glycan strands substituted by partly cross-linked tri- or tetrapeptides. However, *N*-glycolylmuramic acid is present instead of the usual *N*-acetylmuramic acid (see Chapter 1) and there are two kinds of interpeptide linkages, namely D-Ala–meso-DAP and meso-DAP–meso-Dap (D-Ala representing D-alanine, and meso-DAP being α,ε-diaminopimelic acid).

The arabinogalactan is a highly branched polymer containing D-arabinose and D-galactose (approximate ratio 5:2) and about 1 in 10 of the arabinose residues is esterified by a molecule of mycolic acid (an α-branched β-hydroxy acid containing 60–90 carbon atoms). Arabinogalactan molecules are covalently linked to peptidoglycan by phosphodiester linkages.

Free lipids account for about 25–30% of the weight of the cell walls of mycobacteria. These comprise wax D and cord factors. Wax D, which is probably an autolysis product of the cell wall of *M. tuberculosis* strains, consists of an arabinogalactan esterified by mycolic acids that is linked to a peptidoglycan that contains *N*-acetylglucosamine and *N*-glycolylmuramic acid and L-Ala, D-Ala, meso-DAP and D-glutamic acid. Cord factors, so named because of the tendency of pathogenic mycobacteria to form 'cords' when grown on the surface of a liquid medium, are dimycolates of α,α^1-D-trehalose.

2.7.3 *Biocide resistance*

There are wide responses to biocides within the mycobacteria. Against *M. tuberculosis*, QACs and chlorhexidine are inhibitory (tuberculostatic) but not tuberculocidal. Alcohols, glutaraldehyde, formaldehyde, formaldehyde–alcohol and iodine–alcohol are tuberculocidal.

Another significant pathogen, predominantly with AIDS patients, is the *M. avium intracellulare* group (or MAIS group). The MAIS group may be more than 10 times more resistant to glutaraldehyde than *M. tuberculosis*. *M. smegmatis* is more susceptible than *M. tuberculosis* to chemical disinfectants, whereas *M. terrae* has a similar resistance to *M. tuberculosis*. The mechanism of high intrinsic resistance to biocides amongst mycobacteria is not precisely known, but the hydrophobic nature of the cell wall (see Section 2.7.2) is believed in some way to exclude many hydrophilic compounds. Few investigations have yet been made, however, to correlate particular components with expression of intrinsic resistance to biocides. Nevertheless, it has been demonstrated that chlorhexidine and cetylpyridinium chloride are more effective against MAIS in the presence of ethambutol, an inhibitor of mycobacterial wall arabinogalactan biosynthesis. Although such a combination, of biocide plus chemotherapeutic agent, could clearly not be used in practice, the results are sufficiently encouraging to suggest ways of enhancing the antimycobacterial activity of agents that are normally not lethal towards such organisms. The findings also suggest a role for arabinogalactan in providing an impermeability barrier but do not exclude the possibility of other factors being involved.

Recently, considerable progress has been made in understanding the nature and composition of mycobacterial cell walls. It is hoped that this will enhance knowledge of the mechanisms of biocide resistance and suggest ways to circumvent this resistance.

2.8 Enzymatic degradation as a basis for intrinsic resistance to biocides

In only a few cases is enzymatic degradation of biocides responsible for intrinsic biocide resistance.

Several types of preservatives and disinfectants are readily metabolized by many bacteria. They include QACs, benzoic acid, *para-* (4-) hydroxybenzoic acid, phenols, chlorhexidine and phenylethanol but this metabolism usually occurs only at concentrations well below inhibitory or 'in-use' concentrations. It is thus unlikely that metabolism of biocides normally confers intrinsic resistance on a bacterial cell. However, resistance to chlorhexidine has been described in *Achromobacter xylosoxidans* isolated from an ultrasonic hand washer which involves degradation of the biguanide. Intrinsic formaldehyde resistance in some *Pseudomonas* spp. is linked to expression of an aldehyde dehydrogenase. Other aldehydes are also reduced, to the corresponding acid, by aldehyde dehydrogenase but there is no evidence to suggest that intrinsic resistance to the most important aldehyde, glutaraldehyde, occurs by this mechanism.

The occasional failure of preservatives in pharmaceutical products has been ascribed to their degradation when used as substrates for bacterial growth. Both aerobic and anaerobic metabolism has been demonstrated. However, there is also the possibility of adsorption of a biocide, e.g. a QAC, onto surfaces so that disappearance from solution has occasionally been misleadingly considered as biodegradation and thus erroneously described as resistance.

3
Acquired biocide resistance

Acquired resistance to biocides results from genetic changes in a cell and arises either by mutation or by the acquisition of genetic material from another cell as described for antibiotics in Chapter 5.

3.1 Plasmid-mediated resistance

Plasmid-encoded resistance to antibiotics has been widely studied (Chapter 5). Resistance to antibiotics in bacteria causing hospital infections is frequently determined by transmissible plasmids. Much research has also been conducted on the role of plasmids and transposons in resistance of bacteria to metals, including inorganic and organic mercury compounds. There is, however, little information about the role of plasmids in resistance to other biocides, with the exception of studies demonstrating that antiseptic resistance in staphylococci may be plasmid linked.

3.1.1 *Heavy metal resistance*

Genetic determinants of resistance to heavy metals are often found on plasmids and transposons and this resistance occurs with high frequency. Heavy metal

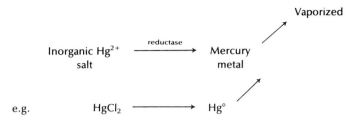

Figure 6.12 Biochemical mechanism of resistance to inorganic mercury compounds.

resistance may be associated with antibiotic resistance but this does not necessarily always occur.

3.1.1.1 Resistance to mercury

Because of its toxicity, mercuric chloride is no longer widely used as a disinfectant. Some organomercury compounds such as phenylmercuric nitrate (PMN), phenyl-mercuric acetate (PMA) and thiomersal are, however, widely used as preservatives in injectable and ophthalmic preparations (PMN, PMA) and in immunological products (thiomersal). Merbromin (mercurochrome) is a weak disinfectant.

Mercury resistance is inducible, is plasmid borne, and may be transferred from donor to recipient cells by conjugation or transduction. Inorganic (Hg^{2+}) and organomercury resistance is common in clinical isolates of *S. aureus* containing penicillinase plasmids and plasmids in Gram-negative bacteria may also carry genes conferring resistance to antibiotics and in some cases to cobalt (Co^{2+}), nickel (Ni^+), cadmium (Cd^{2+}) and arsenate (AsO_4^{3-}).

Plasmids conferring resistance to mercurials are of two types.

(a) 'Narrow-spectrum' plasmids are responsible for resistance to Hg^{2+} (by reduction to, and vaporization of, metallic mercury: see Fig. 6.12) and to the organomercury compounds merbromin and fluorescein mercuric acetate (probably by exclusion) in *E. coli*. Such plasmids do not, however, confer resistance to methylmercury, ethylmercury, PMN, PMA, *p*-hydroxymer-curibenzoate (PHMB) and thiomersal.

(b) 'Broad-spectrum' plasmids specify resistance to all the compounds listed in (a). Hydrolysis of an organomercury compound by a hydrolase (lyase) to inorganic ionic mercury (Hg^{2+}) may be followed by rapid enzymatic reduction to metallic mercury which is readily vaporized (Fig. 6.13). This volatilization does not, however, occur with all organomercury compounds (Fig. 6.13, Table 6.5). Table 6.5 summarizes these data.

Considerable progress has been made in examining the genes responsible for various functions. The most widely studied plasmid is R-100 which confers

Table 6.5 Plasmid-encoded resistance to mercury compounds

Organism	Plasmid-specified resistance to		Comment
	Hg^{2+}	Organomercurials	
E. coli	+	+	Narrow- or broad-spectrum plasmids
Salm. typhimurium	+	−	
Proteus spp.	+	−	
Providencia spp.	+	−	
Ps. aeruginosa	+	+	Narrow- or broad-spectrum plasmids
S. aureus	+	+	Broad-spectrum plasmids

(1) Host cell background might affect resistance pattern.
(2) Although Hg^0 may be formed by volatilization from a number of organomercury substrates, this does not necessarily indicate that resistance is conferred. Seemingly, a threshold level of Hg^0 must be formed which, if exceeded, confers resistance.
(3) Resistance to an organomercury compound does not necessarily involve volatilization of Hg^0: cell impermeability responsible?

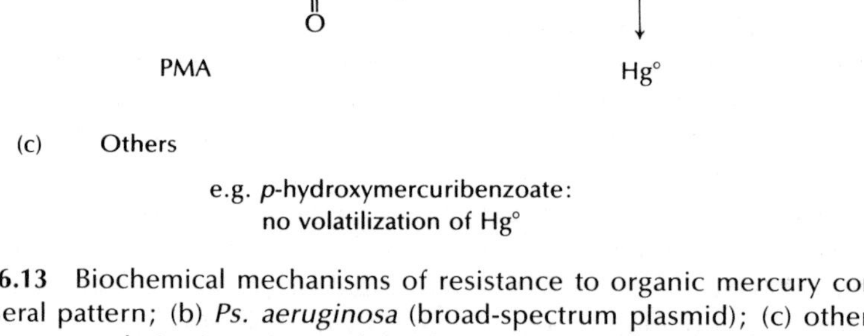

Figure 6.13 Biochemical mechanisms of resistance to organic mercury compounds: (a) general pattern; (b) *Ps. aeruginosa* (broad-spectrum plasmid); (c) other organomercury derivatives. Permeability barriers may play a role in resistance of Gram-negative bacteria. Note that Hg^0 formation does not necessarily confer resistance. PMA, phenylmercuric acetate.

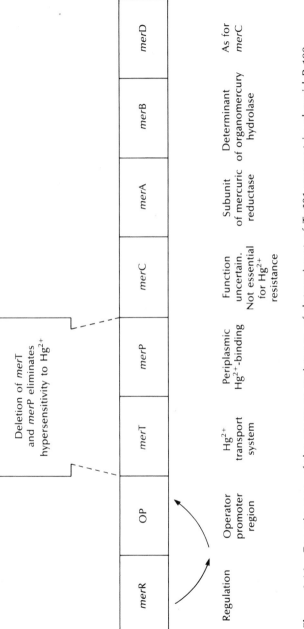

Figure 6.14 Genetic map of the mercury resistance of determinant of Tn501 present in plasmid R-100.

Hg^{2+} but not organomercury resistance. The genes are as follows (see Fig. 6.14 for genetic map).

  (i) *mer*R is a regulatory gene, mediating both positive and negative regulation, whose product is an inducer–repressor. This is followed by a promoter–operator region.
  (ii) *mer*T is responsible for an Hg^{2+} transport system that brings extracellular mercury into the cell.
  (iii) *mer*P produces a periplasmic Hg^{2+}-binding protein (encoded by Tn501)
  (iv) *mer*C is of unknown function but is not considered to be essential for Hg^{2+} resistance.
  (v) *mer*A produces a subunit of mercuric reductase.
  (vi) *mer*B determines the production of organomercury lyase. This gene, if present, lies between *mer*A and *mer*D and confers resistance to phenyl-mercury and other organomercurials.
  (vii) *mer*D is a gene defined by mutations distal to *mer*A. Like *mer*C, its function is unknown, but loss of activity leads to decreased Hg^{2+} resistance.

3.1.1.2 Resistance to silver

In the context of hospital infection, plasmid-mediated resistance to silver salts is particularly interesting because silver nitrate and silver sulphadiazine (AgSu) have been used topically for preventing infections in severe burns.

Plasmid-encoded resistance to Ag^+ occurs in clinical isolates of *Enterobacter* spp., *Pseudomonas* spp. and *Citrobacter* spp. The mechanism of resistance has not been elucidated but does not appear to be due to efflux or silver reduction. However, a pseudomonad from photographic sludge accumulates silver as Ag^0, Ag_2O or Ag^+ but not as silver sulphide (Ag_2S) or silver chloride. From this study, it was postulated that silver had been detoxified (a) by its reduction to the metallic form (Ag^0) and (b) by its complexation with cellular components. Cell-free extracts did not reduce Ag^+ to Ag^0. The current hypothesis remains that sensitive cells bind silver so tightly that they extract it from silver chloride whereas resistant cells do not compete successfully with Ag^+–halide complexes for Ag^+. It is unclear whether resistance in this case is plasmid encoded.

3.1.1.3 Resistance to other cations and to anions

Plasmid-encoded resistance to cations other than mercury and to anions may occur as described in Table 6.6.

Resistances to arsenate (AsO_4^{3-}), arsenite (AsO_3^{3-}) and antimony (III) are encoded by an inducible operon-like system in both *E. coli* and *S. aureus*. Interestingly, any of the three ions induces resistance to all three. The mechanism of arsenate resistance involves energy-dependent efflux of inhibitor, producing a

Table 6.6 Plasmid-encoded resistance to cations and anions

Anion or cation	Plasmid-specified resistance in
Ag^+	*E. coli, Salm. typhimurium*
Cd^{2+}	*S. aureus*
Co^{2+}	*E. coli*
Ni^+	*E. coli*
Zn^{2+}	*S. aureus*
Pb^{2+}	*S. aureus*
Cu^{2+}	*E. coli*
Arsenate, arsenite, antimony(III)	*E. coli, S. aureus*
CrO^{2-}	*Pseudomonas* strains, *Strep. lactis*
Tellurate, tellurite	*Alcaligenes* strains

reduced net accumulation. This efflux system is mediated by an ATPase transport system.

The plasmid-located genes conferring resistance to arsenicals are known as *ars*. In *E. coli*, phosphate transport systems are responsible for accumulating arsenate, and this organism possesses two such constitutive systems, Pit (Pi transport) and Pst (phosphate specific transport). Both are responsible for arsenate uptake although Pit has a lower affinity for phosphate. Three *ars*-encoded polypeptides are involved in expression of resistance to arsenicals in *E. coli*: ArsA (molecular weight 63 000), a catalytic subunit of arsenical-transducing ATPase; ArsB (molecular weight 46 000), a membrane-located component of the arsenic pump; ArsC (molecular weight 16 000) which modifies ArsA and ArsB to allow efflux of arsenite. Consequently, imported arsenate is rapidly pumped out of resistant cells by a system that behaves like an ATPase (Fig. 6.15). It must be pointed out that this ATPase differs from that involved in cadmium resistance (this section, below).

In contrast, plasmid-mediated chromate (CrO_4^-) resistance which occurs in several *Pseudomonas* strains is expressed at the level of uptake rather than efflux, i.e. a decreased uptake, since there is no difference in efflux between sensitive and resistant cells.

Tellurite and tellurate resistances are plasmid encoded, but the resistance mechanisms are as yet unknown.

At least four plasmid-determined systems confer cadmium (Cd^{2+}) resistance. The first two, and the most widely studied, are the *cad*A and *cad*B systems unique to staphylococcal plasmids. Cd^{2+} is transported into the cell by an energy-dependent, chromosomally determined manganese (Mn) transport system which is highly specific for Cd and Mn ions (Fig. 6.16(a)). The *cad*A gene specifies an approximately 100-fold increase in Cd^{2+} resistance, whereas the *cad*B locus provides a smaller (10-fold) increase detectable in *cad*A$^-$ mutants. Resistance

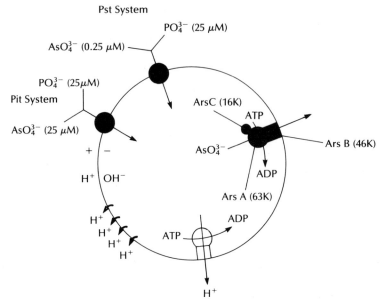

Figure 6.15 Accumulation of phosphate and arsenate by *E. coli*. The upper left-hand side of the diagram shows the Pst (phosphate specific transport) and Pit (Pi transport) systems, both of which can accumulate phospate and arsenate ions. The values of 0.25 μM or 25 μM where indicated are the K_m values for phosphate, or the K_i values for arsenate as a competitive inhibitor of phosphate transport. Beneath the Pit system is illustrated the electrogenic extrusion of protons, catalysed by the respiratory chain, which establishes the electrochemical proton gradient with the indicated polarity. The lower portion of the diagram shows the FOF1 proton translocating ATPase; above this the ATPase mediating arsenical efflux is illustrated. It is believed to consist of three polypeptides ArsA, ArsB and ArsC.

mediated by *cad*A results from energy-dependent Cd^{2+} efflux via a specific efflux ATPase, involving a Cd^{2+}–$2H^+$ exchange (Fig. 6.16(b)). As noted above, this ATPase differs from that involved in arsenate resistance.

   *cad*A and *cad*B systems also confer resistance to several other heavy metal ions. The third system has a *cad*A-type mechanism but differs in that it confers Cd^{2+} resistance only. A fourth system, found in an *Alcaligenes* strain, involves simultaneous plasmid-mediated resistance to Cd^{2+}, Zn^{2+} and Co^{2+}. The mechanism of resistance is unknown.

   Plasmid-determined copper (Cu^{2+}) resistance has been reported in some Gram-negative bacteria. In *E. coli* plasmid Rtsl encodes resistance to copper ostensibly by a decreased accumulation process although the exact mechanism is unknown. In *M. scrofulaceum*, two resistance mechanisms have been proposed, involving removal of copper from culture media by (a) a sulphate-dependent

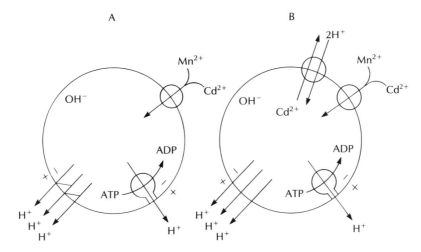

Figure 6.16 Accumulation of manganese and cadmium ions by *S. aureus*. (a) Cadmium and manganese co-transport into a cadmium-sensitive cell; (b) transport of these cations, but in addition shows the *cad*A-encoded cadmium efflux protein in a cadmium-resistant cell which promotes electroneutral cadmium–proton exchange. For other details see the text and the legend to Fig. 6.15. (From Tynecka *et al.* (1981): reproduced with permission from *Journal of Bacteriology* **147**: 313–319.)

precipitation as copper sulphide and (b) a sulphate-independent mechanism. In *Ps. syringae* pv tomato, possible copper-binding sites in proteins implicated in resistance have been identified. Clearly, further studies are necessary to elucidate plasmid-mediated mechanisms of resistance to Cu^{2+}.

3.1.2 *Resistance to other biocides*

The role of plasmids in bacterial resistance to biocides has not been studied extensively. However, it is convenient to consider the available data by examining first Gram-negative and then Gram-positive bacteria.

3.1.2.1 *Gram-negative bacteria*

Strains of *Prov. stuartii* isolated from paraplegic patients often harbour plasmids conferring resistance to Hg^{2+} and several antibiotics and the organisms may also express resistance to cationic biocides. However, attempts to transfer chlorhexidine and QAC resistance to suitable recipients have failed and the occurrence of a plasmid-linked association between antibiotic and antiseptic resistance has not been shown (see also Chapter 8 for a fuller discussion).

Table 6.7 Plasmid-mediated resistance to cationic bactericides in *Staphylococcus aureus* and *Escherichia coli*[a]

Bactericide	S. aureus MIC ratio (P$^+$:P$^-$)	E. coli MIC ratio (P$^+$:P$^-$)[b]
Chlorhexidine gluconate	2	4–8
Benzalkonium chloride	2	4
Acriflavine	128	8
Ethidium bromide	64	16

[a]Based on data of Yamamoto *et al.* (1988). P$^+$ and P$^-$ are plasmid-bearing and isogenic plasmidless strains, respectively.
[b]*E. coli* P$^+$ strain is strain carrying recombinant plasmid with genetic material from *S. aureus* resistance plasmids.

High-level resistance to biocides has been observed in hospital isolates of other Gram-negative bacteria but no clear role for plasmid-mediated biocide resistance has emerged in

(1) chlorhexidine-, antibiotic-resistant *P. mirabilis*,
(2) chlorhexidine-resistant strains of *Ps. cepacia* and *Achromobacter zylosoxidans*, or
(3) chlorhexidine- and QAC-resistant *Ps. aeruginosa* and several members of the Enterobacteriaceae.

Apart from metallic ions (Section 3.1.1), very few examples of plasmid-encoded resistance to biocides have been described in Gram-negative bacteria. These include hexachlorophane (hexachlorophene) and *Ps. aeruginosa*, mechanism of increased resistance unknown, and transferable resistance to formaldehyde and formaldehyde-releasing agents in *Ser. marcescens*, as a consequence of surface changes in, or reduced uptake or enhanced aldehyde metabolism by, resistant strains.

E. coli cells that have acquired, by recombinant DNA techniques, a plasmid from *S. aureus* that confers low-level resistance to various biocides (Section 3.1.2.2, Table 6.7) can expel, by a biocide efflux system, such agents. Such a system does not appear to be widely available in Gram-negative bacteria.

In conclusion, it is clear that plasmids are not generally involved in resistance of Gram-negative bacteria to biocides. Intrinsic resistance (Section 2) is of much greater relevance with these organisms.

3.1.2.2 *Gram-positive bacteria*

S. aureus is a major cause of surgical sepsis, septicaemia and bacteraemia in hospitals. Methicillin-resistant *S. aureus* (MRSA) strains first appeared in the 1960s

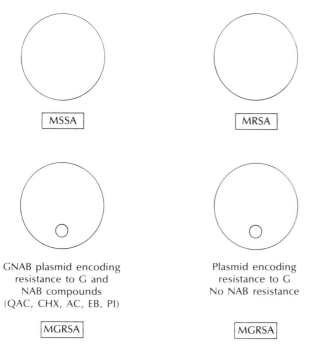

Figure 6.17 Plasmids and resistance of *Staphylococcus aureus* to biocides: MSSA, methicillin-sensitive *S. aureus*; MRSA, methicillin-resistant *S. aureus*; MGRSA, methicillin-, gentamicin-resistant *S. aureus*; G, gentamicin; NAB, nucleic acid binding; CHX, chlorhexidine; AC, acridine; EB, ethidium bromide; PI, propamidine isethionate; QAC, quaternary ammonium compound.

but by the mid-1970s the 'hospital staphylococcus' was considered to be in decline. The re-emergence in 1976 of MRSA strains which were in addition resistant to gentamicin led to staphylococcal outbreaks throughout Europe and Australia (see Chapter 8 for further details).

In Australia an analysis of MRSA strains showed them to be closely related and to contain only two classes of R plasmids:

(a) small (4.5 kb) chloramphenicol resistance plasmids, varying in the carriage of additional determinants for resistance to aminoglycoside antibiotics (genta-micin, kanamycin, tobramycin), penicillins and trimethoprim;

(b) larger (20–36 kb) plasmids encoding resistance to antiseptics, disinfectants and dyes such as acriflavine, QACs, ethidium bromide (EB) and diamidines (e.g. propamidine isethionate, PI).

The majority of the gentamicin R plasmids also possessed a determinant encoding resistance to QACs and this was originally referred to as QA-r. This determinant conferred resistance to the other cationic agents referred to in (b) above, all of

Table 6.8 Antiseptic and disinfectant resistance determinants in *Staphylococcus aureus*

Multidrug resistance determinant	Location of gene	Resistance encoded
*qac*A gene	Predominantly on pSKI family of multiresistance plasmids Also on β-lactamase and heavy metal resistance plasmids	Intercalating dyes (ethidium, acriflavine) QACs, e.g. benzalkonium chloride, cetrimide Diamidines, e.g. propamidine Biguanides, e.g. chlorhexidine
*qac*B gene	β-Lactamase and heavy metal resistance plasmids	Intercalating dyes QACs
*qac*C gene	Small (<3 kb) plasmids or large conjugative plasmids	Ethidium bromide, some QACs

which bind to nucleic acids so that it is now termed a nucleic-acid-binding resistance (NAB-r) determinant. The QAC cetyltimethylammonium bromide (CTAB) precipitates anionic macromolecules from solution at critical ionic strengths. Plasmid DNA may thus be isolated from *S. aureus* strains by a rapid method, the principle of which is the precipitation of DNA from cleared lysates by CTAB at low salt concentration.

The association of resistance to EB with β-lactamase plasmids was observed several years ago and more recently it has become associated with plasmids encoding gentamicin resistance. It has been suggested that the extensive use in hospitals of NAB compounds has been responsible for the selection of NAB-resistant strains. The NAB resistance determinants are usually found in large plasmids in association with other phenotypic markers, the most common of which is gentamicin. They have also, however, been found on the chromosome, associated with other plasmid markers or on small plasmids which carry no other known phenotypic markers.

Genetic analysis of *S. aureus* plasmids (Fig. 6.17) encoding resistance to NAB agents has identified distinct genes designated *qac*A–*qac*E, of which the first three (*qac*A, *qac*B and *qac*C) are summarized in Table 6.8. Of these, *qac*A and *qac*B share restriction site identity and DNA sequence homology, but the former determines resistance to a broader spectrum of compounds. The *qac*C gene is located typically on small plasmids or on large conjugative plasmids. Genes *qac*D and *qac*E are both carried on conjugative aminoglycoside resistance plasmids and share some similarity with *qac*C. Despite the phenotypic and genetic differences between the various *qac* genes, the resistance mechanism encoded by each is associated with an efflux system involving the PMF. A high proportion of hospital

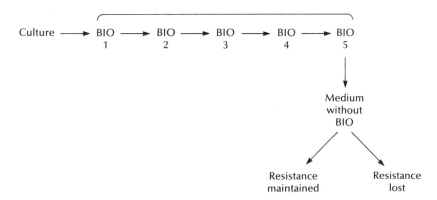

Figure 6.18 Laboratory-acquired resistance to a biocide by stepwise subculture. This is assumed to occur by a series of mutations in one or more chromosomal genes. In this case, expression of resistance is unstable and removal of selection pressure usually leads to back-mutations and re-expression of a sensitive phenotype. BIO, biocide.

isolates of coagulase-negative staphylococci (CNS) contain both *qac*A and *qac*C, a combination uncommon in *S. aureus* isolates; it has been suggested that such a combination confers a selective advantage on CNS. The prevalence of such multiexport genes in clinical isolates of *S. aureus* and CNS results from the widespread use of some NAB agents such as QACs and chlorhexidine as hospital antiseptics and disinfectants.

Resistance to some biocides has been transferred in laboratory experiments from *S. aureus* to *E. coli* by recombinant techniques. This has been expressed as high-level QAC resistance, although more frequently low level plasmid-mediated resistance to chlorhexidine, QACs, acriflavine and ethidium bromide has been transferred (Table 6.7).

Clearly, reports of resistance towards NAB compounds need to be put into perspective. Acridines and ethidium bromide are not employed for their anti-microbial properties and the diamidines have limited, specific uses. It is possible, even likely, that QACs and chlorhexidine, which are widely used in the hospital environment could select for resistant strains but the concentrations of these agents employed in practice are considerably higher than the MIC values recorded for these strains. Accordingly, strains resistant to NAB agents (Fig. 6.17) probably do not constitute a clinical problem to biocides under most circumstances.

3.2 Resistance acquired by transformation

There has been one report of transferability of chlorhexidine resistance by genetic transformation. DNA from chlorhexidine-resistant mutants of *Streptococcus sanguis* (isolated by stepwise inoculation of chlorhexidine-containing media: see Fig. 6.18) transformed competent sensitive *Strep. sanguis* to chlorhexidine resistance. The basis of resistance is unknown and its clinical significance unproven.

3.3 Resistance determined by chromosomal gene mutation

Chromosomal mutation to antibiotic resistance has been recognized in bacteria for many decades (Chapter 5). In contrast, fewer studies have been made with antiseptics, disinfectants and preservatives to determine whether chromosomal mutations confer resistance. However, some 50 years ago it was demonstrated that *Ser. marcescens*, normally inhibited by a QAC at <100 μg/ml, could adapt to grow in the presence of 100 mg/ml of that compound. Resistant and sensitive cells showed different surface properties, the former possessing an increased lipid content. Resistance was unstable, however, being lost when the resistant cells were grown in QAC-free media, presumably by back mutation.

Resistance to chlorhexidine can develop in some bacteria, e.g. *E. coli*, *P. mirabilis*, *Ps. aeruginosa* and *Ser. marcescens*, but may or may not be stable when the resistant cells are incorporated into biocide-free media (Fig. 6.18). Chlorhexidine-resistant strains may also show increased resistance to QACs. Chloroxylenol-resistant strains of *Ps. aeruginosa* have been isolated by repeated subculture in media containing gradually increasing concentrations of the xylenol. Again, however, resistance is unstable.

Chromosomal mutants of *Ps. aeruginosa* produced by stepwise exposure (Fig. 6.18) to polymyxin are resistant to both polymyxin and EDTA. They have a defective self-promoted uptake pathway and contain increased amounts of a major outer membrane protein (H1) with a corresponding decrease in envelope Mg^{2+}. Identical phenotypes appear in cells growing in Mg^{2+}-deficient media and it has been proposed that protein H1 may replace Mg^{2+} at cross-bridging sites with LPS, these sites normally being those at which interaction occurs with Mg^{2+} (e.g. EDTA) or at which displacement of Mg^{2+} takes place (polymyxin).

Although resistance to cadmium is usually plasmid mediated (see Section 3.1.1.3), examples of chromosomal mutation to resistance are also known. A chromosomal mutation in *B. subtilis* involves the membrane manganese (Mn^{2+}) transport system, which normally transports Mn^{2+} and Cd^{2+}, so that Cd^{2+} is no longer accumulated.

The lipid bilayer of the cytoplasmic membrane is the target for alcohols and other low molecular weight solvents. Resistant *E. coli* mutants have been isolated in which resistance is due to a decrease in the ratio of inner membrane phosphatidylethanolamine to anionic phospholipids (phosphatidylglycerol and diphosphatidylglycerol). Resistance to acridines can also develop as a result of mutation, but the basis of this is unknown.

Chromosomal mutation to chlorhexidine resistance has been described in *Prov.*

Table 6.9 Possible mechanisms[a] of resistance to biocides found in non-sporing bacteria

Biocide(s)	Intrinsic resistance		Acquired resistance	
	Impermeability	Enzyme inactivation	Plasmid-encoded	Mutation
Acridines			Efflux in MRSA	
Alcohols	OM?			Altered phospholipids in inner membrane
Anions				
Arsenate			Efflux by ATPase pump	
Chlorhexidine	OM, GCX		Efflux in MRSA?	Prov. stuartii: periplasmic protective proteins?
Chlorine	SL			
Crystal violet	OM		Efflux in MRSA	
Diamidines	OM		Efflux in MRSA	
Ethidium bromide			Efflux in MRSA	
EDTA				Altered HI OM protein in Ps. aeruginosa
Formaldehyde		Dehydrogenase		
Hexachlorophane			Mechanism unknown	
Iodine	GCX			
Metals				
Cadmium			cadA system (S. aureus): efflux by ATPase pump	Cd^{2+} not accumulated
Mercury (inorganic)			Reduction to Hg^0 and vaporization	
Mercury (organic)			Hydrolase then reductase	
Silver			Decreased uptake	
Parabens	OM	(+)		
Phenols	OM	(+)		
QACs	OM		Efflux in MRSA	Altered lipid content

[a]OM, outer membrane of Gram-negative bacteria; GCX, glycocalyx; SL, slime layer; MRSA, methicillin-resistant S. aureus strains.

(+), not conclusively established as a basis for resistance.

stuartii, but there is no evidence that an efflux mechanism is responsible, or that the biguanide is inactivated. An osmotic shocking procedure, which removes periplasmic proteins, sensitizes the cells to the biocide, resistance being restored when the cells are allowed to revive in growth medium. It is tentatively concluded that mutant periplasmic protective proteins bind or trap chlorhexidine preventing it from reaching its target site.

3.4 Acid habituation

A long-held view has been that bacteria cannot adapt to low pH values. However, it has now been demonstrated that bacteria such as *E. coli* grown in a medium of moderate acid pH ($\approx$5) are more resistant to subsequent acid exposure than are cells grown at neutral pH. Acid-pH-grown organisms are more resistant at acid pH to lactic, propionic, benzoic, sorbic and acetic acids. Changes in the outer membrane occur at mildly acid pH, e.g. the porin *OmpC* gene is regulated by the pH of the growth medium so that genes involved in adaptation may affect the structure of the outer membrane. This form of acid habituation or resistance can therefore be classified as phenotypic adaptation within the intrinsic resistance mechanism previously defined.

4
General conclusions

From the foregoing, it is apparent that several mechanisms of resistance might occur in non-sporing bacteria that can be classified as intrinsic or acquired (Table 6.9).

Examination of Table 6.9 demonstrates that studies on the biochemical mechanism of resistance to biocides are not as advanced as those on antibiotics (see Chapter 5).

Further reading

General reviews on antiseptics, disinfectants and preservatives

Fleurette, J., Freney, J. & Reverdy, M. E. (1995). *Antisepsie et Désinfection*. Editions Eska, Paris.

Russell, A. D. (1991). Principles of antimicrobial activity. In *Disinfection, Sterilization and Preservation* (ed. S. S. Block). Fourth edition, pp. 29–58. Lea & Febiger, Philadelphia.

Russell, A. D., Hugo, W. B. & Ayliffe, G. A. J. (eds) (1992). *Principles and Practice of Disinfection, Preservation and Sterilization*. Second edition. Blackwell Scientific Publications, Oxford.

Reviews on bacterial surfaces

Benz, R. (1988). Structure and function of porins from Gram-negative bacteria. *Annual Review of Microbiology* **42**: 359–393.

Denyer, S. P., Gorman, S. P. & Sussman, M. (eds) (1993). *Microbial Biofilms: Formation and Control.* Society for Applied Bacteriology Technical Series No. 30. Blackwell Scientific Publications, Oxford.

Poxton, I. R. (1993). Prokaryote envelope diversity. *Journal of Applied Bacteriology (Symposium Supplement)* **74**: 1S–11S.

Reviews on bacterial resistance

Al-Masaudi, S. B., Day, M. J. & Russell, A. D. (1991). Antimicrobial resistance and gene transfer in *Staphylococcus aureus*. *Journal of Applied Bacteriology* **70**: 279–290.

Brown, M. R. W. & Gilbert, P. (1993). Sensitivity of biofilms to antimicrobial agents. *Journal of Applied Bacteriology (Symposium Supplement)* **74**: 87S–97S.

Carpentier, B. & Cerf, O. (1993). Biofilms and their consequences with particular reference to hygiene in the food industry. *Journal of Applied Bacteriology* **75**: 499–511.

Chopra, I. (1988). Efflux of antibacterial agents from bacteria. *Homeostatic Mechanisms of Microorganisms*. FEMS Symposium No. 44, pp. 146–158. Bath University Press, Bath.

Costerton, J. W., Cheng, K.-J., Geesey, G. G., Ladd, T. I., Nickel, J. C., Dasgupta, M. & Marrie, T. J. (1987). Bacterial biofilms in nature and disease. *Annual Review of Microbiology* **41**: 435–464.

Heinzel, M. (1988). The phenomena of resistance to disinfectants and preservatives. In *Industrial Biocides*. Critical Reports on Applied Chemistry, Volume 23 (ed. K. R. Payne) pp. 52–67. John Wiley & Sons, Chichester.

Hugo, W. B. (1991). The degradation of preservatives by microorganisms. *International Biodeterioration* **27**: 185–194.

Lyon, B. R. & Skurray, R. A. (1987). Antimicrobial resistance of *Staphylococcus aureus*: genetic basis. *Microbiological Reviews* **51**: 88–134.

Russell, A. D. (1991). Mechanisms of bacterial resistance to non-antibiotics: food additives and food and pharmaceutical preservatives. *Journal of Applied Bacteriology* **71**: 191–201.

Russell, A. D. (1992). Mycobactericidal agents. In *Principles and Practice of Disinfection, Preservation and Sterilization* (eds A. D. Russell, W. B. Hugo & G. A. J. Ayliffe). Second edition, pp. 246–253. Blackwell Scientific Publications, Oxford.

Russell, A. D. & Day, M. J. (1993). Antibacterial activity of chlorhexidine. *Journal of Hospital Infection* **25**: 229–238.

Silver, S. & Misra, S. (1988). Plasmid-mediated heavy metal resistances. *Annual Review of Microbiology* **42**: 717–743.

Silver, S., Nucifora, G., Chu, L. & Misra, T. K. (1989). Bacterial ATPases: primary pumps for exporting toxic cations and anions. *Trends in Biochemical Sciences* **14**: 76–80.

Bacterial resistance: selected papers

Cookson, B. D., Bolton, M. C. & Platt, J. H. (1991). Chlorhexidine resistance in methicillin-resistant *Staphylococcus aureus* or just an elevated MIC? An *in vitro* and *in vivo* assessment. *Antimicrobial Agents and Chemotherapy* **35**: 1997–2002.

Gandi, P. A., Sawant, A. D., Wilson, L. A. & Ahearn, D. G. (1993). Adaptation and growth of *Serratia marcescens* in contact lens disinfectant solutions containing chlorhexidine gluconate. *Applied and Environmental Microbiology* **59**: 183–188.

Leelaporn, A., Paulsen, I. T., Tennent, J. M., Littlejohn, T. G. & Skurray, R. A. (1994). Multidrug resistance to antiseptics and disinfectants in coagulase-negative staphylococci. *Journal of Medical Microbiology* **40**: 214–220.

Littlejohn, T. G., DiBerardino, D., Messerotti, L. J., Spiers, S. J. & Skurray, R. A. (1991). Structure and evolution of a family of genes encoding antiseptic and disinfectant resistance in *Staphylococcus aureus*. *Gene* **101**: 59–66.

Midgley, M. (1986). The phosphonium ion efflux system of *Escherichia coli*: a relationship to the ethidium efflux system and energetic studies. *Journal of General Microbiology* **132**: 3187–3193.

Midgley, M. (1987). An efflux system for cationic dyes and related compounds in *Escherichia coli*. *Microbiological Sciences* **4**: 125–127.

Nies, D. H. & Silver, S. (1995). Ion efflux systems involved in bacterial metal resistances. *Journal of Industrial Microbiology* **14**: 186–199.

Rastogi, N., Goh, K. S. & David, H. L. (1990). Enhancement of drug susceptibility of *Mycobacterium avium* by inhibitors of cell envelope synthesis. *Antimicrobial Agents and Chemotherapy* **34**: 759–764.

Rouch, D. A. Cram, D. S., DiBerardino, D., Littlejohn, T. G. & Skurray, R. A. (1990). Efflux-mediated antiseptic resistance gene *qac*A from *Staphylococcus aureus*: common ancestry with tetracycline- and sugar-transported proteins. *Molecular Microbiology* **4**: 2051–2062.

Russell, A. D. (1993). Microbial cell walls and resistance of bacteria and fungi to antibiotics and biocides. *Journal of Infectious Diseases* **168**: 1339–1340.

Russell, A. D., Broadley, S. J., Furr, J. R. & Jenkins, P. A. (1994). Potentiation of the antimycobacterial activity of biocides. *Journal of Infection* **28**: 108–109.

Stickler, D. J., Dolman, J., Rolfe, S. & Chawla, J. (1989). Activity of some antiseptics against urinary *Escherichia coli* growing as biofilms on silicone surfaces. *European Journal of Clinical Microbiology and Infectious Diseases* **8**: 974–978.

Stickler, D. J., Dolman, J., Rolfe, S. & Chawla, J. (1991). Activity of antiseptics against urinary tract pathogens growing as biofilms on silicone surfaces. *European Journal of Clinical Microbiology and Infectious Diseases* **10**: 410–415.

Tennent, J. M., Lyon, B. R., Midgley, M., Jones, I. G., Purewal, A. S. & Skurray, R. A. (1989). Physical and biochemical characterization of the *qac*A gene encoding antiseptic and disinfectant resistance in *Staphylococcus aureus*. *Journal of General Microbiology* **135**: 1–10.

Van Klingeren, B. & Pullen, W. (1993). Glutaraldehyde resistant mycobacteria from endoscope washers. *Journal of Hospital Infection* **25**: 147–149.

Yamamoto, T., Tamura, Y. & Yokota, T. (1988). Antiseptic and antibiotic resistance plasmid in *Staphylococcus aureus* that possesses ability to confer chlorhexidine and acrinol resistance. *Antimicrobial Agents and Chemotherapy* **32**: 932–935.

CHAPTER SEVEN

Mechanisms of spore resistance to biocides

1
Introduction

Bacterial spores are generally considerably more resistant to biocides than are germinated spores or non-sporulating bacteria (Fig. 7.1). As demonstrated in Chapter 4, there are several stages during sporulation subject to inhibition by antibacterial agents. Conversely, there are also several stages where resistance of spores to chemicals may arise. This is undoubtedly of potential significance in the

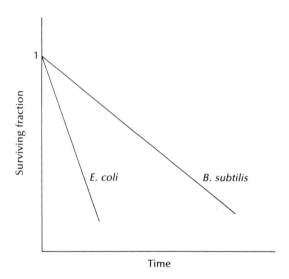

Figure 7.1 Comparative responses of non-sporing (*Escherichia coli*) and sporing (*Bacillus subtilis*) organisms to a bactericidal and sporicidal agent. In practice, *E. coli* would be killed rapidly by a low concentration of the biocide, whereas a much higher concentration would be needed for a sporicidal action to be achieved, especially if large numbers of spores were present (Chapter 4: Table 4.2).

Table 7.1   Sporulation and resistance to biocides: experimental procedures

Method	Comment
(1) Sample removal during sporulation	Criticism: cells at different stages of sporulation
(2) Cultures treated with subinhibitory concentrations of biocide at commencement of sporulation, then as (1)	Little studied; spore development should be linked to electron microscopy
(3) Spo⁻ mutants	Mutants unable to develop beyond a genetically determined sporulation stage
(4) Dap⁻ mutants	Conditional spore cortexless mutants of *B. sphaericus*: possible changes elsewhere in spore do not appear to have been studied
(5) Step-down procedure	Probably synchronous spore development, thus improvement on (1)
(6) Coatless spores	Use of UDS[a] to remove outer and inner spore coats (cortex may also be removed to some extent)
(7) Coatless and cortexless spores	Use of UDS[a] with lysozyme
(8) Spores ($\alpha^-\beta^-$) deficient in α/β-type SASPs	Studied to date only with hydrogen peroxide

[a]Urea + dithithreitol + sodium dodecyl sulphate

context of food and medical microbiology. Thus, this chapter will consider those factors that are deemed to be responsible for the high resistance of bacterial spores to chemical biocides. Reference has already been made in Chapters 1 (Section 3), 3 (Section 3.1) and 4 to the nature and composition of spores, the uptake of biocides and the mechanisms of action of sporicidal and sporistatic agents.

2
Experimental aspects

Various techniques have been employed to investigate the mechanism by which spores resist chemical inhibitors. These include the use of sporulation (Spo⁻), $\alpha^-\beta^-$ and other mutants, an examination of the changes in sensitivity that occur during sporulation and the use of specific agents that affect the spore coat(s) or cortex. It is important to consider the theoretical principles underlying some of these procedures because they enable us to achieve a better understanding of the mechanisms involved in spore resistance to biocides.

A summary of these procedures is presented in Table 7.1, together with some

Table 7.2 Use of sporulation (Spo⁻) mutants of *Bacillus subtilis* in studying development of resistance to biocides

B. subtilis strain	Characteristics
Wild type	Develops into mature spores
IV mutants	Do not develop beyond stage IV
V mutants	Do not develop beyond stage V
VI mutants	Do not develop into fully mature spores

Table 7.3 Onset of resistance to antibacterial agents during the sporulation process

Agent	Sporulation stage	
	At which resistance develops	Where resistance is fully developed
Toluene	Late stage III	Early stage IV
Chlorhexidine	Stage IV	Stage V
Heat	Stage V	Stage IV
Lysozyme	Middle of stage V	Stage VI
Glutaraldehyde	Late stage V	Stage VI completed

comments about their relative usefulness. Theoretical aspects are considered in more detail below from which some general conclusions may be reached.

2.1 Use of Spo⁻ mutants

The use of Spo⁻ mutants of *B. subtilis* strain 168 for studies on resistance is increasing. These mutants are unable to develop beyond a certain stage in the sporulation process (Table 7.2) and are consequently of value in correlating structural changes and biochemical characteristics with response to antibacterial compounds (Table 7.3) or to physical processes such as heat, ultraviolet or ionizing radiations. For example wild-type and stages IV, V and VI mutants are exposed to a test biocide of appropriate concentration under carefully standardized conditions and samples removed at appropriate intervals to determine the number of survivors (Fig. 7.2).

Studies with these Spo⁻ mutants reveal that resistance to toluene develops early in sporulation, whereas resistance to lysozyme is a late event. Toluene cannot, of course, be considered as a useful antibacterial agent and lysozyme is rarely used

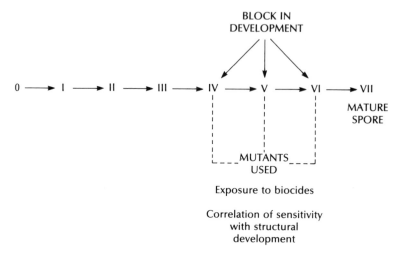

Figure 7.2   Spore mutants of *Bacillus subtilis* strain 168.

as such. Both can, however, be regarded as useful markers. Resistance to chlorhexidine occurs later than toluene and just before heat resistance, whereas glutaraldehyde resistance is a very late event, occurring after the development of lysozyme resistance (Table 7.3). This view is reinforced by studies on wild-type (Spo$^+$) cultures of *B. subtilis* 168 (see Section 2.3 and Figs 7.4 and 7.5).

A wide range of antibacterial agents has now been studied with these Spo$^-$ mutants. The resistance of *B. subtilis* during sporulation to various compounds develops in the following order: toluene (first), formaldehyde, sodium lauryl sulphate, phenol, phenylmercuric nitrate, *m*-cresol, chlorocresol, chlorhexidine, cetylpyridinium chloride, mercuric chloride, moist heat, sodium dichloro-isocyanurate, sodium hypochlorite, lysozyme and finally glutaraldehyde.

2.2   Use of Dap$^-$ mutants

Conditional spore-cortexless mutants of a strain of *B. sphaericus* have been described. These are deficient in the synthesis of meso-diaminopimelic acid (Dap), and the muramic lactam and hence cortex content increase with an increase in the external concentration of Dap (see Chapter 1 for details of muramic lactam). Spores with varying cortical contents can thus be obtained by growth in media containing different Dap concentrations. Characteristic spore properties are associated with different amounts of cortex, e.g. 25% of maximal cortex content to show octanol resistance but 90% is needed to demonstrate heat resistance.

Unfortunately changes may occur elsewhere in the spore and thus conclusions reached by this approach must be made with caution. Nevertheless, it is becoming increasingly clear that the cortex, as well as the spore coats, might be involved

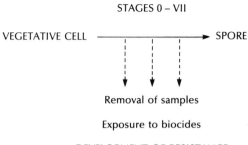

STAGES 0 – VII

VEGETATIVE CELL ⟶ SPORE

Removal of samples

Exposure to biocides

DEVELOPMENT OF RESISTANCE

Figure 7.3 Non-synchronous sporulation and development of resistance to biocides.

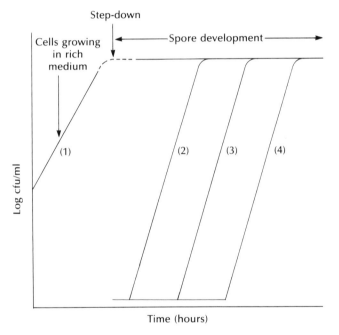

Figure 7.4 Diagrammatic representation of sporulation and development of resistance. (1) Cells growing in nutritionally rich medium are suddenly transferred to a nutritionally poor medium ('step-down' procedure). During sporulation, samples are removed and exposed to various inhibitors. Early, intermediate and late development of resistance to inhibitors is shown by the increased number of survivors in curves (2), (3) and (4), respectively.

in spore resistance to biocides (Section 2.4). Findings obtained with Dap⁻ mutants should thus be seen in the overall context and could be re-examined with a broader range of antibacterial agents.

2.3 Development of resistance during sporulation

Useful information can be obtained by attempting to correlate resistance to chemicals (or physical agencies) with structural and other changes that occur during sporulation. Three types of methods can be used (Sections 2.3.1–2.3.3).

2.3.1 Sample removal during sporulation

If vegetative cells of a spore-forming organism such as *B. subtilis* are inoculated into a liquid broth medium then, after a period of vegetative cell growth and division, spores will develop. Samples can be removed during the sporulation process to measure response to a test biocide (Fig. 7.3).

This procedure suffers from the criticism that cells at different stages of spore development may be present so that it could be difficult to correlate biocide sensitivity or resistance with a particular sporulation stage.

2.3.2 Step-down procedure

In this method (Fig. 7.4), *B. subtilis* cells growing in a nutritionally rich medium are rapidly transferred to a nutritionally poor medium. About 90–95% of the cells form spores in a synchronous manner. During sporulation, samples can be removed and responses to test biocides (or to physical agencies such as heat and radiation) determined. Appropriate markers are used simultaneously to demonstrate early resistance (toluene resistance), intermediate (moist heat resistance) and late resistance (lysozyme and glutaraldehyde resistance), as depicted in Fig. 7.5.

2.3.3 Sporulation in presence of biocide

In this procedure (Fig. 7.6), cells are incubated in sporulation medium in the presence of a subinhibitory and sublethal biocide concentration and the sporulation stage reached determined, e.g. by electron miscroscopy. This approach has not been widely used but could generate data to substantiate those obtained with Spo⁻ mutants (Section 2.1).

2.4 Coatless and cortexless spores

Spores remain viable even after removal of the spore coats and cortex. Thus, the role of the coats and cortex in resistance to biocides can be examined by comparing

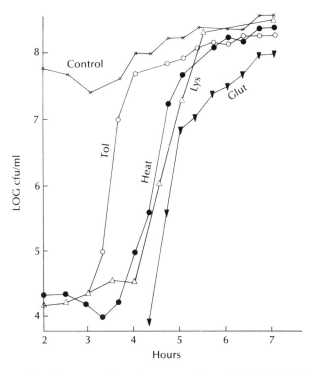

Figure 7.5 Development of resistance to glutaraldehyde (Glut) and other agents during sporulation of *B. subtilis* strain 168: Tol, toluene; Lys, lysozyme.

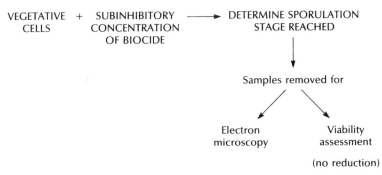

Figure 7.6 Sporulation in presence of a subinhibitory concentration of a biocide.

Table 7.4 Removal of outer and inner spore coats and cortex

Chemical agent(s)[a]	Properties	Function
DTT	Disulphide-bond-reducing agent	Removal of outer spore coat
SDS	Dissociates polypeptides	Dissociation of inner spore coat
UDS	Urea + DTT + SDS	Removal of inner and outer spore coats and of some cortex
UDS(L)	UDS + lysozyme	Additional extraction of cortex

[a]DTT, dithiothreitol; SDS, sodium dodecyl sulphate; L, lysozyme

Table 7.5 Extraction of spore coat protein and cortex peptidoglycan from *B. subtilis* by various treatments

Treatment	Total coat protein extracted (%)	Cortex hexosamine extracted (%)
NaOH		
0.2%	10	0
0.4%	17.5	0
1.0%	24.5	0
UDS	67.5	50
UDS + lysozyme	—	75

From Bloomfield & Arthur (1994).

the sensitivity of intact spores with that of spores from which these structural components have been removed.

UDS, a combination of urea, dithiothreitol (DTT) and sodium dodecyl sulphate (SDS), employed at a pH of about 10 removes spore coats. DTT, a disulphide-bond-reducing agent, substantially removes the outer coat; it can be replaced by another disulphide-bond-reducing agent, mercaptoethanol. SDS, an anionic surfactant, dissociates acidic polypeptides in the inner coat. UDS removes outer and inner coat protein as well as a substantial amount of cortex hexosamine (Tables 7.4 and 7.5), and additional cortex hexosamine is extracted if lysozyme is subsequently used (Table 7.5). Sodium hydroxide used alone extracts some coat protein (Table 7.5).

By selective use of these agents, therefore, it is possible to produce spores lacking outer coat as well as spores devoid of both coats and a substantial amount

Table 7.6 Pretreatment of spores and subsequent sensitivity to halogens

Pretreatment	Chlorine-releasing agents	Iodine-releasing agents
Sodium hydroxide	NaOCl and NaDCC: increased sporicidal activity Chloramine: no effect	Slight increase
UDS	Increased activity to all	Increased activity
UDS then lysozyme	Increased activity to all	Marked increased activity

Table 7.7 Mechanism of spore resistance to antibacterial agents

Antibacterial agent	Spore component(s)	Comment[a]
Alkali	Cortex	
Lysozyme	Coat(s)	
Hypochlorites, chlorine dioxide	Coat(s), cortex	UDS (±lysozyme) spores highly sensitive
Glutaraldehyde	Coat(s), cortex (?)	UDS spores highly sensitive
Iodine	Coat(s), cortex	UDS spores highly sensitive
Hydrogen peroxide	Coat(s)	Varies with strain
Chlorhexidine	Coat(s), cortex (?)	
Ethylene oxide	Coat(s)?	Exact relationship unclear
Octanol	Cortex	DAP⁻ mutants of
Xylene		B. sphaericus used
Ozone	Coat(s), cortex (?)	UDS spores highly sensitive

[a]UDS, urea + dithiothreitol + sodium lauryl sulphate.

of cortex, also. UDS-treated spores are rendered highly sensitive to glutaraldehyde, iodine, hydrogen peroxide, ozone, chlorine dioxide and chlorine.

Pretreatment of *B. subtilis* spores with NaOH, to extract alkali-soluble coat protein, increases activity of NaOCl and NaDCC, but not of chloramine, and has only a slight effect on iodine-releasing agents. Increased activity of all agents occurs when spores are pretreated with UDS, and the activity of iodine-releasing agents is further enhanced when spores are pre-exposed to UDS + lysozyme (Table 7.6). The cortex, as well as the coats, thus plays a part in determining spore resistance to halogen-releasing agents and possibly to other types of biocides (Table 7.7).

Whether spore coats play a role in the resistance of spores to ethylene oxide is unclear. Ethylene oxide, $(CH_2)_2O$, is a comparatively small molecule (molecular weight 44) that might be expected to enter spores freely. Generally, however, molecular size may be an important factor in governing spore permeability, since the coats play an important role in limiting entry to other small molecule inhibitors, as noted above. The comparatively high resistance of bacterial spores to ethylene oxide is not lost during germination, so that hydration of the spore core and alteration of spore coat layers do not appear to be linked to sensitivity to this gaseous disinfectant.

In some organisms, the spore coats offer better protection than in others. For example, the spore coat offers a protective barrier against peroxide in *Clostridium bifermentans* but is much less effective in conferring resistance in *B. cereus*. This probably results from differences in the composition of the coats in different species.

2.5 $\alpha^- \beta^-$ Spores

It was pointed out in Chapters 1 and 4 that small, acid-soluble proteins (SASPs) constituted about 10–20% of the protein in the dormant spore, that they existed in two forms (α/β and γ) and that they were degraded during germination. The SASPs are essential for expression of spore resistance to ultraviolet radiation and also appear to be involved in resistance to hydrogen peroxide.

As pointed out in Chapter 4 (Section 5.2.7) spores ($\alpha^- \beta^-$) deficient in α/β-type SASPs are much more sensitive to H_2O_2 than are wild-type spores. It has been proposed that, in the latter, DNA is saturated with α/β-type SASPs and is thus protected from attack by hydroxyl radicals. Such protection of DNA from free radical damage may be a major factor in spore longevity.

$\alpha^- \beta^-$ spores have not yet been used in studies with other sporicidal or sporistatic agents. Such investigations might shed further light on the role of SASPs in protecting spore DNA from damage by hitherto unrecognized mechanisms.

3
Revival of injured spores

It was stated in Chapter 4 (Section 5.5) that sublethal spore injury (damage) may be manifested as an increased susceptibility to 'stressing agents', such as alkali and various types of surface-active agents that are not sporicidal. This has been demonstrated conclusively with spores injured by exposure to aldehydes (formaldehyde, glutaraldehyde) and halogens (chlorine- and iodine-releasing agents).

It is possible to revive some spores of *Bacillus* species that have been exposed to high concentrations of sporicides even for prolonged periods. The dialdehyde glutaraldehyde has been most widely studied in this context and it has been demonstrated that alkali (NaOH or KOH) increases the ability of some spores exposed to glutaraldehyde to germinate. Alkali inhibits the outgrowth stage. The exact mechanism of the repair process associated with alkali treatment is unknown, although five possibilities are considered in Table 7.8. Glutaraldehyde is an

Table 7.8 Possible mechanisms of alkali-induced revival of glutaraldehyde-treated *Bacillus subtilis* spores

Mechanism	Comment
(1) High pH dissolves alkali-soluble protein components from spore coat	Unlikely: only very small amount of protein released from glutaraldehyde-treated spores
(2) Alkali acts as trigger for germination, substituting for, for example, L-alanine	Untreated spores: no germination in buffer + D-glucose + NaOH. However, germination is involved in revival process[a]
(3) Alkali may desorb glutaraldehyde	Not found, although experiments with labelled dialdehyde would be helpful
(4) Simple pH effect	Unlikely: high pH inhibits germination
(5) Small proportion of spores may be superdormant	Require extreme conditions for germination. Role of NaOH unknown

[a]Addition of NaOH to glutaraldehyde-treated spores may increase potential for germination in a small proportion of spores whilst outgrowth is inhibited.

electron microscope fixative, and thus spores that have survived exposure to this agent might be in a 'superdormant' state; the addition of alkali may then, in an unknown manner, increase their potential for germination. However, alkali is incapable of reviving formaldehyde-treated spores, or spores exposed to halogen-releasing agents.

The revival of injured spores, as manifest by their decreased susceptibility to stressing agents, is depicted in Fig. 7.7. In this procedure, injured spores are held at 37 °C in nutrient broth and their ability to form colonies on agar containing a stressing agent is determined. Thus, repair of injury is reflected by an increase in colony numbers. Repair occurs primarily during outgrowth and is initiated soonest for iodine-releasing agents and latest for glutaraldehyde: this is logical because, of the four biocides (iodine, chlorine, formaldehyde and glutaraldehyde), iodine causes the least and glutaraldehyde the most injury.

4
Conclusions

Comparative resistance to some sporicides develops during sporulation and is lost during germination and/or outgrowth (Chapter 4). Resistance is not associated with biodegradation of antibacterial agents by sporulating cells or by mature spores. An alternative explanation would be alteration of the target site during sporulation.

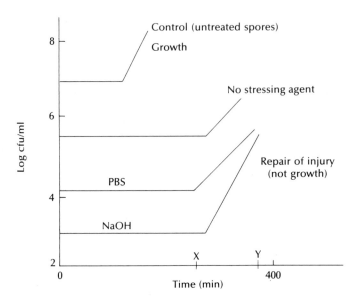

Figure 7.7 Revival of spores of *Bacillus subtilis* following exposure to sublethal biocidal injury. Following exposure to a biocide, spores were held in nutrient broth at 37 °C and plated on to agar with or without a stressing agent (polymyxin B sulphate (PBS) or sodium hydroxide). Over the period X to Y, the cells regain the ability to form colonies on agar containing a stressing agent, the increasing number of cfu/ml denoting repair of injury.

Although there is little evidence for this, it should be noted that at the level of DNA organization, spore DNA *in vivo* (but not *in vitro*) occurs in the A form rather than the normal B form (see Chapter 1). Possibly the A conformation is associated with resistance of spores to some agents interacting with DNA.

The sporicides discussed in this chapter are quite distinct from antibiotics and chemotherapeutic agents. The latter tend to have very specific sites of action (Chapter 2) and target site mutations that lead to resistance in vegetative bacteria do indeed occur (Chapter 5). Sporicides, however, are much less specific in their actions (see, for example, aldehydes and alkylating agents already referred to in the present chapter), and inaccessibility of target sites is the most likely mechanism responsible for the comparative resistance to spore inhibitors. Obviously, spore coats have an important role to play here, and synthesis of specific spore coat proteins is associated with development during sporulation of resistance to lysozyme. The even later development of resistance to glutaraldehyde is, however, unlikely to be associated with specific spore coat proteins but rather to the presence of the coat *per se* because the dialdehyde interacts significantly and rapidly with various types of proteins. The spore cortex is also likely to act as a barrier to at least some antibacterial compounds, notably halogen-releasing agents (Fig. 7.8).

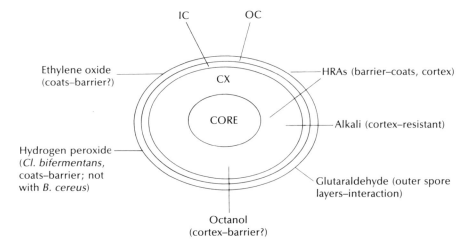

Figure 7.8 Possible spore barriers to specific non-antibiotic agents: OC, outer spore coat; IC, inner spore coat; CX, cortex.

Finally, the dehydration of the spore core itself might slow the reaction of biocidal agents with core components.

Further reading

General works on spore resistance to biocides

Bloomfield, S. F. (1992). Resistance of bacterial spores to chemical agents. In *Principles and Practice of Disinfection, Preservation and Sterilization* (eds A. D. Rusell, W. B. Hugo & G. A. J. Ayliffe). Second edition, pp. 230–245. Blackwell Scientific Publications, Oxford.

Bloomfield, S. F. & Arthur, M. (1994). Mechanisms of inactivation and resistance of spores to chemical biocides. *Journal of Applied Bacteriology (Symposium Supplement)* **76**: 91S–104S.

Foegeding, P. M. (1983). Bacterial spore resistance to chlorine compounds. *Food Technology* **37**(11): 100–104.

Gould, G. W. (1985). Modification of resistance and dormancy. In *Fundamental and Applied Aspects of Bacterial Spores* (eds G. J. Dring, D. J. Ellar & G. W. Gould) pp. 371–382. Academic Press, London.

Hurst, A. & Gould, G. W. (eds) (1983). *The Bacterial Spore*, Volume 2. Academic Press, London.

Russell, A. D. (1982). *The Destruction of Bacterial Spores*. Academic Press, London.

Russell, A. D. (1990). Bacterial spores and chemical sporicidal agents. *Clinical Microbiology Reviews* **3**: 99–119.

Stevenson, K. E. & Shafer, B. D. (1983). Bacterial spore resistance to hydrogen peroxide. *Food Technology* **37**(11): 111–114.

Spore resistance to biocides: selected papers

Bloomfield, S. F. & Arthur, M. (1989). Effect of chlorine-releasing agents on *Bacillus subtilis* vegetative cells and spores. *Letters in Applied Microbiology* **8**: 101–104.

Dadd, A. H. & Daly, G. M. (1982). Role of the coat in resistance of bacterial spores to inactivation by ethylene oxide. *Journal of Applied Bacteriology* **53**: 109–116.

Jenkinson, H. F. (1981). Germination and resistance defects in spores of a *Bacillus subtilis* mutant lacking a coat of polypeptide. *Journal of General Microbiology* **127**: 81–91.

Jenkinson, H. F., Sawyer, W. D. & Mandelstam, J. (1981). Synthesis and order of assembly of spore coat proteins in *Bacillus subtilis*. *Journal of General Microbiology* **123**: 1–16.

Knott, A. G., Russell, A. D. & Dancer, B. N. (1995). Development of resistance to biocides during sporulation of *Bacillus subtilis*. *Journal of Applied Bacteriology* **79**: 492–498.

Power, E. G. M., Dancer, B. N. & Russell, A. D. (1988). Emergence of resistance to glutaraldehyde in spores of *Bacillus subtilis* 168. *FEMS Microbiology Letters* **50**: 223–226.

Shaker, L. A., Dancer, B. N., Russell, A. D. & Furr, J. R. (1988). Emergence and development of chlorhexidine resistance during sporulation of *Bacillus subtilis* 168. *FEMS Microbiology Letters* **51**: 73–76.

Shaker, L. A., Furr, J. R. & Russell, A. D. (1988). Mechanism of resistance of *Bacillus subtilis* spores to chlorhexidine. *Journal of Applied Bacteriology* **64**: 531–539.

Waites, W. M. & Bayliss, C. E. (1979). The effect of changes in the spore coat on the destruction of *Bacillus cereus* spores by heat and chemical agents. *Journal of Applied Biochemistry* **1**: 71–76.

Williams, N. D. & Russell, A. D. (1992). The nature and site of biocide-induced sublethal injury in *Bacillus subtilis* spores. *FEMS Microbiology Letters* **99**: 277–280.

Williams, N. D. & Russell, A. D. (1993). Injury and repair in biocide-treated spores of *Bacillus subtilis*. *FEMS Microbiology Letters* **106**: 183–186.

Williams, N. D. & Russell, A. D. (1993). Revival of biocide-treated spores of *Bacillus subtilis*. *Journal of Applied Bacteriology* **75**: 69–75.

Williams, N. D. & Russell, A. D. (1993). Revival of *Bacillus subtilis* spores from biocide-induced injury in the germination process. *Journal of Applied Bacteriology* **75**: 76–81.

CHAPTER EIGHT

Impact on society of bacterial resistance to antibiotics and biocides and ways of counteracting it

1
Introduction

Previous chapters have dealt with the genetic and biochemical basis of resistance to antibiotics and biocides expressed by bacteria and their spores. In this chapter the social implications of bacterial resistance, particularly in the contexts of human medicine and hygiene, are considered. Later sections deal with strategies for counteracting resistance to antibacterial agents.

2
Impact of bacterial resistance to chemotherapeutic antibiotics

2.1 Consequences for therapy of infectious diseases: overview

As mentioned in Chapter 5, acquired rather than intrinsic antibiotic resistance usually poses the greatest threat to successful chemotherapy. Table 8.1 gives specific examples in which the emergence of acquired antibiotic resistance has either eliminated a number of previously valuable treatments, or made treatment more difficult or more costly because alternative agents must now be used. Three of the examples in Table 8.1 are considered in more detail below.

2.1.1 *Penicillin resistance in* Neisseria gonorrhoeae

Until the mid-1970s single-dose oral therapy with penicillins such as ampicillin or amoxycillin was invariably the preferred choice for treatment of *N. gonorrhoeae* infections. However, in 1976, β-lactamase-producing organisms, with a high level of resistance to penicillins and causing infections refractory to penicillin therapy, emerged in the United Kingdom and United States. These strains have now spread throughout the world and possess plasmids that encode the TEM-1 β-lactamase. Infections with such organisms are now frequently treated with β-lactamase-stable cephalosporins such as cefoxitin, cefuroxime and cefotaxime. However, these

Table 8.1 Valuable treatments under threat or no longer available

Type of infection	Treatments under threat	Treatments no longer available
Meningococcal meningitis and septicaemia	Several β-lactams	Sulphonamides (for initial treatment)
H. influenzae infections	Chloramphenicol, several β-lactams	Ampicillin (for initial treatment)
Urinary tract infections	Ampicillin, trimethoprim, quinolones	
Gonorrhoea	'High dose' penicillin, tetracyclines	'Low dose' penicillin
Pneumococcal infections	Penicillin, macrolides	
Salmonella infection	Chloramphenicol, cotrimoxazole, amoxycillin	
Methicillin-resistant staphylococcal infection	All but vancomycin	
Enterococcal infections	Many antibiotics	
Tuberculosis	Aminoglycosides, ethambutol, isoniazid, pyrazinamide, rifampicin	
Hospital coliform infection	Many antibiotics	Ampicillin
Shigellosis		Sulphonamides, ampicillin

Based on Lambert (1994) and Neu (1992).

cephalosporins are considerably more expensive than the penicillins that could be used previously, they have to be given intramuscularly and none is very effective in dealing with pharyngeal infections.

The incidence of β-lactam-resistant strains of *N. gonorrhoeae* that do not produce β-lactamase has also increased in recent years. Resistance in such strains is due to mutations in chromosomal genes which either result in the production of altered forms of penicillin-binding proteins (PBPs) that have decreased affinity for β-lactams or cause reduced uptake of the antibiotics across the gonococcal outer membrane. The combined effect of such mutations can result in a 1000-fold increase in resistance levels to β-lactams. This situation has further undermined the use of β-lactam antibiotics for treatment of gonococcal infections, necessitating the use of other antibiotics which are either more costly or have more pronounced side-effects on the patient than β-lactams.

2.1.2 *Methicillin-resistant staphylococcal infections*

As already noted in Chapter 6, staphylococci are members of a group of invasive Gram-positive pathogens known as pyogenic cocci that can cause acute to chronic infections in man ranging from surgical sepsis to generalized septicaemia and bacteraemia.

Prior to the introduction of antibiotics in clinical medicine the prognosis for patients with severe staphylococcal infections was very poor. However, the introduction of benzylpenicillin in the 1940s offered effective treatment for severe infections caused by invasive staphylococci, e.g. *Staphylococcus aureus*. Unfortunately, within a few years of the introduction of penicillin the majority of hospital isolates were resistant to the antibiotic, the strains expressing β-lactamase activity. Thus, soon after the introduction of penicillin for clinical use, a large-scale World Health Organization survey showed that approximately 8% of strains were resistant; by 1956 the value was about 70%. The introduction of other types of antibiotics (e.g. streptomycin, chloramphenicol, tetracycline) for the therapy of staphylococcal infections also resulted in the emergence of strains specifically resistant to these compounds. Furthermore, strains which had acquired resistance to the new antibiotics were also often resistant to penicillin because of β-lactamase production. Such multiply resistant *S. aureus* strains were responsible for many outbreaks of hospital infection during the 1950s.

The predominance of β-lactamase-producing staphylococci in the 1950s led to an urgent search for β-lactamase-stable penicillins that could be used for chemotherapy. The discovery and introduction of such compounds, e.g. methicillin, caused a major decline in the incidence of multiply resistant *S. aureus* strains during the 1960s. However, during the late 1970s and early 1980s strains of *S. aureus* resistant to multiple antibiotics including methicillin and gentamicin emerged that were responsible for outbreaks of hospital infections throughout the world. Such strains, referred to as MRSA (methicillin-resistant *S. aureus*) not only cause difficulty in hospitals but spread from them to nursing homes and to surrounding communities. The pattern of resistance exhibited by MRS imposes serious constraints on the choice of antibiotics for therapy since the organisms involved are resistant to virtually all the antibiotics available to clinicians. Vancomycin, which is a somewhat toxic antibiotic requiring intravenous administration, is often the only drug effective against such staphylococci. Clearly this antibiotic is suitable for use only in hospitals.

2.1.3 *Multiple drug resistance in* Mycobacterium tuberculosis

In recent years there has been a global resurgence of tuberculosis. This trend is closely associated with the pandemic of the acquired immune deficiency syndrome (AIDS), whereby the depressed cell-mediated immunity of such individuals leads either to reactivation of a previously latent *M. tuberculosis* infection or susceptibility to a newly acquired infection.

Treatment of tuberculosis in patients with AIDS usually involves therapy with isoniazid, rifampicin, pyrazinamide and ethambutol for 9–12 months. Indeed, the major problem associated with such therapeutic regimens concerns the length of treatment required for a successful outcome. Although compliance can be maintained for a patient who has been hospitalized, many AIDS patients in the community fail to complete a course of therapy. The great number of medications that AIDS patients must take plus the encephalopathy which is a common component of the syndrome are factors which lead to patient confusion and decreased compliance with treatment regimens. Non-compliance results not only in continued infectivity but also in the selection of drug-resistant organisms, leading to the emergence of multiple drug resistance in *Mycobacterium tuberculosis* (MDRTB) strains in the community. These organisms are spread to the hospital environment when AIDS patients are admitted to hospital for acute care. Some MDRTB clinical isolates have acquired resistance to as many as seven agents used in the chemotherapy of tuberculosis, including resistance to five of the so-called 'first-line' agents described in Chapter 2.

3
Strategies for counteracting resistance to chemotherapeutic antibiotics

From the foregoing examples it is clear that the emergence of acquired antibiotic resistance in bacteria is having a profound impact on the treatment of bacterial infections with antibiotics: resistance has rendered useless a number of previously valuable treatments and in other cases has made treatment more difficult or more expensive. Consequently, strategies for counteracting and/or minimizing resistance to antibiotics have been sought. A number of these are described in the following sections.

3.1 Development of analogues of existing drugs stable to enzymatic inactivation (Mechanism 1, Table 5.3)

As noted in Chapter 5, enzymatic inactivation is an important mechanism of resistance in the case of β-lactams, chloramphenicol, AGAC and MLS group antibiotics. In several cases enzyme-stable analogues have been developed, most notably with the β-lactams.

3.1.1 β-Lactam antibiotics

As mentioned in Section 2.1.2, the increase in the frequency of penicillin-resistant strains of *S. aureus* throughout the world during the 1950s led to the development of methicillin (Fig. 8.1) a β-lactam of the penam class (Chapter 2) stable to attack by staphylococcal β-lactamases. Methicillin (a derivative of 6-aminopenicillanic acid; 6-APA), is stable to attack by staphylococcal β-lactamase because its side chain (Fig. 8.1) causes the antibiotic to have very poor affinity with the enzyme. Further work with penicillins stable to staphylococcal β-lactamase led to the development of other 6-APA derivatives. Particularly important are the so-called isoxazolyl series comprising oxacillin, cloxacillin, dicloxacillin and flucloxacillin (Fig. 8.1).

Agents exhibiting stability to enterobacterial β-lactamases have also been developed, e.g. cefoxitin and temocillin (Fig. 2.27). The presence of methoxy side chains in these compounds results in a very high degree of stability to the β-lactamases produced by Gram-negative bacilli. Monobactams (Fig. 2.27) also display stability to enterobacterial β-lactamases.

The discovery and development of the carbapenems (Fig. 2.27) represent one of the most important recent advances in the synthesis of β-lactam antibiotics stable to degradation by β-lactamases. The first members of the carbapenem class, olivanic acid and thienamycin (Fig. 2.27), were discovered in the mid-1970s. Both compounds have broad-spectrum antibacterial activity and are stable to the majority of β-lactamases described in Chapter 5, with the exception of the group 3 metallo-β-lactamases (Table 5.5). However, olivanic acid and thienamycin are both chemically unstable and it has not been possible to develop these antibiotics for use in the clinic. Nevertheless, the *N*-formimidoyl derivative of thienamycin, now known as imipenem (Fig. 2.27, Chapter 5; Fig. 8.2(a)), was much more stable than olivanic acid or thienamycin, permitting development of the compound for clinical use.

The stability of the carbapenems to hydrolysis by β-lactamases results from the presence of side chains in the *trans* (α) configuration at the C6 position of the molecule, contrasting with the penams and cephems which have side chains in the *cis* (β) configuration at positions 6 and 7 (Fig. 2.27, Chapter 5).

Imipenem, which has a C6 hydroxyethyl side chain, lacks a substituent at C1 (Fig. 8.2). The absence of a C1 substituent renders the molecule susceptible to the enzyme dehydropeptidase 1 which is found in the brush border of mammalian renal tubular cells and other tissues. Consequently, imipenem has been developed for use in humans in conjunction with cilastatin, an efficient inhibitor of dehydropeptidase 1, which is co-administered with the antibiotic.

Meropenem (Fig. 8.2(b)) which has recently received market approval in a number of countries (see Chapter 1 for antibiotic development process) retains the 6-α-hydroxyethyl group of imipenem (conferring β-lactamase stability), but unlike imipenem possesses a C1 methyl substituent that confers stability to dehydropeptidase 1. Therefore meropenem does not need to be co-administered with a dehydropeptidase 1 inhibitor.

3.1.2 AGAC group antibiotics

As discussed in Chapter 5, resistance to these antibiotics can result from the production of enzymes that acetylate, adenylylate or phosphorylate the antibiotics. Compounds stable to individual, but not all, modifying enzymes have been developed. These compounds lack certain hydroxyl and amino groups so that complex patterns of resistance may exist in individual strains depending on the

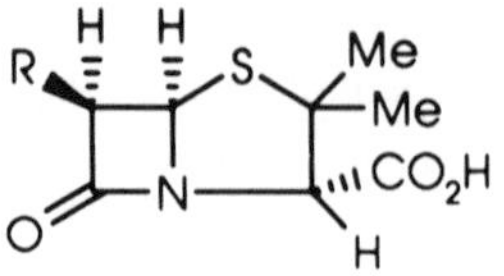

R	β-lactam
NH$_2$	6-aminopenicillanic acid (6-APA)
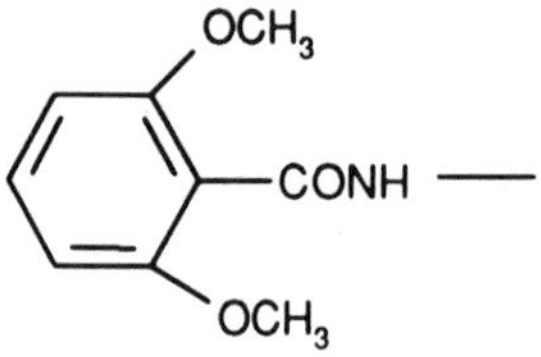	Methicillin
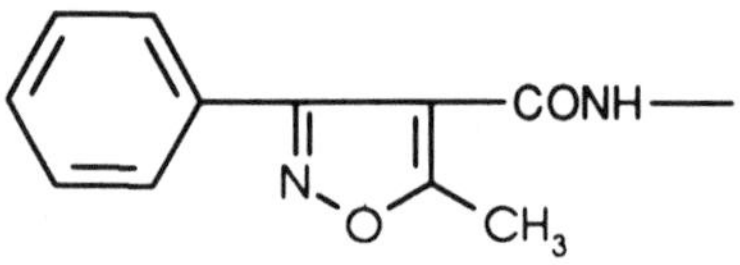	Oxacillin
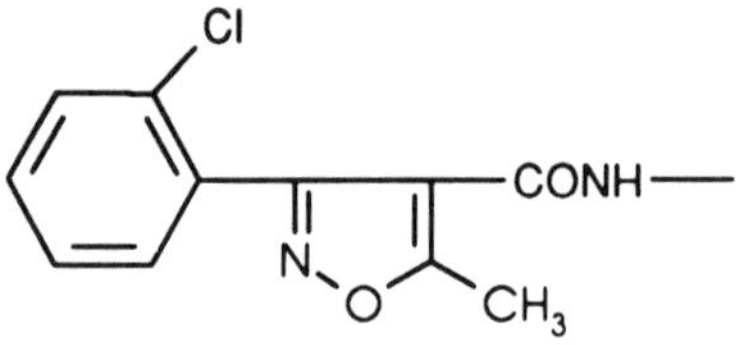	Cloxacillin
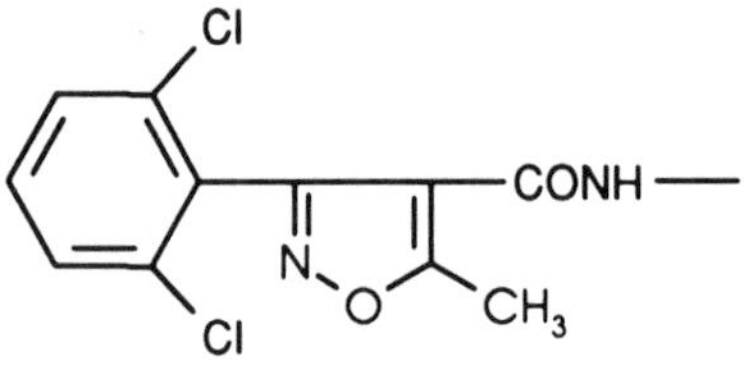	Dicloxacillin
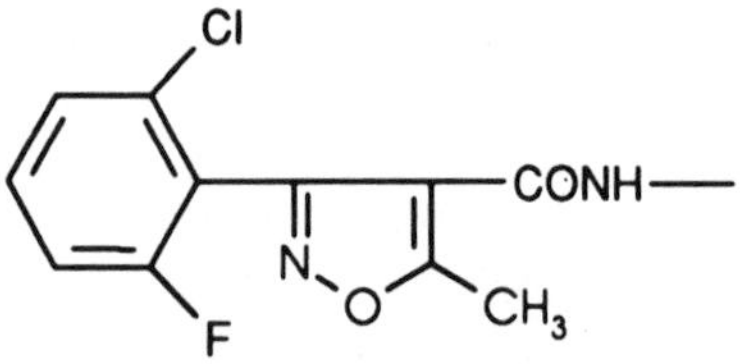	Flucloxacillin

Figure 8.1 Antibiotics of the penam class, derived from 6-aminopenicillinanic acid (6-APA), that exhibit stability to staphylococcal β-lactamases.

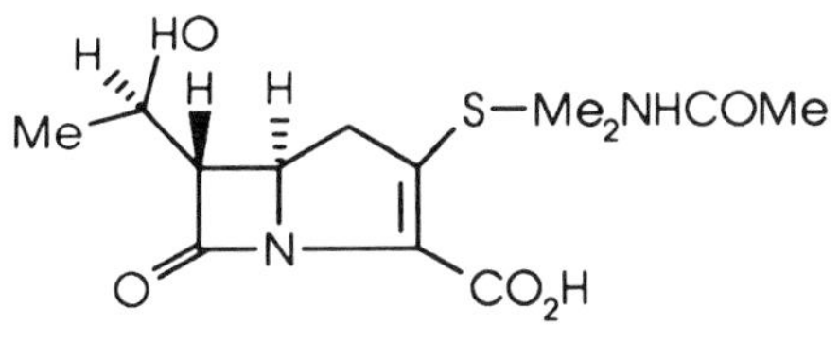

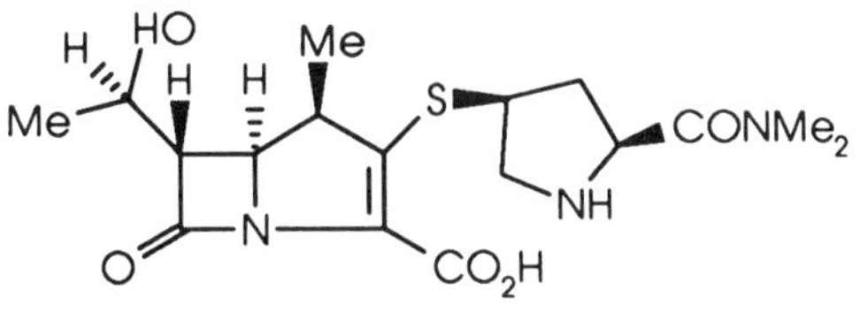

(a)   **(b)**

Figure 8.2   Structures of (a) imipenem and (b) meropenem.

enzymes involved (Table 5.4). Therefore the ability to administer an enzyme-stable AGAC antibiotic for therapy depends upon the prevalence and type of AGAC resistance encountered.

3.1.3   Chloramphenicol

As noted in Chapter 5, chloramphenicol is inactivated by chloramphenicol acetyltransferases. Chemical modification of chloramphenicol to produce antibiotically active, enzyme-resistant molecules has proved difficult. However, 3-fluoro-3-deoxy derivatives have been synthesized which are resistant to modification by chloramphenicol acetyl transferases. Unfortunately, these derivatives may be toxic.

3.2   Enzyme inhibitors (mechanism 1, Table 5.3)

The principle of using one agent to inhibit an enzyme that would otherwise inactivate a partner drug has been successfully applied to the β-lactam antibiotics.

The suggestion that β-lactamase inhibitors might extend the action of penicillin to organisms not otherwise susceptible first arose during the 1940s. However, it was not until the 1970s that such inhibitors were discovered. Clavulanic acid (Fig. 2.27), first described in 1977, exhibits weak antibacterial activity, but binds with high affinity and essentially irreversibly to many bacterial β-lactamases (see Table 5.5). Clavulanic acid protects many β-lactam antibiotics from destruction and has now been introduced commercially in combination with amoxycillin (Augmentin) for oral and parenteral use and ticarcillin (Timentin) for parenteral use only.

Other β-lactamase inhibitors have also been introduced. Sulbactam (Fig. 2.27) (a penicillanic acid sulphone) is marketed in combination with ampicillin, for both oral and parenteral use, and tazobactam has been combined with piperacillin for parenteral use.

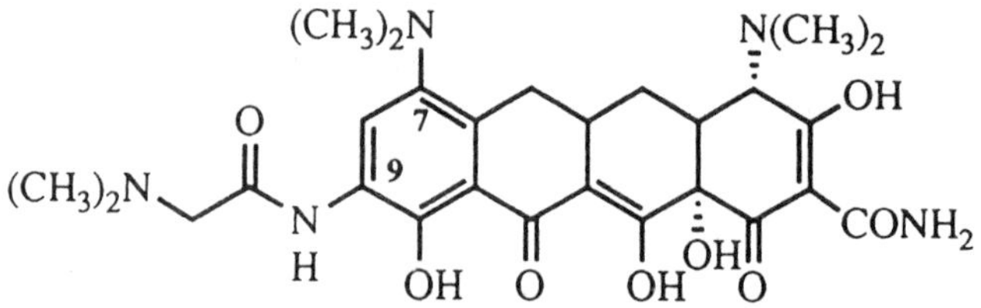

Figure 8.3 Structures of two tetracycline analogues, which are members of the new glycylcycline group of antibiotics:
(a) N,N-dimethylglycylamido-6-demethyl-6-deoxytetracycline;
(b) *N*,*N*-dimethylglycylamidominocycline.

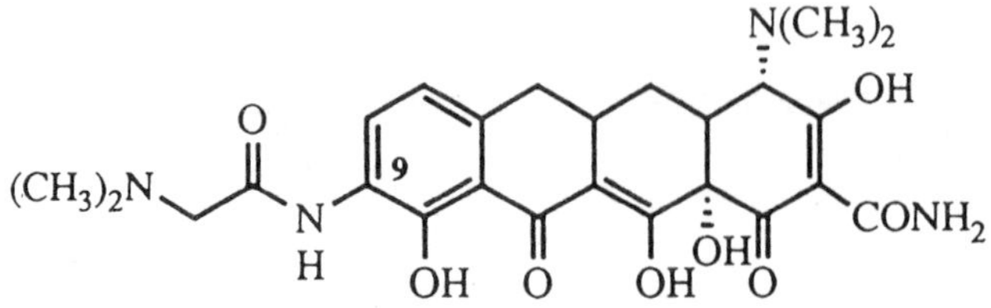

3.3 Development of analogues of existing drugs able to circumvent efflux mechanisms (mechanism 3b, Table 5.3)

As noted in Chapter 5, efflux mechanisms mediate bacterial resistance to the quinolones, tetracyclines and macrolides. Clearly, the development of analogues within the above groups that are not recognized by the efflux mechanisms provides a plausible method to counteract efflux-based resistance systems.

 Recently, progress has been made in this area by the discovery of the glycylcyclines which represent a new generation of tetracycline analogues. The glycylcyclines are novel tetracyclines substituted at the C9 position of the molecule with a dimethylglycylamido side chain. Figure 8.3 illustrates the N,N-dimethylglycylamido derivatives of minocycline and 6-demethyl-6-deoxytetracycline.

 The glycylcyclines possess activity against organisms expressing resistance to the older tetracyclines mediated by the eight determinants (*tet*A through *tet*F, *tet*K and *tet*L) that encode tetracycline efflux proteins (see Chapter 5, Section 3.6.1). The glycylcyclines therefore represent a significant advance within the tetracycline group of antibiotics because they are not recognized by the efflux proteins that recognize older members of this antibiotic class.

3.4 Development of analogues of existing drugs able to bind to modified target sites (mechanism 2, Table 5.3)

The glycylcyclines described in Section 3.3 also possess activity against organisms expressing the *tet*M and *tet*O determinants which probably mediate resistance to the older tetracyclines by modifying the tetracycline binding site on the bacterial 30S ribosomal subunit (see Chapter 5, Section 3.6.2). Therefore the affinity, or mechanism of binding of the glycylcyclines to ribosomes modified by the *tet*M or *tet*O proteins, is presumably sufficient to prevent aminoacyl-tRNA binding despite expression of the resistance determinant in the cell.

The synthesis of modified macrolides which are able to bind to ribosomes expressing resistance to other macrolides (Chapter 5, Section 3.5.1) represents another example of this approach to overcoming existing antibiotic resistance mechanisms.

3.5 Antibiotic hybrid molecules

This approach has involved the synthesis and evaluation of cephalosporin–quinolone hybrid molecules in an attempt to circumvent the problems associated with expression of β-lactamases. It has been known since the mid-1960s that certain side chains at position 3 in the cephem nucleus (see Fig. 2.27, Chapter 2) can be dislodged (ejected) when the β-lactam ring is hydrolysed by a β-lactamase. Based on this principle a number of cephalosporin–quinolone hybrid molecules have been synthesized which have alternative modes of action depending on the presence of β-lactamases. Against bacteria that do not express β-lactamases, the hybrid molecules act as cephalosporins inhibiting peptidoglycan synthesis. In contrast, expression of β-lactamase results in release of the quinolone moiety and the organisms are killed by its interaction with DNA gyrase (see Section 2.4.2.2, Chapter 2). Therefore, an organism should be susceptible to the hybrid antibiotic irrespective of whether it expresses β-lactam resistance mediated by β-lactamases.

The above approach is still at the experimental research evaluation phase and has not yet resulted in agents for human use.

3.6 Enhancement of permeability

The concept of using one antibiotic to promote entry of another to an otherwise inaccessible target site could, in principle, be applied to overcome acquired and intrinsic resistance due to mechanism 3a described in Table 5.3. Agents interfering with bacterial peptidoglycan synthesis or outer membrane integrity are the most likely antibiotics to facilitate entry of other agents normally excluded.

This approach has proved useful in the treatment of streptococcal endocarditis where penicillin, by promoting cell envelope damage, enhances uptake of AGAC antibiotics. However, the use of outer-membrane-disrupting agents, e.g. polymyxin B nonapeptide, to enhance uptake of other antibiotics into bacteria has not proved promising in terms of likely clinical application (see the article by Lam and coworkers listed in 'Further Reading' at the end of this chapter).

Nevertheless, this approach, using specific inhibitors of cell wall synthesis, may prove to be of value in developing new combinations of chemotherapeutic agents effective against mycobacteria.

3.7 Other strategies for counteracting antibiotic resistance

As already noted in Chapter 5, the emergence of acquired resistance to antibiotics results from the selective pressure imposed by antibiotic usage. This alters the natural ecological balance which otherwise favours the predominance of antibiotic-susceptible bacteria. Because the use of antibiotics is related to the emergence of bacterial resistance, the ways in which these drugs are prescribed has been closely scrutinized. In some cases underusage (e.g. the poor compliance with TB drug regimens) is responsible for resistance, but other studies indicate that unnecessarily excessive use of antibiotics is a particular risk factor for the emergence of antibiotic-resistant organisms.

A consensus is now emerging that greater effort must be devoted to limiting antibiotic usage for essential therapeutic purposes. Various antibiotic management systems have been proposed and many hospitals now exert some degree of control over the prescribing of antibiotics. Control of antibiotic usage also applies to agricultural meat production where the practice of using therapeutic antibiotics as growth promoters in animal feeds has been restricted in many countries for fear that antibiotic-resistant organisms arising in animals may be transferred to humans.

In addition to controls on antibiotic use, it is clear that effective measures to prevent cross-infection between hospital patients limit the spread of antibiotic-resistant organisms in the hospital environment. Various procedures can be adopted (for further details see the article by Lambert listed at the end of this chapter).

4
Impact of bacterial resistance to antiseptics, disinfectants and preservatives

4.1 Biocide resistance

As already noted in Chapter 3, non-antibiotic antibacterial agents are widely used as antiseptics, disinfectants and preservatives. Furthermore, they may also be utilized as so-called chemosterilizer systems for delicate medical equipment that cannot be sterilized by physical procedures such as heat, e.g. endoscopes which are disinfected between patient usage. Both intrinsic and acquired transferable resistance to biocides can significantly influence the effectiveness of these agents as inhibitors of bacterial growth or killing agents. Some examples are given below.

Compared with other isolates, Gram-negative bacteria recovered from the hospital environment often show decreased susceptibility to disinfectants, which may reflect the extensive usage of these agents in the hospital. In particular, disinfectants of the QAC type have been contaminated with such bacteria. This has required the introduction of more hygienic methods of preparation and storage of formulated solutions. The widespread use of chlorhexidine and QACs may be correlated with the emergence of resistant strains of Gram-negative bacteria in paraplegic patients; these bacteria may also be resistant to multiple antibiotics. Such organisms can be difficult to control, e.g. a hospital outbreak caused by a strain of *P. mirabilis* that was resistant to chlorhexidine and to several antibiotics, including gentamicin, has been described.

Chlorhexidine bladder washouts are currently believed to be unsuitable for eliminating established infections with Gram-negative bacteria that occur in patients with indwelling bladder catheters. Such organisms are often able to grow as microcolonies embedded in a polysaccharide matrix and thus resist the biguanide, as described in Fig. 6.10 (Fig. 6.10(a), biofilm; cf. Fig. 6.10(b), chlorhexidine in solution). Industrially, too, biofilms are frequently a problem and have been held responsible for resistance of *S. aureus* to chlorine in poultry-processing plants, of various types of biofilm bacteria to chlorhexidine, hypochlorites and monochloramine and of *Ser. marcescens* to chlorhexidine. *Ps. cepacia* is frequently highly resistant to biocides *in vivo*, but less so *in vitro*, and *L. pneumophila* also is more sensitive under laboratory conditions than in cooling towers. The problems of resistance associated with biofilm development have necessitated the incorporation of biocides into biomaterials. Biocide molecules leach from these materials thereby decreasing bacterial adhesion and subsequent biofilm formation. A better understanding of the effects of biocides on bacteria within biofilms is clearly needed.

Gram-positive bacteria (other than mycobacteria) are generally more sensitive to biocides than are Gram-negative organisms, although, as pointed out above, *S. aureus* in biofilms may show a reduced sensitivity. As noted earlier, enterococci are frequently resistant to antibiotics but do not appear to be particularly resistant to biocides. Some MRSA strains, however, are more resistant to cationic-type disinfectants than are other staphylococci. It has been claimed that this property confers a selective advantage, i.e. survival, when these disinfectants are employed clinically. However, the in-use concentrations of these agents are several times higher than those required to inhibit the growth of MRSA or other anti-biotic-resistant *S. aureus* strains. Too much emphasis has been placed on growth-inhibitory concentrations (MICs) and insufficient attention devoted to staphylococcal inactivation. Thus, the claim that such organisms have a selective advantage has yet to be fully substantiated.

Patients with AIDS (acquired immune deficiency syndrome) caused by HIV (human immunodeficiency virus) are highly susceptible to bacterial (and fungal) infections. Transmission of such infection may be prevented by disinfection of inanimate objects. In this context, *M. avium intracellulare* is a potentially problematic organism because it is even more resistant to disinfectants than other mycobacteria. The possible transmission of mycobacterial infection via endoscopes is thus a potentially serious clinical problem.

Because of the importance of choosing appropriate biocidal agents in the hospital environment, disinfection policies are clearly essential and must be rigorously adhered to, otherwise there is the risk of transmitting infections caused by resistant bacteria.

4.2 Possible relationship between antibiotic and biocide resistance

In the majority of cases, the genetic determinants responsible for acquired resistance to antibiotics and biocides are unrelated. There have been specific instances, however, when biocides have been claimed to select for antibiotic-resistant strains. This potentially alarming situation was first suggested when it was found that about 15% of Gram-negative strains (*Ps. aeruginosa, P. mirabilis* and *Prov. stuartii*) isolated from urinary tract infections in a paraplegic unit expressed resistance to cationic bactericides (QACs, chlorhexidine) and concomitantly to at least five antibiotics. This led to the proposal that the widespread use of chlorhexidine might be responsible for selecting antibiotic-resistant strains, i.e. that the various resistance determinants might reside on a common plasmid. However, all attempts to demonstrate a plasmid-linked association between antibiotic and chlorhexidine resistance have been unsuccessful. Furthermore, chlorhexidine-resistant mutants have been derived from chlorhexidine-sensitive *E. coli*, but they do not show enhanced resistance to antibiotics. The association between chlorhexidine and multiple antibiotic resistance in *Prov. stuartii* strains isolated from paraplegic patients has yet to be fully explained. However, it is possible that chlorhexidine-resistant strains act as more efficient recipients of plasmids conferring antibiotic resistance.

Bacteria expressing multiple antibiotic resistance have been isolated from drinking-water. It has already been pointed out that disinfection and purification of water may augment the occurrence of antibiotic-resistant bacteria and that chlorination may select or induce such changes. The finding that *E. coli* containing a virulence plasmid (ColV) is better able to attach to particles and exhibits increased chlorine resistance is another example of a potential public health hazard. Also, in this context, natural waters exposed to toxic chemical wastes show a higher incidence of antibiotic-resistant and plasmid-bearing strains than samples of clean ocean waters. Moreover, treated sewage contains large numbers of bacteria that simultaneously possess antibiotic and biocide resistances together with multiple plasmids. Obviously, as in the case of chlorhexidine and antibiotic resistance, the basis of 'linked' biocide–antibiotic resistance in organisms isolated from aquatic sources is of potential clinical and public health importance.

Multiple-antibiotic-resistant *S. aureus* strains that exhibit resistance to biocides were alluded to in Section 4.1. Although the mechanisms of biocide resistance in these strains (often by efflux) are similar to those responsible for antibiotic resistance, the significance of biocide resistance in these strains is still contentious.

5
Strategies for counteracting resistance to biocides

5.1 Combined systems

The principal method for counteracting resistance to biocides usually involves combination systems. The following systems are efficacious.

(1) An agent that enhances permeability (cf. Section 3.6) can be included. Agents such as EDTA, polylysine, lactoferrin and transferrin all potentiate antibiotic activity *in vitro* (Table 3.3). EDTA also potentiates the efficacy of various biocides against Gram-negative bacteria, but the other compounds have not yet been examined in detail for possible synergistic activity with biocides. Nevertheless, it is expected that some of the newer permeabilizers might have a role to play in this context.

   Agents that enhance the mycobactericidal activity of biocides are also a possibility. The cell wall of mycobacteria is complex, consisting mainly of three insoluble macromolecular components, i.e. arabinogalactan, peptidoglycan, and mycolic acid that make up the mycolarabinogalactanpeptidolglycan core of the wall (Fig. 1.9). The major structural component consists of the mycolic acids which constitute about 50%, by weight, of this core. The mycobacterial cell wall is highly hydrophobic in nature and the mycolic acids (Fig. 1.10) have an important role to play in reducing permeability to hydrophilic molecules. Thus, a possible strategy is to consider as permeabilizers those chemicals that inhibit the biosynthesis of, or have a direct action on, mycolic acids. An alternative is to examine compounds that affect arabinogalactan biosynthesis; in this context it is of interest to note that the chemotherapeutic drug ethambutol potentiates the growth-inhibitory effects of chlorhexidine and cetylpyridinium chloride (CPC) against mycobacteria. An ethambutol–chlorhexidine/CPC combination is not a practical clinical proposition, but it does illustrate that the antimycobacterial activity of biocidal agents can be enhanced by an agent such as ethambutol that acts as a cell wall synthesis inhibitor.

(2) Preservatives that rely on the combined effects of physical factors such as

suboptimal pH, temperature and water activity, as well as the chemical preservative itself, to inhibit microbial growth can be used in foods. Citric acid, a naturally occurring acidulant in many foods, can also act synergistically with other added biocides. Many of these combination systems act by placing additional energy demands on cells through interference with energy-requiring homeostatic mechanisms.

(3) A combination of preservatives can be used in some pharmaceutical and other products.

(4) The addition of α,β-unsaturated and aromatic aldehydes to glutaraldehyde gives what is claimed to be an enhanced mycobactericidal effect.

5.2 Prevention of transmission via endoscopes of infection caused by resistant mycobacteria

Some manufacturers have developed autoclavable endoscopes, but most endoscopes are unable to withstand repeated heat sterilization processes. Thus, the use of a high-level biocidal agent, such as glutaraldehyde, is essential for disinfection of endoscopes between patients and at the end of a working day or week in an endoscopy unit. Although all patients should be considered at risk in terms of acquiring an infection, the actual transmission of infection is low, despite the marked increase in the use of flexible fibre optic endoscopes. Nevertheless, there is concern at the spread of tuberculosis at bronchoscopy and mycobacteria are considered to be problematic organisms, so that suitable precautions must be adopted.

Mycobacteria generally are more resistant than other non-sporulating bacteria to glutaraldehyde. Preliminary cleaning of bronchoscopes is essential, after which they should be soaked in 2% alkaline glutaraldehyde for 30 min when the presence of mycobacteria is suspected. Other disinfectants may be used provided that they are equivalent in activity. However, glutaraldehyde-resistant *M. avium* and *M. chelonae* (*M. chelonei*) strains have recently been isolated. The mechanism of resistance is unknown. In view of the emergence of glutaraldehyde-resistant isolates, it has recently been proposed that peracetic acid might be a suitable replacement in such circumstances.

6
Impact of spore resistance on society

Under conditions of carbon, nitrogen or phosphorus limitation, some bacteria, notably the genera *Bacillus* and *Clostridium*, can form highly resistant, dehydrated spores. These spores are amongst the most resistant forms to biocides and to physical agents such as heat, radiation, drying and freezing and are well adapted for long periods of survival under adverse conditions. Medically, spores are important because they are responsible for the dissemination of some serious diseases, e.g. botulism, tetanus, gas gangrene, anthrax and food poisoning. In foods, inhibition by food preservatives of spore germination and outgrowth is of primary importance.

It is particularly important that spores are excluded from medical appliances intended for introduction into the human or animal body. Since certain medical equipment of this type cannot be sterilized by physical processes, chemical sporicides must be used. However, the high resistance of bacterial spores to biocides has meant that comparatively few chemicals are sufficiently toxic against spores to be employed in this context. Indeed, glutaraldehyde, ethylene oxide and formaldehyde (the last, sometimes with low-temperature steam) are essentially the only sporicides available for sterilization of such medical equipment.

7
Strategies for counteracting resistance of spores to chemicals

As already noted, bacterial spores are amongst the most resistant forms of microbial life to both chemical and physical processes. There are, however, various procedures for counteracting the high tolerance of spores, although not all have practical applications.

7.1 Use of heat treatment with biocides

It was pointed out in Chapter 3 (Section 2.3) that the activity of most antibacterial agents is potentiated at high temperatures. Until 1988 certain parenteral and ophthalmic products were sterilized by heating at 98–100 °C in the presence of a specified phenolic or organomercury compound. Although this method had been widely used in the UK for many years, doubts had frequently been expressed about its efficiency as a true sterilization procedure. Consequently, heating in an autoclave (in the absence of biocide), which employs a temperature of 121 °C, is now the only recommended pharmacopoeial method for sterilizing thermostable solutions.

In the food industry, a process known as acid-heat treatment has long been used as a sterilizing procedure. This depends on spores being more heat sensitive at low, rather than high, pH.

7.2 Use of chemical combinations

Two or more biocides (or antibiotics) in combination may produce a synergistic response against non-sporing bacteria. It is logical, therefore, to consider whether the same principle applies to bacterial spores. Although the subject has not been approached in a systematic or rational manner, the following provide some examples of this principle.

(1) *Combinations of aldehydes.* Some disinfectant formulations are available which contain more than one aldehyde. Their sporicidal activity is claimed to be greater than that observed with a single aldehyde. It is difficult to explain this observation unless there is greater overall uptake into the spore with the combined formulation.

(2) *Glutaraldehyde plus surface-active agents and metals.* (a) The sporicidal action of the dialdehyde may be potentiated by non-ionic surfactants and by metal divalent cations; (b) inorganic cation–anionic surfactant combinations greatly increase dialdehyde activity at acid pH, possibly as a result of effects on the spore surface resulting in greater aldehyde uptake.

(3) *Hypochlorite plus methanol.* The hypochlorites are sporicidal, but this activity is enhanced in the presence of methanol or other alcohols. Methanol is claimed to modify the spore coats, thereby allowing increased hypochlorite penetration. This hypothesis has yet to be substantiated and the converse could apply.

(4) *Acid–alcohol treatment.* Alcohol is not sporicidal, and only high concentrations (9%) of hydrochloric acid are sporicidal. Acid alcohol (1% HCl in 70% alcohol) will, however, kill spores within a few hours. The reason for this is unknown, but spore permeability is probably affected by some, as yet unknown, mechanism.

It is clear from the above that little is known about the basis of improved sporicidal activity when combinations of chemical agents are used. Increased penetration of one or both agents is an obvious possibility, but evidence to support this contention is often lacking. It is not yet known how to design specific sporicidal molecules that would be able to penetrate efficiently the spore coats.

7.3 Chemical plus ionizing radiation

Radiation as a means of sterilizing certain foods or of reducing microbial contamination is viewed with alarm by the general public. Radiation doses for inactivating spores or for preventing spore germination or outgrowth can be minimized when appropriate preservatives are present.

7.4 Chemical plus ultraviolet radiation

Ultraviolet light and hydrogen peroxide are synergistic when used in combination. This probably results from the formation of hydroxyl ($^{.}$OH) radicals that damage spore DNA.

8
Conclusions

The development of acquired resistance to antibiotics is a major factor complicating the use of chemotherapeutic agents and the control of infectious diseases. Indeed, in recent years the serious medical problems associated with the widespread emergence of acquired resistance to antibiotics have received unprecedented worldwide attention.

Therefore the concepts described in this chapter, which illustrate how resistance can be circumvented, or controlled, are likely to assume even greater importance in coming years. In addition to the chemical and biochemical approaches for counteracting resistance mechanisms described here, the identification of novel agents with unique modes of action which are not susceptible to existing resistance mechanisms obviously provides another general strategy to overcome resistant organisms.

Inhibition of resistance gene transfer between donor and recipient cells might provide a further means of controlling the spread of resistance. Molecular understanding of conjugal transfer mechanisms is now probably sufficient to examine the feasibility of inhibiting such processes.

Further reading

Books

Levy, S. B. (1992). *The Antibiotic Paradox. How Miracle Drugs are Destroying the Miracle.* Plenum Press, New York and London.

Russell, A. D., Hugo, W. B. & Ayliffe, G. A. J. (1992). *Principles and Practice of Disinfection, Preservation and Sterilization.* Second edition. Blackwell Scientific Publications, Oxford.

Review articles and reports

Appelbaum, P. C. (1992). Antimicrobial resistance in *Streptococcus pneumoniae*: an overview. *Clinical Infectious Diseases* **15**: 77–83.

Armstrong, D., Neu, H., Peterson, L. R. & Tomasz, A. (1995). The prospects of treatment failure in the chemotherapy of infectious diseases in the 1990s. *Microbial Drug Resistance* **1**: 1–4.

Brown, M. R. W. & Gilbert, P. (1993). Sensitivity of biofilms to antimicrobial agents. *Journal of Applied Bacteriology (Symposium Supplement)* **74**: 87S–97S.

Carpentier, B. & Cerf, O. (1993). Biofilms and their consequences, with particular reference to hygiene in the food industry. *Journal of Applied Bacteriology* **75**: 499–511.

Chopra, I. (1994). Glycylcyclines—third generation tetracycline analogues. *Expert Opinion in Investigational Drugs* **3**: 191–193.

Coates, D. & Hutchinson, D. N. (1994). How to produce a hospital disinfection policy. *Journal of Hospital Infection* **26**: 57–68.

Coleman, K., Athalye, M., Clancey, A., Davison, M., Payne, D. J., Perry, C. R. & Chopra, I. (1994). Bacterial resistance mechanisms as therapeutic targets. *Journal of Antimicrobial Chemotherapy* **33**: 1091–1116.

Easmon, C. S. F. (1985). Gonococcal resistance to antibiotics. *Journal of Antimicrobial Chemotherapy* **16**: 409–412.

Gould, G. W., Russell, A. D. & Stewart-Tull, D. E. S. (eds) (1994). *Fundamental and Applied Aspects of Bacterial Spores. Journal of Applied Bacteriology (Symposium Supplement)* **76**: 1S– 138S.

Gould, I. M. (1988). Control of antibiotic use in the United Kingdom. *Journal of Antimicrobial Chemotherapy* **22**: 395–397.

Greenwood, D. (1986). Strategies for counteracting resistance to antibacterial agents. *Journal of Antimicrobial Chemotherapy* **18** (Supplement B): 141–151.

Gustafson, R. H. & Kiser, J. S. (1985). Nonmedical uses of the tetracyclines. In *The Tetracyclines*. Handbook of Experimental Pharmacology. Volume 78 (eds J. J. Hlavka & J. H. Boothe) pp. 405–446. Springer-Verlag, Berlin.

Hamilton-Miller, J. W. T. (1994). Dual-action antibiotic hybrids. *Journal of Antimicrobial Chemotherapy* **33**: 197–200.

Kunin, C. M. (1993). Resistance to antimicrobial drugs—a worldwide calamity. *Annals of Internal Medicine* **118**: 557–561.

Lambert, H. P. (1984). Impact of bacterial resistance to antibiotics on therapy. *British Medical Bulletin* **40**: 102–106.

Moellering, R. C. (1991). The enterococcus: a classic example of the impact of antimicrobial resistance on therapeutic options. *Journal of Antimicrobial Chemotherapy* **28**: 1–12.

Moellering, R. C., Eliopoulos, G. M. & Sentochnik, D. E. (1989). The carbapenems: new broad spectrum β-lactam antibiotics. *Journal of Antimicrobial Chemotherapy* **24** (Supplement A): 1–7.

Neu, H. C. (1992). The crisis in antibiotic resistance. *Science* **257**: 1064–1073.

Report (1969). Joint Committee on the Use of Antibiotics in Animal Husbandry and Veterinary Medicine. HMSO, London.

Report (1986). Guidelines for the control of epidemic methicillin-resistant *Staphylococcus aureus. Journal of Hospital Infection* **7**: 193–201.

Rolinson, G. N. (1988). The influence of 6-aminopenicillanic acid on antibiotic development. *Journal of Antimicrobial Chemotherapy* **22**: 5–14.

Russell, A. D. & Day, M. J. (1993). Antibacterial activity of chlorhexidine. *Journal of Hospital Infection* **25**: 229–238.

Russell, A. D. & Russell, N. J. (1995) Biocides: activity, action and resistance. *Fifty Years of Antimicrobials*. Symposium No. 53 of the Society for General Microbiology (eds P. A. Hunter, G. K. Darby & N. J. Russell) pp. 327–365. Cambridge University Press, Cambridge.

Silver, L. L. & Bostian, K. A. (1993). Discovery and development of new antibiotics: the problems of antibiotic resistance. *Antimicrobial Agents and Chemotherapy* **37**: 377–383.

Sudre, P., tenDam, G. & Kochi, A. (1992). Tuberculosis: a global overview of the situation today. *Bulletin of the World Health Organisation* **70**: 149–159.

Tally, F. T., Ellestad, G. A. & Testa, R. T. (1995). Glycylcyclines: a new generation of tetracyclines. *Journal of Antimicrobial Chemotherapy* **35**: 449–452.

Tomasz, A. (1994). Multiple-antibiotic-resistant pathogenic bacteria. *New England Journal of Medicine* **330**: 1247–1251.

Vaara, M. (1992). Agents that increase the permeability of the outer membrane. *Microbiological Reviews* **56**: 395–411.

Viljanen, P. & Boratynski, J. (1991). The susceptibility of conjugative resistance transfer in Gram-negative bacteria to physiochemical and biochemical agents. *FEMS Microbiology Reviews* **88**: 43–54.

Young, L. S. (1993). Mycobacterial diseases in the 1990s. *Journal of Antimicrobial Chemotherapy* **32**: 179–194.

Research papers

Goldman, R. C. & Kadman, S. K. (1989). Binding of novel macrolide structures to macrolide-lincosamide-streptogramin B-resistant ribosomes inhibits protein synthesis and bacterial growth. *Antimicrobial Agents and Chemotherapy* **33**: 1058–1066.

Gordon, M. D., Ezzell, R. J., Bruchner, N. I. & Ascenzi, J. M. (1994). Enhancement of mycobactericidal activity of glutaraldehyde with α,β-unsaturated and aromatic aldehydes. *Journal of Industrial Microbiology* **13**: 77–82.

Jarlier, V. & Nikaido, H. (1990). Permeability barrier to hydrophilic solutes in *Mycobacterium chelonae*. *Journal of Bacteriology* **172**: 1418–1423.

Lam, C., Hildebrandt, J., Schutze, E. & Wenzel, A. F. (1986). Membrane-disorganizing property of polymyxin B nonapeptide. *Journal of Antimicrobial Chemotherapy* **18**: 9–15.

Leelaporn, A., Paulsen, I. T., Tennent, J. M., Littlejohn, T. G. & Skurray, R. A. (1994). Multidrug resistance to antiseptics and disinfectants in coagulase-negative staphylococci. *Journal of Medical Microbiology* **40**: 214–220.

Nikaido, H., Kim, S.-H. & Rosenberg, E. Y. (1993). Physical organization of lipids in the cell wall of *Mycobacterium chelonae*. *Molecular Microbiology* **8**: 1025–1030.

Snider, D. E. & Roper, W. L. (1992). The new tuberculosis. *New England Journal of Medicine* **326**: 703–705.

Testa, R. T., Petersen, P. J., Jacobus, N. V., Sum, P.-E., Lee, V. J. & Tally, F. P. (1993). *In vitro* and *in vivo* antibacterial activities of the glycylcyclines, a new class of semisynthetic tetracyclines. *Antimicrobial Agents and Chemotherapy* **37**: 2270–2277.

Watt, S. R. & Clarke, D. J (1994). Role of autolysins in the EDTA-induced lysis of *Pseudomonas aeruginosa*. *FEMS Microbiology Letters* **124**: 113–120.

Index